COGNITIVE THERAPY TECHNIQUES FOR CHILDREN AND ADOLESCENTS

Cognitive Therapy Techniques for Children and Adolescents

TOOLS FOR ENHANCING PRACTICE

Robert D. Friedberg
Jessica M. McClure
Jolene Hillwig Garcia

THE GUILFORD PRESS
New York   London

Library of Congress Cataloging-in-Publication Data

Friedberg, Robert D., 1955–
   Cognitive therapy techniques for children and adolescents : tools for enhancing practice / Robert
D. Friedberg, Jessica M. McClure, Jolene Hillwig Garcia.
     p. cm.
   Includes bibliographical references and index.
   ISBN 978-1-60623-313-9 (hardcover: alk. paper)
   1. Cognitive therapy for children. 2. Cognitive therapy for teenagers. I. McClure, Jessica
M. II. Garcia, Jolene Hillwig. III. Title.
   RJ505.C63F755 2009
   618.92′89142—dc22
                                                                  2009018760

About the Authors

Robert D. Friedberg, PhD, ABPP, is Associate Professor, Director of the Cognitive Behavioral Therapy Clinic for Children and Adolescents, and Director of the Psychology Post-Doctoral Fellowship program in the Department of Psychiatry at Milton S. Hershey Medical Center, Penn State University College of Medicine. A clinical psychologist, Dr. Friedberg is author of five other books, and his scholarly publications and national and international presentations span the globe. Dr. Friedberg also supervises trainees at the Beck Institute for Cognitive Therapy and Research. He is a Founding Fellow of the Academy of Cognitive Therapy and a board-certified diplomate in cognitive-behavioral therapy.

Jessica M. McClure, PsyD, is a clinical psychologist at Cincinnati Children's Hospital Medical Center. She is coauthor, with Robert Friedberg, of the book *Clinical Practice of Cognitive Therapy with Children and Adolescents*. She has also written articles and book chapters and given presentations on cognitive-behavioral therapy with children and adolescents. Her expertise includes cognitive-behavioral treatment of children and adolescents with anxiety, depression, behavioral disorders, and pervasive developmental disorders. Dr. McClure is currently active in an initiative at Cincinnati Children's Hospital Medical Center to help clinicians translate evidence-based treatment protocols to everyday practice as a way of spreading evidence-based care for children and adolescents.

Jolene Hillwig Garcia, MD, is completing psychiatry residency training in the Department of Psychiatry at Milton S. Hershey Medical Center, Penn State University College of Medicine, and has completed a fellowship in child and adolescent psychiatry. She received an MD from Penn State University College of Medicine and a BS in Biology and BA in Art–Commercial Design from Lycoming College. Dr. Garcia has been involved in scholarly research and publications, as well as professional presentations on topics of interest in child and adolescent psychiatry. In addition, she continues her work in graphic and fine art.

Acknowledgments

As always, "props" must be fully directed to my wonderful wife, Barbara, whose giving and loving nature makes me a better person. A big "shout out" is also merited to my now grown daughter, Rebecca, whose evanescent mind and wit ("Oh c'mon Dad!") persistently amaze me. My prime coauthor, Jessica, "rocks" and is simply the best collaborator ever! Jolene, a new and valued colleague, kept the material real and fresh with her illustrations and insight. A project like this one reminds me that I stand on the shoulders of my mentors: Christine A. Padesky and Raymond A. Fidaleo. Special thanks go to Penn State University Milton S. Hershey Medical Center and College of Medicine for providing me the opportunity to pursue my clinical service and research. Finally, I am honored to have the privilege of caring for the many children, adolescents, and families who entrusted their well-being to me in my work at the Cognitive Behavioral Therapy Clinic for Children and Adolescents at the Milton S. Hershey Medical Center.

ROBERT D. FRIEDBERG

Thank you to my husband, Jim, and daughters, Lydia and Juliana, for their encouragement and support. I am grateful to my coauthor, Bob, for his creativity and collaboration. I would also like to acknowledge the children and their families who have inspired the techniques in this book.

JESSICA M. MCCLURE

Thank you to my family for their love, support, and consistent example of faith, especially to my husband for his undying patience and continued encouragement to follow my calling. Thank you to my colleagues and friends for their humor and inspiration during this process. I am grateful to my teachers and mentors for their knowledge and advice, and of them, a very special thanks to Robert Friedberg and Jessica McClure for inviting me along and shepherding me through the duration of this endeavor. And to my patients and their families, thank you for the honor of learning from you and the joy of caring for you.

JOLENE HILLWIG GARCIA

Contents

CHAPTER 1. Beginnings   1

CHAPTER 2. Using Assessment Efficiently   12

CHAPTER 3. Psychoeducation   55

CHAPTER 4. Behavioral Interventions   79

CHAPTER 5. Self-Instructional and Cognitive Restructuring Methods   121

CHAPTER 6. Rational Analysis   189

CHAPTER 7. Performance, Attainment, and Exposure   240

CHAPTER 8. Final Points   291

References   297

Index   319

The reproducibles are also provided in a large-size format on Guilford's website (www.guilford.com/p/friedberg2) for book buyers to download and use in their clinical practice.

CHAPTER 1

Beginnings

This book offers practicing cognitive-behavioral clinicians a wide range of techniques and procedures to make practice easier and more effective for both children and therapists. It is designed to serve as a companion to our previous book, *Clinical Practice of Cognitive Therapy with Children and Adolescents: The Nuts and Bolts* (Friedberg & McClure, 2002). The first book presented the basics of treatment. Here, we go beyond to present more techniques and approaches to target those hard-to-reach clients, difficult-to-treat problems, and more complex cases. We offer a modular approach to help clinicians choose the right technique to fit the client. The book is also designed to bridge the gap between empirically supported treatment manuals and what we find in typical clinical practice.

In this chapter, we present some of the findings from the literature to help orient clinicians to ways to use components found effective in empirically supported or informed treatment. In addition, we explore the modular approach to treatment, and how it can offer benefits to working in typical clinical settings.

Research supporting cognitive-behavioral therapy (CBT) with children is methodologically rigorous and has yielded significant efficacy results. These promising findings have led to calls for empirically supported or at least empirically informed practice. Yet many practitioners remain skeptical about using research protocols in clinical practice (Southam-Gerow, 2004; Weisz, 2004). Indeed, efforts at disseminating effective treatment to the community have been largely unsuccessful (Addis, 2002; Carroll & Nuro, 2002; Chambless & Ollendick, 2001; Edwards, Dattilio, & Bromley, 2004; Gotham, 2006; Schulte, Bochum, & Eifert, 2002; Seligman, 1995). There are a number of reasons for this situation.

Clinicians confront many challenges that research protocols work hard to avoid. For example, clinicians generally treat severely distressed patients with greater comorbidity who are highly likely to drop out of treatment (Weisz, 2004). Yet participants recruited into research protocols are often volunteers and are often paid for their participation. In typical clinics, parents seeking treatment for their children rarely recognize their problems, commonly disagree with treatment goals, and infrequently seek services on their own (Creed & Kendall, 2005; Shirk & Karver, 2003). Clinical populations generally suffer from greater family psychopathology, and sadly many of these children may suffer from some form of abuse (Weisz, 2004). In addition, clinicians are often deluged by burdensome productivity demands, bureaucratic requirements, forms, and paperwork (Southam-Gerow, 2004; Weisz, 2004). Southam-Gerow (2004) astutely noted that manual developers incorrectly view clinicians as passive consumers or "end users." He asserted that clinicians should be viewed as creative codevelopers who are able to make intelligent decisions. As Jones and Lyddon (2000, p. 340) wrote, "Developing practice guidelines is not a process carved in stone, rather a continually evolving one." In other words, research can point clinicians in the right direction but individual clinicians working in the real world must find specific ways to get to the destination.

The modular approach to CBT offered in this book gives clinicians an attractive alternative to manuals by balancing the precision of the protocol with flexibility and clinical creativity. We cannot say with certainty that a modular approach is a better path than a manual-driven therapy. The data are not yet in on this issue. However, the promise of a modular approach lies in its potential for real-world practicality.

A MODULAR APPROACH TO CBT

A modular approach to intervention is skills based and applicable to a variety of children and adolescents presenting with multiple complaints (Van Brunt, 2000). Chorpita, Daleiden, and Weisz (2005b, p. 142) defined *modularity* as "breaking complex activities into simpler parts that function independently." The modular approach we have used for this book consists of distilling individual techniques and procedures from empirically supported treatment manuals and grouping them by therapy task into modules (Chorpita, Daleiden, & Weisz, 2005a; Curry & Wells, 2005; Rogers, Reinecke, & Curry, 2005). The techniques and procedures in this volume are organized into six modules covering the following areas: psychoeducation, assessment and behavioral interventions, self-monitoring, cognitive restructuring, rational analysis, and exposure/experiential methods. All of the techniques within a module share a common therapeutic purpose (e.g., psychoeducation), but they may differ in developmental appropriateness (child or adolescent), target population, and modality (individual, group, or family therapy).

Constructing an individualized case formulation is a key step in implementing the modular approach presented in this book. Kendall, Chu, Gifford, Hayes, and Nauta (1998) correctly asserted that CBT with children is directed by a theoretical rationale rather than by techniques. Readers from different theoretical orientations will likely recognize some techniques traditionally associated with other therapeutic paradigms. The ties that bind the diverse techniques in this book are conceptual ones. Remember: what makes a technique cognitive is its theoretical context and proposed conceptual mechanism of change (J. S. Beck, 1995).

Figure 1.1 shows the modules and their relation to each other over the course of a treatment. Assessment and psychoeducation are the first two modules. While you begin with assessment and psychoeducation, the bidirectional arrows allow you to return to these techniques throughout the treatment process as you proceed to behavioral, cognitive restructuring, rational analysis, and performance attainment procedures.

FIGURE 1.1. Modular approach to CBT.

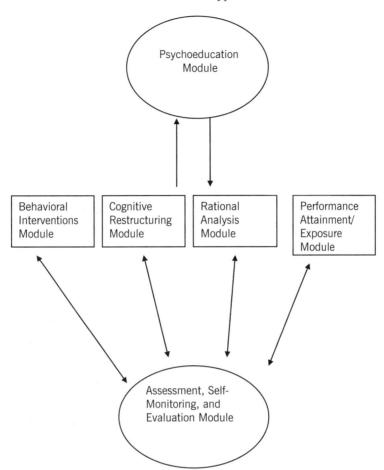

The techniques in the assessment, self-monitoring, and evaluation module direct patients and therapists to appropriate clinical targets as well as provide data on how treatment is going. For instance, if the patient is high in anhedonia, pleasant activity scheduling may be initiated. If social skills are lacking, then training in these areas is a logical treatment strategy. In some instances, self-monitoring and other assessment methods may indicate the need for a cognitive restructuring intervention. A technique can then be tried and evaluated. If the data indicates the intervention was successful, the therapist may move on to a more advanced cognitive restructuring procedure, or to a procedure in the subsequent rational analysis or exposure modules. If evaluation reveals lack of success, then another cognitive restructuring technique may be selected or an intervention from the preceding behavioral module. Chapter 2 presents various assessment and self-monitoring methods.

Psychoeducation gives children, adolescents, their families, and therapists a common understanding of the therapy process. Frank (1961) aptly stated that all psychotherapies include a rationale that explains illness and recovery. More specifically, Frank stated:

The therapeutic rationale finally enables the patient to make sense of his [or her] symptoms. Since he [or she] often views them as inexplicable which increases their ominousness, being able to name and explain them in terms of an overarching conceptual scheme is powerfully reassuring. The first step in gaining control of any phenomenon is to give it a name. (1961, p. 328)

Chapter 3 offers many specific psychoeducational techniques.

There are four intervention modules: behavioral interventions, cognitive restructuring, rational analysis, and performance attainment/exposure. The modules are sequenced according to how skill building proceeds: from simple task to complex task. In general, behavioral interventions (Chapter 4) are easier for children to acquire and apply whereas the more cognitive interventions such as cognitive restructuring (Chapter 5) or rational analysis (Chapter 6) are somewhat more sophisticated skills. Exposure and other performance attainment methods (Chapter 7) are placed later in the sequence to allow the building of coping skills that can facilitate progress toward experiential/exposure tasks.

CASE CONCEPTUALIZATION IS CRUCIAL

Reliance on case conceptualization separates clinicians from technicians (Freeman, Pretzer, Fleming, & Simon, 1990). A case conceptualization increases the flexibility of treatment strategies, allows the therapist to recognize what techniques work and which procedures fall flat, and facilitates productive troubleshooting when treatment is stymied. Although a full discussion of case conceptualization is beyond the scope of this chapter, we will nonetheless provide a rubric for conceptualizing patients. For readers who require more background on the fundamentals of case conceptualization, we recommend work by J. S. Beck (1995), Friedberg and McClure (2002), Kuyken, Padesky, and Dudley (2009), and Persons (2008).

Friedberg and McClure (2002) outlined the critical elements of case conceptualization, which include developmental history, cultural context, behavioral antecedents, cognitive structures, and presenting problems. Presenting problems are the issues that bring young people into treatment. While these are crucial and often urgent, they represent only part of the picture. In our model, presenting problems are best understood in the context of past learned history, cultural factors, systemic influences, and developmental variables. These variables have a bidirectional influence on the presenting problems. They shape and in turn are shaped by the presenting complaints. In order to conceptualize a case and successfully implement a treatment package, you will need to obtain relevant patient data as follows.

Developmental milestones regarding self-regulation (e.g., eating, sleeping, toileting), responsiveness to changes in routines, and adjustment to school should be considered. Further, a youngster's *school functioning* should also be queried (e.g., academic performance; attendance; disciplinary history such as detention, suspension, and expulsions; and experiences in the cafeteria, gym, and recess). *Social functioning* is also very important (Who are the patient's friends? How are friends acquired? How long do the friendships last? What is the patient's dating/sexual history? Does the patient go to birthday parties? Sleepovers? Dances?). You should collect specific data on the *family functioning* (parents'/siblings' psychiatric and medical history; What disciplinary techniques are employed?; Is domestic violence present?; Do parents agree on discipline?; How does the child see the family organization?; Who is in charge?; Who is peripheral?). Of course, the child's *substance use* (illicit drugs, alcohol, food, laxatives, over-the-counter medicines), *medical conditions*, and *legal history* should be obtained.

Ethnocultural data should also be collected. Levels of acculturation, ethnocultural identity, and specific ethnocultural beliefs should be considered. You should ask about cultural beliefs about the presenting problem and treatment. Any experiences of prejudice, discrimination, oppression, and marginalization should be funneled into the conceptualization.

After collecting and synthesizing all this data, you begin the inferential process. We agree with Persons (1995) that simple formulations are preferred to complex ones. A simple rubric suggested by Persons is to use patient data to formulate a view of the self (e.g., "I am ... "), a view of the world ("The world is ... ," "The environment is ... "), and a view of other people ("People are ... "). These pieces combine into a whole picture that reads "I am _____ in a world _____ where other people are _____."

The "world" and "other people" components directly affect the way the young patient sees therapy and the therapist. For instance, a patient who sees others as rejecting, critical, uncaring, and/or controlling will fear negative evaluation and coercion by the therapist. On the other hand, a young patient who sees others as inferior, subordinate, and/or undeserving will devalue the therapist, see treatment as a waste of time, and act to "get one over" on the therapist.

USING THE CASE CONCEPTUALIZATION TO GUIDE MODULAR CBT

In order to see how the case conceptualization impacts modular CBT, let's look at some examples. Consider a 10-year-old girl who sees herself as ineffective ("I am helpless.") in a world where others are coercive and the world is rejecting. These beliefs about the world and other people will fundamentally shape the child's perception of the therapist and therapy. This youngster will be prone to interpret interventions as coercive, and Socratic questions as implicit criticism. Your initial challenge is to place the modular interventions in a context that fosters autonomy, control, and collaboration, and that communicates understanding. Hence, psychoeducation is pivotal. The modular interventions themselves should focus on decreasing this patient's sense of hopelessness. As treatment progresses, you can move toward addressing her views of others and the world. As you achieve treatment success, her views of others as coercive and the world as being rejecting will be disconfirmed.

In another case example, a 17-year-old held the view "Unless I am always in perfect control of myself, others, and the world, I am incompetent because the world is dangerous and others are both unpredictable and domineering." For this patient, absolute control equals safety and competence. Consistent session structure and collaboration will ease his harsh views of others and the world. However, to prove his competence, he must preserve absolute and certain control of everything. Modular interventions aimed at looking at the advantages and disadvantages of perfect control, evaluating alternate determinants of "competence," testing the evidence of whether competence is related to control, and behavioral experiments where the client "loses" some control yet maintains competence are recommended.

We believe theoretical coherence is essential to good clinical practice. The choice of procedures and techniques needs to be guided by cognitive-behavioral theory. Cognitive-behavioral case conceptualization prevents theoretical drift. Moreover, reliance on conceptualization allows you to access mechanisms of change. You can then see why treatment works well or is moving slowly or not at all. In this way, obstacles can be overcome.

INTEGRATING PROCEDURES WITH PSYCHOTHERAPEUTIC PROCESSES

As any clinician readily recognizes, psychotherapy is fundamentally an interpersonal enterprise (Southam-Gerow, 2004). We believe that the relationship is essential but not sufficient for therapeutic change. Accordingly, we recommend that each procedure be mindfully integrated with psychotherapeutic processes (Shirk & Karver, 2006). The treatment relationship and intervention are not independent. Procedures and relationship building are contemporaneous tasks. They work in concert to establish powerful working alliances. Simply, interventions build good relationships and strong alliances make interventions effective.

Collaboration between patient and therapist enhances the therapeutic alliance. Creed and Kendall (2005) found that rushing the patient and behaving too formally predicted lower alliance ratings. Therapists' curiosity often stimulates collaboration. Curious therapists often induce curiosity in their young patients and behavioral experimentation is dependent on curiosity. Kingery et al. (2006) encouraged therapists to invite young people to integrate aspects of their personal life (friends, interests, hobbies) into therapy. Gosch, Flannery-Schroeder, Mauro, and Compton (2006) recommended that therapists employ appropriate self-disclosure with their young patients. The disclosure not only enhances rapport but also sets the therapist up as a coping model.

Friedberg and McClure (2002) designed a clinically useful rubric for integrating psychotherapeutic structure, process, and content variables, as shown in Table 1.1. *Structure* refers to the procedures and techniques that characterize CBT. These elements include, but are not limited to, session structure, psychoeducation, assessment, self-monitoring, behavioral tasks, social skills training, cognitive restructuring, rational analysis, and exposure. For example, Beckian cognitive therapy uses a consistent session structure (A. T. Beck, Rush, Shaw, & Emery, 1979; J. S. Beck, 1995) that involves mood check-in, feedback from previous sessions, homework review, agenda setting, processing session content, homework assignment, and feedback/summaries. It is important to remember that session structure should be maintained over the course of therapy when employing the procedures described in this text.

Content is the direct therapeutic material elicited via the structure. The individual patient's automatic thoughts, emotions, responses on assessment measures, coping thoughts, and results from behavioral experiments all represent content.

Process adds a third dimension. It refers to the way children respond to the structure and content of the session. No one reacts identically to the same procedure. Children's

TABLE 1.1. Examples of Therapeutic Structure, Content, and Process

Structure	Content	Hypothesized process
Agenda setting	"I don't know—you decide."	Submissiveness, passivity, perfection, fear of negative evaluation, fear of change.
Feedback	"You stink as a therapist. Did you even graduate from high school?"	Provocation, competitiveness, independence seeking.
Homework assignment/ review	"Perfect completion" with no cross-outs or mistakes.	Fear of negative evaluation, approval seeking.
Self-monitoring/ assessment	Ripped up the forms and said, "You are more interested in these forms than me."	Patient sees the therapist as mechanical, uncaring, and lacking in understanding.
Cognitive restructuring	Platitudinous and pollyannaish coping thoughts: "Nothing bad will happen to me."	Avoidance, intolerance of negative affect.
Behavioral experiments/exposure	"It's silly. Why would I want to get more worried or nervous?"	Avoidance, low self-efficacy.

idiosyncratic reactions to cognitive-behavioral procedures are important aspects of understanding the treatment process. Pos and Greenberg (2007) noted that patients display problematic cognitive, behavioral, and emotional states while in session. Attending to the therapeutic process facilitates recognition of these markers, which are opportunities for intervention. Yontef (2007, p. 23) rightly recommended, "The therapist has to recognize openings and learn the sequence of what must come before what." Children's process markers can include responses such as teariness, flushing, a shifting posture, a shaking foot, changing topics, climbing under a table, cynicism, smugness, irritation, pessimism, eagerness to please, dismissiveness, and superficiality.

Weaving procedures and process into a coherent psychotherapeutic fabric is key. Consider a few clinical examples. An aggressive 13-year-old girl named Tanya believed she was under siege from most other people. She routinely misinterpreted benign actions as deliberate threats. Since the possibility of assault always seemed imminent, she was primed for preemptive counterattacks. In session, she responded to an innocuous comment ("It must be hard to think you are totally on your own.") with a stinging angry response ("You are really pissing me off. You are insulting. Go _____ yourself."). With this clear process marker, the therapist intervened by asking, "What went through your mind just when I said that?" In a moment of insightful awareness, Tanya commented that she saw it as a criticism implying she was too weak to handle the stresses in her life.

In another example, Chloe, a 16-year-old patient with anorexia, habitually inhibited her thoughts and feelings. She believed power was best attained through secrecy. Thus, sharing her thoughts and feelings with a therapist was a tough task made even more difficult by her sense that disclosure was defeating. Chloe brought very superficial thought diaries to her sessions. They lacked emotional meaningfulness and were overly intellectual and impersonal. The therapist then used the thought diaries to capture dysfunctional beliefs about disclosure and expressing feelings. Chloe identified beliefs such as

"People will reject and coerce me. If I hide myself, I am less of a target"; "Being secretive gives me control and the more control I have, the more acceptable I am"; and "No one will give me what I want. I have to trick them into it." Once these beliefs were recorded, the therapist progressed toward a test of evidence ("What convinces you I will reject or coerce you?"; "What makes you doubt I will reject and coerce you?") and reattribution procedures ("What are other ways to be competent and acceptable in addition to hiding away your thoughts and feelings?"). By weaving together Chloe's process (where she inhibited thoughts and feelings as protection against potential coercion, and believed deception is the best way to get what I want) with therapeutic procedures (such as test of evidence and reattribution), the therapist was able to test Chloe's assumptions.

APPLY TECHNIQUES
IN THE CONTEXT OF PATIENTS' EMOTIONAL AROUSAL

It is vital that clinicians apply techniques and procedures in the context of patients' negative affective arousal. Emotional arousal is the lifeblood of CBT. Procedures lay lifeless when they are delivered in an emotionally sterile environment. The recommendation to apply therapy in an emotional context has been made often (Burum & Goldfried, 2007; Castonguay, Pincus, Agras, & Hines, 1998; Frank, 1961; Friedberg & McClure, 2002; Goldfried, 2003; Greenberg, 2006; Greenberg & Paivio, 1997, 2002; Robins & Hayes, 1993; Samoilov & Goldfried, 2000). Gosch et al. (2006, p. 259) noted, "A key ingredient to successful CBT is making the therapy content child-focused and the process experiential." Good therapy is like live theater (Kraemer, 2006): it reveals and deals with the drama of patients' lives. At their most inspiring, both theater and therapy form an experiential bond between audience (therapist) and performer (patient) forged in an emotional furnace sparked by genuine expression, sound reflection, and true creative action.

Clinicians need to use procedures when patients are experiencing problematic emotions—otherwise therapy becomes an abstract intellectual exercise. When therapists elicit and sensitively process patients' deeply felt emotions, treatment takes off. The challenge and excitement of CBT with young people is to make use of intensely charged emotional moments in the present (Friedberg & Gorman, 2007).

Enduring change is facilitated when treatment is embedded in emotional arousal (Robins & Hayes, 1993). Indeed, we argue that when properly executed, CBT is a truly experiential form of therapy. Kraemer (2006, p. 245) emphasized that "learning from experience means being affected by the here and now." Thus, CBT with children is not an intellectual exercise.

Hayes and Strauss (1998) employ the concept of destabilization in processing patients' in-session emotional arousal. *Destabilization* refers to creating dramatic shifts in beliefs, behavior, and feelings. Samoilov and Goldfried (2000) suggested that destabilization is fostered by narrowing patients' attention to their here-and-now experience and amplifying their emotional arousal. This intense experience leads to greater change in meaning structures and changes in depressive symptoms (Hayes & Strauss, 1998).

Cotterell (2005) has likened CBT to sculpting steel. In order to bend steel and create change, intense heat and fire are necessary. Emotions represent the "heat" in CBT. Cognitions that are associated with increased emotional arousal are referred to as "hot cognitions" (Samoilov & Goldfried, 2000). Recent advances in affective neuroscience also support this view of emotional arousal. Brain changes in CBT for obsessive–compulsive disorder are "due to activation of relevant basal ganglia, cingulate, and OFC [orbito-frontal cortex] circuits during exposure and habituation to anxiety-provoking stimuli, thereby permitting the formation of novel (and more adaptive) cortical and subcortical neural patterns of stimulus-linked information processing" (Ilardi & Feldman, 2001, p. 1077).

The proper use of many of the techniques and methods described in this book requires emotional arousal. The more procedures are applied in moments of affective arousal, the more they will take hold or stick.

APPLYING THE TECHNIQUES IN GROUP AND FAMILY FORMATS

Most of the procedures in this book can be readily applied in group and family formats as well as in individual therapy. Individual case formulations need to dictate if and when a group and/or family format will be used. As with individual therapy, integrating the procedures with therapeutic processes is essential, as is applying them in the context of emotional arousal. However, cognitive therapy becomes more complicated when there are more people in the room. In such cases, it is important that each person be an active participant. Everyone should be involved! This requires you to be able to divide your attention between the various people in the room.

When there are multiple people in the room, each person's thoughts, feelings, and behaviors have an impact on those of the others. Family CBT recognizes the reciprocal interaction of family members' cognitions, emotions, actions, and relationships (Dattilio, 1997, 2001). Friedberg (2006, p. 160) noted that the "family environment is the milieu where children and parents' cognitions are played out." Family processes initiate, exacerbate, and maintain dysfunctional thinking, feeling, and action patterns. More specifically, families may collude to avoid negative affect (Barrett, Dadds, & Rapee, 1996; Ginsburg, Siqueland, Masia-Warner, & Hedtke, 2004). Ginsburg et al. (2004) commented that parents may see anxiety as catastrophic, view their parental value and competence in being able to protect their child, and inadvertently undermine their youngsters' fragile sense of self-efficacy.

Because all the family or group members have thoughts and feelings about what is going on in the room, comparing thought records is an excellent idea. Some people may have similar records while others may have records that are uniquely personal. Dealing with points of convergence and divergence makes group and/or family CBT come alive.

The group or family context is a robust circumstance for testing, modifying, and/or problem solving dysfunctional beliefs. For example, children with interpersonal anxieties about negative evaluation, humiliation, and/or embarrassment will emit characteristic cognitions, emotions, and behaviors in the group context. This allows for the immediate therapeutic processing and modification of these problematic states. Similarly, families challenged by an identified patient will show the therapist their distress and reveal dysfunctional patterns. When problems become more transparent, you can more readily intervene with cognitive and behavioral procedures to help patients change their actions, thoughts, and feelings. The family therapy context allows the members to collectively witness and participate in each other's change process. Finally, applying CBT with groups and families may further the generalization process by teaching patients to use their skills in relevant circumstances.

A WORD ABOUT OUR TRANSCRIPTS

In order to protect the confidentiality of our patients, all of the case examples are fictionalized or disguised clinical accounts. They represent a combination of our many cases.

CONCLUSION

This book's modular format offers some of the guidance of a manualized approach, with flexibility for selecting and modifying interventions to match individual clients' case conceptualizations. Each module's techniques and procedures can be applied to numerous symptom sets at various points in therapy. This approach allows clinicians to choose interventions based on patients' age, developmental level, presenting problem, severity of symptoms, interests, intervention modality, and skill set. We outline tools for clinicians to make informed choices about how to proceed in treatment. The creativity in the drawings and presentation style of these interventions keeps patients interested and engaged in treatment, as well as gives clinicians more options to choose from, adding to the individualization of the treatment protocol. By using eye-catching illustrations and interesting metaphors, the ideas come alive for clinicians and patients.

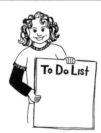

BOX 1.1. Tips for Using the Techniques in This Book

- Embed *everything* in a cognitive-behavioral case conceptualization.
- Maintain the traditional session structure.
- Integrate procedures with psychotherapeutic processes such as therapeutic alliance, collaboration, and guided discovery.
- Remain emotionally alert and present when implementing procedures.
- Apply the techniques in the context of emotional arousal.

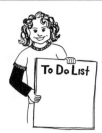

BOX 1.2. Tips for Using These Techniques with Families and Groups

- Get everyone actively participating by dividing your attention among the individuals.
- Each person's thoughts, feelings, and behaviors affect those of everyone else.
- Be wary of individuals colluding to avoid negative affect.
- Make effective use of the interpersonal contexts by applying thought diaries, cognitive restructuring methods, and experiential learning.

CHAPTER 2

Using Assessment Efficiently

Assessment and evaluation in psychotherapy are ongoing procedures used to form hypotheses about patients, scaffold treatment strategies, judge progress, and evaluate outcome (Nelson-Gray, 2003; Peterson & Sobell, 1994; Schroeder & Gordon, 2002). The formal and informal measures described in this chapter provide data for hypotheses regarding case formulation. Based on the information gleaned from the various instruments described here, you can identify specific mood symptoms, dysfunctional beliefs, problematic behaviors, behavioral contingencies, and maladaptive schemas. All these factors are central ingredients in putting together your case formulation.

The measures in this chapter also allow you to monitor treatment progress. You can repeatedly administer and score the instruments to track treatment gains. If you use a formal measure like the Beck Depression Inventory–II (BDI-II), you can elect standard markers for progress (e.g., a 3-point change) or judge differences in scores on an individualized case-by-case basis. Based on the scores, you can make treatment planning decisions regarding the frequency of sessions, termination/discharge, and referrals for medication.

The majority of assessment instruments presented in this chapter are self-report measures. We also present some teacher, parent, and clinician report measures. Self-report inventories are a tradition in child assessment (Reynolds, 1993), but they possess both advantages and limitations. Their use should be tempered by considering the problem being assessed and the developmental abilities of the individual child.

We begin this chapter with our recommendations for the initial session and for ongoing monitoring, including issues of interpretation and clinical process. Next, we review selected formal measures for assessing depression, anxiety, anger, disruptive behavior disorders, pervasive developmental disorders (PDD), and eating disorders. Cognitive content measures that tap automatic thoughts and schemas are also presented. The second part of the chapter offers idiographic or highly individualized self-monitoring procedures grouped by the domain monitored: emotion, behavior, and cognition. Many of these self-monitoring techniques set the stage for treatment techniques presented in later chapters.

RECOMMENDATIONS FOR THE INITIAL SESSION

Assessment in the initial session provides important background information, parameters of the presenting problems, and baseline data. Moreover, the data obtained forms the basis for a preliminary case formulation. A good clinical interview that yields data is essential; using children's self-report measures helps guide this initial interview. You can follow up on salient issues (e.g., "I don't like myself"; "I am a worrier") and query for specific examples. In addition, we recommend screening measures for mood and anxiety symptoms. Generally, we use the Child Depression Inventory (CDI; Kovacs, 1992) and the Screen for Child Anxiety Related Emotional Disorders (SCARED; Birmaher et al., 1997), with children 14 years and younger. With older patients, we recommend the BDI-II (A. T. Beck, 1996) and the Multidimensional Anxiety Scale for Children (MASC; March, Parker, Sullivan, Stallings, & Conners, 1997). We also add the parent report version of the SCARED and the CDI to the assessment. If the child presents with complaints associated with attention-deficit/hyperactivity disorder (ADHD), we will add a SNAP-IV (Swanson, Sandman, Deutsch, & Baren, 1983), Connors' Parent Rating Scales, or Connors' Teaching Ratings Scales (CPRS; CTRS; Connors, 2000). Finally, if a child or adolescent presents with suicidal ideation, we will also add a Beck Hopelessness Scale (BHS) or the Hopelessness Scale for Children (HSC).

The above measures provide immediate information on pivotal issues regarding suicidality and hopelessness (e.g., items 2 and 9 on both the CDI and the BDI-II). Self-reports offer several additional advantages in the first session. First, you clearly communicate the message that you take the children's subjective reports seriously. Second, the initial evaluation shows that you are going to integrate assessment and treatment. Not only is the data fundamental to your understanding and treatment of the patient, the mere fact of completing these forms has purpose. Third, children endorse the items themselves, so they play a central role in identifying their own symptoms. Consequently, they are less likely to be defensive about the ultimate content of the evaluation. Fourth, and finally, many youngsters welcome the emotional distance provided by completing a paper-and-pencil measure, and thus the task offers a way for them to be somewhat dispassionate about their symptoms.

Obtaining both parents' and children's reports yields useful comparative data. By identifying points of convergence and divergence, you conceptualize other critical factors, such as Are the parents attuned to their child's distress? Does the child or parent magnify or minimize the distress? In addition, you can note how these are subsequently processed: "What do you make of the fact that your mother's score for you is less than yours?"; "How do you explain that Johnny's score is far below your score for him?" Piacentini, Cohen, and Cohen (1992) rightly noted that when both parents and child endorse the same item, you can be confident that the problem is present.

Parents tend to be more reliable reporters of externalizing and disruptive behavior problems than children themselves (Bird, Gould, & Staghezza, 1992; Loeber, Green, Lahey, & Stouthamer-Loeber, 1991). In fact, there are limited data supporting the validity of children's self-report of ADHD symptoms (Pelham, Fabiano, & Massetti, 2005). On the other hand, children better chronicle their own emotional distress compared to their parents. Further, parents' reports are subject to their own mood states (De Los Reyes & Kazdin, 2005; Krain & Kendall, 2000; Silverman & Ollendick, 2005). A depressed parent may inaccurately magnify a child's problems and give an overly critical or catastrophic assessment. Maternal depression creates a negative bias in the way mothers describe their child's internalizing and externalizing problems (Chi & Hinshaw, 2002; Najman et al., 2000; Youngstrom, Loeber, & Stouthamer-Loeber, 2000).

Informant discrepancies are clinical facts of life. De Los Reyes and Kazdin (2005) offer a commonsense rubric for understanding these discrepancies based on sound empirical data and astute conceptual reasoning. First, they argue that various informants, including children, parents, and teachers, have differing motivations and goals for completing the assessment process. For instance, parents may view the assessment process as a way to identify and understand their children's problems. Children, on the other hand, may want to minimize their problems and avoid treatment. In other situations, parental psychopathology may lead to an exaggeration of the child's distress and impairment to shift the focus away from their own difficulties. Or the child may be accurately reflecting his or her own low level of distress and impairment.

De Los Reyes and Kazdin (2005) noted that parents are prone to seeing children's problems as dispositional, whereas children see their difficulties as more contextual. In other words, observers may see problems as residing within the child, whereas children locate their problems in situations and environments. De Los Reyes and Kazdin state that the point of assessment is to collect negative information about the child's behavior. If both the child and the parent are attuned to this goal, consistent information is more likely.

De Los Reyes and Kazdin's (2005) model has different implications for how you conduct the interview. First, balance questions for assessing dispositional characteristics with questions about situations and environmental circumstances. Second, try to identify each informant's motivations for his or her report. Third, if discrepancies emerge, they do not necessarily have to be resolved. They may represent the child's functioning in multiple contexts. Finally, differing reports should elicit questions about how the parent and the child view assessment and treatment.

Assessment is a process. You should be curious not only about the actual scores, but also about how the scores were obtained. For example, did the child complete his or her own CDI independently or did the parent complete or correct it? What was the reason the parent completed the form (reading ability, mistrust, etc.)? You should not be shy about asking for clarification on specific items. This is particularly important when inquiring about responses to items 2 and 9 on both the CDI and the BDI-II which assess suicidality. Querying particular items adds more to the assessment and also communicates that you take the patients' reports seriously.

Total scores, factor scores, and responses to individual items should be considered starting points rather than end points. Pelham et al. (2005) compellingly emphasized this point when discussing ADHD assessment. A child's or parent's response to an individual item (e.g., "Often does not seem to listen when spoken to directly") may mean different things. Item endorsement says nothing about the causing, maintaining, or exacerbating factors. Pelham et al. (2005) rightly stated that the problem could be due to poor parental commands, child avoidance of aversive tasks, and/or an auditory processing problem. They urge us to identify areas and levels of impairment, operationalize target behaviors, and determine antecedents, discriminative stimuli, and consequences of the problem behavior.

Curious findings during the assessment are common. They are important data sources and you should be "nosy" about them. For example, some children may omit specific items. For distracted and careless children, this omission may be fairly benign (e.g., they simply missed it). On the other hand, the child may feel uncomfortable marking an answer or may be actively deceptive. In still other cases, the omitted items may represent a test the young patient constructs to see what you will do about the omitted items. The patient may be asking: "Will you follow up on omitted responses about hopelessness or suicidality?"; "Do you wonder about the reasons I did not answer the question about liking myself?"; "Do you care if I answered the question about things seeming unreal when I get anxious?"

Many patients edit the self-report measures. We find the revision process useful and encourage this "collaboration." The edits may take the form of adding numbers to the scale or options to the responses provided. Some youngsters write comments in the margins responding to the questions ("This is a stupid question.") or clarifying their choices ("The reason I marked this was … "). The editorial process is a good data source and more importantly shows that the child is making the process his or her own. For example, one young patient added a fourth point to each item on the MASC to illustrate how intensely and frequently his symptoms bothered him.

Clinicians should share the findings and scores from the assessment process. The meaning of the scores should be clearly communicated to the patient and the family. We graph scores and show them to patients. In this way, collaboration is enhanced and assessment is something done *with* rather than *to* the patient.

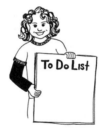

BOX 2.1. Summary Pad for Initial Assessment

- Do a good clinical interview.
- For patients with mood and/or anxiety complaints:
  - 7- to 15-year-olds: consider SCARED and CDI.
  - 15 years and older: consider BDI-II and MASC.
- If suicidal ideation is present, add:
  - Children: Hopelessness Scale for Children, SIQ Jr.
  - Adolescents: BHS and SIQ.
- For ADHD, consider SNAP-IV, CTRS, and CPRS.
- Obtain data from multiple informants.
- Remember that assessment is a process.
- Assessment in CBT is transparent. Share the data with patients!

Showing how these assessment findings are useful and relevant continues the collaborative process and facilitates reliable self-reports (Freeman et al., 1990). For instance, we consistently discuss the way the assessment informs case conceptualization and treatment planning (e.g., "Based on the SCARED findings, it seems Matteo is very concerned with disappointing you and avoiding your disappointment. For this reason, he is slow completing his homework for fear of making a mistake and risking your disappointment."). Both patients and third-party payors respond favorably to using this data for treatment planning.

RECOMMENDATIONS FOR ONGOING MONITORING

Repeated administration of the parent, teacher, and self-report measures is our regular practice. As a general rule, we give the measures on a monthly basis. Yet, if the child is in severe distress or more labile, we may administer the measures more often, such as on a weekly or biweekly basis. We often graph results and invite patients and their families to do the same. This is especially helpful for patients who have repeated acute depressive episodes. Patients can see how their moods have peaks and valleys. Coping skills could be taught to the patients for the different phases of their illness (e.g., low, moderate, high acuity). By regularly monitoring their own symptoms, patients can identify the warning signs of worsening conditions and then attempt to take corrective actions. Finally, charting symptom levels is also helpful for patients and parents who consult with pediatricians and child psychiatrists regarding medications. The data allow patients to authoritatively talk with their prescribing physician about the effects of the medicine on their symptoms. Most physicians welcome the data.

You may have cases in which a patient would benefit from medication but both patient and family are reluctant. By collaboratively sharing the monitoring data with the patient, you can propose to revisit the medication referral in 2 weeks or 4 weeks if symptoms remain at a high level. Thus, rather than forcing or fighting with a patient and family, you can make a medication referral into an "empirical" question.

Regular tracking of patients' symptoms fundamentally shapes your treatment planning decisions and is a particularly pivotal issue, especially if the patient's insurance benefits allow for a limited number of sessions (e.g., 20 per year). You can dose the sessions every week while symptoms are in the high to moderate range, and then taper the frequency of sessions to every 2 weeks, 4 weeks, and so on as the scores dictate.

Many clinicians worry about the effect of frequent administrations on the psychometric integrity of the various instruments. It can be reassuring to see the patient as his or her own baseline or control group. In clinical practice, you are doing idiographic assessment. Noise in the data is clinically useful. If you suspect that the data do not accurately reflect the patient's experience or functioning level, you should investigate further. For instance, the patient may complete the forms and the resulting scores may suggest huge improvement, yet there is little evidence to substantiate the gains. You could ask questions such as "How do you explain your lower scores, but your mom and teacher see your behavior as the same or even a little worse?" or "What do you want to tell me by filling out the scores in this way?" In this way, seamless integration of assessment and treatment is continued.

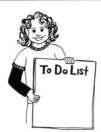

BOX 2.2. Summary Pad for Ongoing Monitoring

- In general, readminister symptom measures every month.
- Use the monitoring to inform treatment planning.
- Like the initial assessment, remember that monitoring is a process.
- Make a graph or other record of the scores.
- Ongoing monitoring is transparent and collaborative.

FORMAL SELF-REPORT AND OTHER-REPORT MEASURES

Depression

Table 2.1 presents a variety of instruments we use for assessing depression in children and adolescents. A full critique for the depression instruments, as well as for all the other measures mentioned in this chapter, is beyond the scope of this book. The interested reader is directed to Klein, Dougherty, and Olino (2005) for an outstanding review. While a number of inventories are listed in Table 2.1, we focus our discussion on the Children's Depression Inventory (CDI), Beck Depression Inventory–II (BDI-II), and the Beck Youth Depression Scale (BYDS).

We most often use the CDI and the BDI-II. The CDI (Kovacs, 1992) is easy to complete and score. The instrument yields a total score and data on five important factor scores (negative mood, interpersonal difficulties, negative self-esteem, ineffectiveness, and anhedonia). The CDI produces raw scores which can be converted to standard scores (*T*-scores). Kovacs (1985) recommends a raw score cutoff of 13. The CDI can be administered in a long or a short form. Additionally, it offers both a child self-report and a parental report of a child's depressive symptoms. Finally, the CDI has English and Spanish versions. The CDI is a useful tool to monitor treatment progress. Fristad, Emery, and Beck (1997) recommended the CDI as a way to assess and track symptom severity. The CDI is also responsive to treatment effects (Brooks & Kutcher, 2001; Myers & Winters, 2002; Silverman & Rabian, 1999).

The CDI factor scores are especially helpful in conceptualization and treatment planning. For example, factor analysis can "unpack" a child's depression to reveal the contributions of anhedonia and interpersonal problems that you can specifically target. In this way, treatment is made more efficient.

The BDI-II is a widely used instrument (A. T. Beck, Steer, & Brown, 1996; Dozois & Covin, 2004; Dozois, Dobson, & Ahnberg, 1998). It generates somewhat different

TABLE 2.1. Selected Formal Standardized Self-Report Measures for Assessing Depressive Mood States

Instrument	Ages	Comments
Children's Depression Inventory (CDI; Kovacs, 1992)	7–17 years	Provides a total score and five factor scores, short and long forms available, self (child) and parent report options, English and Spanish versions
Beck Depression Inventory–II; (BDI; A. T. Beck, 1996)	13–80 years	Measures severity of depression, useful to monitor progress in treatment; has been translated into several languages
Beck Youth Depression Scale (BYDS; J. S. Beck et al., 2001)	7–14 years	Part of the Beck Youth Scales, measures maladaptive cognitions and behaviors
Hopelessness Scale for Children (HSC; Kazdin et al., 1986a, 1986b)	6–13 years	17 items, true/false format, measures the degree of hopelessness
Suicidal Ideation Questionnaire (SIQ; Reynolds, 1987)	Grades 10–12	30 items assessing suicidal ideation
Suicidal Ideation Questionnaire—Jr. (SIQ-Jr; Reynolds, 1988)	Grades 7–9	15 items assessing suicidal ideations
Beck Hopelessness Scale (BHS; A. T. Beck et al., 1974)	Recommended for 16–17 years old and older	20 items assessing hopelessness

cutoff scores than the original BDI. Scores of 20 points or more indicate serious depression. Scores between 13–19 points reflect dysphoria to moderate depression. Female adolescents tend to have higher BDI-II scores than their male counterparts (Kumar, Steer, Teitelman, & Villacis, 2002; Steer, Kumar, Ranieri, & Beck, 1998). Although there is evidence of a subtle factor structure in the measure (Kumar et al., 2002), the BDI-II reveals a clearer factor structure (cognitive, somatic, cognitive/somatic) than the original BDI (Dozois & Covin, 2004). The BDI-II is also translated into several languages. Like the CDI, the BDI-II has been employed in numerous outcome studies supporting its sensitivity to treatment changes. Both the CDI and the BDI-II are responsive to treatment effects. Thus, you can periodically administer them to assess treatment progress.

The Beck Youth Depression Scale (J. S. Beck, Beck, & Jolly, 2001) is part of the Beck Youth Scales and is designed to tap maladaptive cognitions and behaviors associated with depressed mood in children ages 7–14 years (Bose-Deakins & Floyd, 2004). Like the other separate scales in the Beck battery, individual scoring is recommended (Steer, Kumar, Beck, & Beck, 2005). The scale yields a standard score ($T = 50$; $SD = 10$). More specifically, it measures many of the criteria associated with unipolar depressive spectrum disorders (Steer et al., 2005). The sensitivity to treatment effects is currently unclear (Bose-Deakins & Floyd, 2004).

Suicidality is a sometimes tragic symptom of depression and needs to be assessed separately. The CDI and the BDI-II have two items (numbers 2 and 9 in both measures) that specifically assess suicidality. These items should always be reviewed. When you are concerned about a young patient's suicidality, we recommend you add a hopelessness measure. The Hopelessness Scale for Children (HSC; Kazdin, Colbus, & Rodgers, 1986a) and the Beck Hopelessness Scale (BHS; A. T. Beck, Weissman, Lester, & Trexler, 1974) are good options. The HSC is a 17-item self-report scale for children 6 years old to 13 years old that assesses their level of pessimism. The HSC offers a "true or false" response format. Kazdin et al. (1986a) reported a raw score of 7 (67 percentile) indicating high hopelessness.

The BHS is a 20-item measure tapping generalized pessimism (A. T. Beck et al., 1974; Dozois & Covin, 2004). Items are presented in a true–false format. The BHS is best suited to older adolescents (16–17 years) and is a powerful predictor of suicidal ideation in this population (Kumar & Steer, 1995; Steer, Kumar, & Beck, 1993a, 1993b). Cutoffs indicating high hopelessness average from 8 to 15 points. We agree with Dozois and Covin (2004), who recommend using a slightly higher cutoff score than 8 or 9. We suggest 11 as a cutoff score.

The Suicidal Ideation Questionnaire (SIQ) and the SIQ-Jr. (Reynolds, 1987, 1988) are valuable tools for identifying suicidal ideation in adolescents and younger children. The SIQ is a 30-item measure for adolescents in grades 10 through 12. The SIQ-Jr is a 15-item inventory for children in grades seven, eight, and nine. Items are scored on a 7-point scale (0–6), with higher scores reflecting greater suicidality. The cutoff score for the SIQ is 41 and the cutoff score for the SIQ-Jr is 31.

Anxiety

Table 2.2 outlines our preferred tools for assessing anxiety disorders in children and adolescents. The table includes measures giving an overall anxiety score (Beck Youth Anxiety Scale [BYAS], Penn State Worry Questionnaire for Children [PSWQC]), a general score plus specific factor scores (SCARED, MASC, RCMAS, Spence Anxiety), disorder-specific scales (CY-BOCS-CR, CY-BOCS-PR, SPAI-C), and disorder-specific scales with factor scores (FSS-R, SRAS, SASC) that yield an even more refined level of analysis. The psychometrics as well as the pros and cons of each measure can be found in a recent excellent review by Silverman and Ollendick (2005).

The Screen for Child Anxiety Related Emotional Disorders (SCARED; Birmaher et al., 1997) is a favorite tool. Like the CDI, it is easy to complete, score, and interpret. The SCARED yields an overall score for anxiety (raw score = 25) and five factor scores (panic/somatic, generalized anxiety disorder, separation anxiety, social anxiety, and school avoidance). Further, the SCARED has recently undergone a revision (SCARED-R; Muris, Merckelbach, Van Brakel, & Mayer, 1999). More items and additional factors (OCD, PTSD, trauma) were added. The SCARED offers both child and parent report versions.

The Multidimensional Anxiety Scale for Children (MASC; March et al., 1997; March, Sullivan, & James, 1999) is also a preferred instrument. The MASC is somewhat more comprehensive than the SCARED, and the scoring and analysis are slightly more complicated, but the extra effort is worthwhile. The MASC produces an overall anxiety score, factor scores (physiological, harm reduction, social anxiety, separation anxiety), subfactors (tense/restless, perfectionism, anxious coping, humiliation/rejection), an anxiety disorder index, and an inconsistency (lie) scale.

The Beck Youth Anxiety Scale (BYAS; J. S. Beck et al., 2001) measures DSM-IV criteria associated with the anxiety disorders (Steer et al., 2005). Fearfulness, worry,

TABLE 2.2. Selected Measures for Assessing Anxious Mood States

Instrument	Ages	Comments
Screen for Child Anxiety Related Emotional Experiences—Revised (SCARED; Birmaher et al., 1997)	8 years and older	Easy to use and score, provides overall score and five factor scores, offers child and parent report versions
Multidimensional Anxiety Scale for Children (MASC; March et al., 1997)	8–19 years	A more comprehensive measure; provides overall score, factor scores, subfactors, and inconsistency scale; short form is available
Beck Youth Anxiety Scale (BYAS; J. S. Beck et al., 2001)	7–14 years	20-item self-report measure of children's specific worries and DSM-IV criteria for anxiety disorders
Revised Children's Manifest Anxiety Scale (RCMAS; Reynolds & Richmond, 1985)	6–19 years	Contains 37 yes/no items and yields a total score, subscales, and a lie index
Spence Children's Anxiety Scale (SCAS; Spence, 1998)	7–14 years	Measures DSM-IV anxiety disorders
Fear Survey Schedule for Children—Revised (FSSC-R; Ollendick et al., 1989)	7–16 years	80 items, yields five factors, and is useful as a measure of treatment outcomes
Penn State Worry Questionnaire for Children (PSWQC; Chorpita et al., 1997)	6–18 years	Measures frequency and controllability of children's worries
Social Phobia and Anxiety Inventory for Children (SPAI-C; Beidel et al., 1995)	8–17 years	Measures distressing social situations and includes three factor scores
Social Anxiety Scale for Children—Revised (SASC-R; La Greca & Stone, 1993)	8–12 years	Narrow-band measure of social anxiety, includes three subscales
School Refusal Assessment Scale (SRAS; Kearney & Silverman, 1993)	8–14 years	User-friendly tool based on a functional analysis of school refusal; offers parent, teacher, and child report versions
Children's Obsessive–Compulsive Inventory (ChOCI; Shafran et al., 2003)	7–17 years	Offers parent and child reports; measures compulsive symptoms and obsessive symptoms
Children's Florida Obsessive–Compulsive Inventory (C-FOCI; Merlo, Storch, & Geffken, 2007)	8–18 years	17-item scale, with obsessive and compulsive subscales
Children's Yale–Brown Obsessive–Compulsive Scale (CY-BOCS)	8–16 years	Measures obsessive–compulsive symptoms

and bodily symptoms are tapped by this inventory (Bose-Deakins & Floyd, 2004). Like its depression-related counterpart, its sensitivity to treatment changes is still uncertain.

The Revised Children's Manifest Anxiety Scale (RCMAS; Reynolds & Richmond, 1985) consists of 37 yes/no items completed by the child/adolescent. The RCMAS provides a total anxiety score, three factor scores (physiological anxiety, worry/oversensitivity, and social concerns/concentration) and a consistency/lie index. It can be administered individually or in a group setting.

The Spence Children's Anxiety Scale (SCAS; Spence, 1998) is a broad-band measure of DSM-IV anxiety disorders. It assesses the presence and frequency of symptoms associated with separation anxiety, social phobia, obsessive–compulsive disorder, panic disorder with agoraphobia, generalized anxiety disorder, and fears of physical injury. The scale is appropriate for youngsters ages 7–14 years and offers 44 items.

The Fear Survey Schedule for Children—Revised (FSSC-R; Ollendick, 1983; Ollendick, King, & Frary, 1989) is a well-established self-report measure for children ages 7–16 years that can discriminate between clinical and nonclinical populations. It is an 80-item scale with three response options (none, some, a lot). The scale yields five factors including fear of failure and criticism, fear of the unknown, fear of minor injury and small animals, fear of danger/death, and medical fears. The FSSC-R is also quite useful as a pre–post measure of treatment outcome.

The Penn State Worry Questionnaire for Children (PSWQC; Chorpita, Tracey, Brown, Collica, & Barlow, 1997) provides a narrow-band measure of generalized worries. Items yield data on the frequency and controllability of children's worries. The PSWQC consists of 14 items and is appropriate for children ages 6–18 years.

The Social Phobia and Anxiety Inventory for Children (SPAI-C; Beidel, Turner, & Morris, 1995) is a narrow-band measure tapping distressing social situations. The SPAI-C contains three factors including assertiveness/general conversation, traditional social encounters, and public performance. There are 26 items appropriate for children ages 8–17 years.

The Social Anxiety Scale for Children—Revised (SASC-R; La Greca & Stone, 1993) is another narrow-band measure for social anxiety. The SASC-R produces three subscales, including fear of negative evaluation, social avoidance and distress in new situations, and general social avoidance and distress. The children's version consists of 26 items and the new adolescent version (La Greca & Lopez, 1998) has 22 items.

The School Refusal Assessment Scale (SRAS; Kearney & Silverman, 1993) is a very accessible tool based on a functional analysis of school refusal behavior. Kearney and Silverman recognize that school refusal is commonly multiply determined. Thus, the scale assesses and weighs four central factors including avoidance of stimuli-producing negative affectivity (negative reinforcement paradigm), escape from evaluative situations (negative reinforcement paradigm), attention-getting behavior (positive reinforcement), and/or obtaining direct positive reinforcement. Each question is scored on a 7-point scale. The SRAS includes both a parent and a child report version. After the measure is completed, means for each of the four factors are computed. The highest mean is considered the primary maintaining variable.

The Children's Yale–Brown Obsessive–Compulsive Scale (CY-BOCS) is a frequently used instrument for measuring the severity of OCD symptoms and is derived from the Yale–Brown Obsessive–Compulsive Scale (YBOCS; Goodman et al., 1989). It is administered by the clinician through a semistructured interview, and yields separate severity scales for obsessions and compulsions. Based on the parent and/or child responses, a rating is made on a 5-point scale to designate the frequency or duration, interference, distress, resistance to, and control of symptoms. Scores of 15 or higher suggest clinically significant levels of OCD symptoms. Administration time can be lengthy, but the information gained is quite useful (Myers & Winters, 2002). The measure may be readministered to evaluate progress and to determine level of impairment.

There are several new children's self-report and parental reports for OCD (Merlo, Storch, Murphy, Goodman, & Geffken, 2005). The Children's Obsessive–Compulsive Inventory (ChOCI; Shafran et al., 2003) is a 32-item scale that offers both child and parental report scales. Nineteen items are devoted to compulsive symptoms and 13 items are focused on obsessive symptoms. The ChOCI takes about 15 minutes to complete. A cutoff score of 17 is recommended. The Children's Florida Obsessive–Compulsive Inventory (C-FOCI; Merlo, Storch, & Geffken, 2007) is a 17-item scale that contains obsessive and compulsive subscales. It takes about 5–10 minutes to complete. Merlo et al. (2005) recommended the C-FOCI as a screener for OCD.

Storch et al. (2004, 2006) developed a child and a parent report version of the CY-BOCS (CY-BOCS-CR, CY-BOCS-PR). Both the child and the parent report versions are 10-item measures that are rated on a 5-point Likert scale. The CY-BOCS-CR and the CY-BOCS-PR earned satisfactory psychometric properties. The child report version yields lower scores than either the clinician or parent report versions. Storch et al. noted that many children may not find their symptoms distressing. Additionally, they concluded that many children may minimize their distress due to embarrassment, fears regarding treatment, lack of recognition, and family accommodation to symptoms.

Anger

Anger provides energy and motivation for conduct disorders and oppositional defiant disorders as well as adding to a sense of victimization (J. S. Beck et al., 2005). Our recommended measures for assessing anger are discussed below and summarized in Table 2.3.

The Children's Inventory of Anger (ChIA; Nelson & Finch, 2000) is a self-report instrument designed to identify the types of situations that provoke anger and the intensity of anger responses. The ChIA consists of 39 items, can be used with children ages 6–16 years, and yields a total score, a validity index, and four subscale scores (frustration, physical aggression, peer relationships, and authority relations).

The Novaco Anger Scale and Provocation Inventory (NAS-PI; Novaco, 2003) is designed to provide information on children's experience of anger and anger-provoking situations. It is a self-report measure for patients 9 years and older. The NAS-PI consists of two parts, an anger scale (60 items) and a provocation inventory (25 items). The entire scale can be administered, or each scale may be used separately. Separate norms are available for 9- to 18-year-olds and for individuals 19 years and older.

TABLE 2.3. Selected Measures for Assessing Angry Mood States

Instrument	Ages	Comments
Children's Inventory of Anger (ChIA; Nelson & Finch, 2000)	6–16 years	Yields a total score, a validity index, and four subscale scores; identifies the types of situations that provoke anger and the intensity of anger responses
Novaco Anger Scale and Provocation Inventory (NAS-PI; Novaco, 2003)	9–18 years	Consists of anger and provocation scales, which can be administered separately or together
State–Trait Anger Expression Inventory (STAXI; Spielberger, 1988)	13 years–adult	Assesses experience and expression of anger
Beck Anger Inventory for Youth (BANI-Y; J. S. Beck et al., 2001)	7–18 years	Measures perceptions of mistreatment, hostile attributions, negative views of others, and physiological arousal associated with angry affect

The State–Trait Anger Expression Inventory (STAXI; Spielberger, 1988) assesses anger in adolescents through self-report. A 44-item self-report scale, the STAXI taps the experience and expression of anger in ages 13 years through adult.

The Beck Anger Inventory for Youth (BANI-Y; J. S. Beck et al., 2001, 2005; Bose-Deakins & Floyd, 2004; Steer et al., 2005) assesses children's perceptions of mistreatment, hostile attributions, negative views of other, and physiological arousal associated with angry affect.

Disruptive Behavior Disorders

As summarized in Table 2.4, Connors' Parent and Teacher Rating Scales—Revised (CRS-R; Connors, 2000) are widely used behavior rating scales for children exhibiting symptoms of ADHD. The parent versions have seven factors (oppositionality, inattention, hyperactivity–impulsivity, anxious–shy, perfectionism, social problems, and psychosomatic). The teacher report includes six factors (oppositionality, inattention,

TABLE 2.4. Selected Measures for Assessing Disruptive Behavior Disorders

Instrument	Ages	Comments
Connors' Parent and Teacher Rating Scales—Revised (CRS-R; Connors, 2000)	3–18 years	Widely used behavior rating scale for children with ADHD symptoms; includes parent and teacher versions with a number of factors.
Achenbach Scales (ASCBA; Achenbach, 1991a, 1991b, 1991c)	1½ years and older	Parent, teacher, and self-reports available. Yields competency scores, internalizing and externalizing scores, and eight subscale scores.
Behavior Assessment Scale for Children–2 (BASC-2; Reynolds & Kamphaus, 2004)	2–25 years	Parent, teacher, and self-rating scales available. Items include observations of behaviors, thoughts, and emotions. Adaptive and maladaptive functioning are measured.
Beck Disruptive Behavior Inventory (BDBI; J. S. Beck et al., 2001)	7–14 years	Measures delinquent and aggressive behaviors, including aggression toward animals and people, destruction of property, deceitfulness or theft, and serious rule violations. Additionally, the inventory taps arguing, defiance, deliberate annoyance, and vindicativeness.
Eyberg Child Behavior Inventory (ECBI; Eyberg, 1974)	2–16 years	Assesses the frequency and severity of behavior problems. Teacher version available.
SNAP-IV (Swanson et al., 1983)	6–18 years	Assesses symptoms of oppositional defiant disorder, aggression, and ADHD, including DSM-IV criteria. The SNAP-IV is completed prior to the interview.
SKAMP (Pliszka et al., 1999)	6–18 years	Developed to measure ADHD behaviors in the classroom/home. Parent and teacher versions; based on target behaviors for a token system and offers baseline data for school and home behaviors that may be targeted during treatment.
Disruptive Behavior Disorders Rating Scale (DBDRS; Barkley et al., 1999)		Yields scores for ODD, ADHD, and conduct disorder; offers parent and teacher versions.

hyperactivity–impulsivity, anxious–shy, perfectionism, and social problems). Both short and long versions are available in parent, teacher, and self-report forms.

The Achenbach System of Empirically Based Assessment (ASEBA) has been widely used in research concerning multiple childhood internalizing and externalizing problems. The Achenbach scales include the parent form, the Child Behavior Checklist (CBCL; Achenbach, 1991a), the Teacher Report Form (TRF; Achenbach, 1991b), and the Youth Self-Report (YSR; Achenbach, 1991c). Separate forms of the CBCL are available for children in various age groups, ranging from 1½ years to 18 years. The CBCL (excluding the preschool form) yields competency scores in activities, social, and school areas. The higher competency scores indicate better adjustment in the designated areas. The CBCL also asks parents to rate children on a number of problem areas from 0 (not true) to 2 (very or often true). An overall Total Problems score, Internalizing and Externalizing scores, and eight subscale scores provide various levels of analysis, and T-scores indicate severity of impairment. The TRF is completed by the teacher, and items are similar to the CBCL, allowing for comparison of symptoms across environments. The TRF also includes academic and adaptive functioning scales. The YSR follows the basic structure and item content of the CBCL, but is completed by the youth. Achenbach (2007) points out the importance of using multiple informants, as both similarities and discrepancies provide clinically useful information.

The Behavior Assessment Scale for Children–2 (BASC-2; Reynolds & Kamphaus, 2004) is a behavior rating scale that also includes teacher, parent, and self-rating scales. It is a new-generation measure with very solid psychometric properties and is recommended for conduct problems (Kamphaus, VanDeventer, Brueggemann, & Barry, 2006; McMahon & Kotler, 2006). The teacher, parent, and self-ratings each have three forms, depending on the child's age (preschool form for 2- to 5-year-olds, child form for 6- to 11-year-olds, and adolescent forms for 12- to 21-years-olds). Additionally, the self-report scale offers a college form for 18- to 25-year-olds. Items evaluate the rater's observations of behaviors, thoughts, and emotions exhibited by the child or adolescent. Both adaptive and maladaptive functioning are measured by this scale. By utilizing a dimensional classification approach, the BASC-2 provides information on the severity of symptoms (Kamphaus et al., 2006).

The Beck Disruptive Behavior Inventory (BDBI; J. S. Beck et al., 2001) measures delinquent and aggressive behaviors. Like other Beck Youth Inventories, it consists of 20 items. More specifically, the BDBI assesses aggression toward animals and people, destruction of property, deceitfulness or theft, and serious rule violations. Additionally, the inventory identifies arguing, defiance, deliberate annoyance, and vindictiveness.

The Eyberg Child Behavior Inventory (ECBI; Eyberg, 1974) is a parent report of conduct and behavioral problems in youth ages 2–16 years. The ECBI assesses the frequency and severity of behavior problems. The ECBI consists of 36 items on which the parent rates how often the behavior occurs and indicates if the behavior is a problem. A teacher version to measure behavioral functioning at school is also available (Sutter–Eyberg Student Behavior Inventory [SESBI]; Sutter & Eyberg, 1984). The ECBI is a useful measure for screening common disruptive behaviors and parental perception of problem severity. It may also be useful in assessing change throughout treatment (Eyberg, 1992). Eyberg (1992) noted that when problem and intensity scores differ, this discrepancy can be explored and provide additional clinical data.

When measuring behaviors and thoughts consistent with oppositional defiant disorder and conduct disorder, the Beck Disruptive Behavior Inventory for Youth (BDBI-Y; J. S. Beck et al., 2001) is a useful tool. The BDBI-Y is used for children ages 7–18 years, and can be used in combination with the other Beck Youth Inventories (for depression, anxiety, anger, and self-concept) or on its own.

The Swanson, Nolan, and Pelham Rating Scale (SNAP-IV) is a revision of the SNAP Questionnaire (Swanson, Sandman, Deutsch, & Baren, 1983) and is used with children and adolescents ages 6–18 years to assess symptoms of oppositional defiant disorder, aggression, and ADHD. The SNAP-IV is based on DSM-IV criteria. The SNAP-IV is completed prior to the interview, and parent and teacher raters indicate the degree to which the child exhibits each symptom (not at all, just a little, quite a bit, or very much; Pliszka, Carlson, & Swanson, 1999). Collecting this information prior to the clinical interview helps the clinician make efficient use of the interview time. The SNAP-IV yields subscales, and subset averages or item counts may be used to identify "abnormalities" in youth (Pliszka et al., 1999).

The Swanson, Kotkin, Agler, M-Flynn, and Pelham Scale (SKAMP; Swanson, 1992) was developed to measure ADHD symptoms in the classroom, and offers a parent version measuring home behaviors in addition to the teacher version (Pliszka et al., 1999). The SKAMP items are not DSM-IV criteria, but rather reflect how such symptoms may manifest in the classroom or home by interfering with appropriate behaviors (Pliszka, Carlson & Swanson, 1999). SKAMP items are based on a list of 10 behaviors, and offer baseline data for school and home behaviors that may be targeted during treatment (Pliszka et al., 1999). The SKAMP items focus on behaviors targeted for change. The measure is helpful in tracking behaviors that are necessary for functioning at home and at school (e.g., getting ready for school, sticking with tasks, completing assigned work).

The Disruptive Behavioral Disorder Rating Scale (DBDRS; Barkley, Edwards, & Robin, 1999) yields scores for ODD, ADHD, and conduct disorder. The DBDRS offers parent and teacher versions. The parent and teacher report versions contain inattention items (1–9), hyperactivity–impulsivity items (10–18), and ODD items (19–26). To reach clinical threshold, four or more items on the ODD scale must be rated as 2 or 3 on the scale. On the inattentive and hyperactivity scales, six items must be rated as a 2 or 3. The parent version also includes 15 symptom items on the CD subscale, which are circled yes or no.

Pervasive Developmental Disorders

The Child Autism Rating Scale (CARS; Schopler, Reichler, & Renner, 1986) is a clinically useful scale based on direct observation. The CARS, although not diagnostic in and of itself, is useful as part of a broader battery or assessment process (Marcus & Schopler, 1993). The CARS is made up of 15 subscales of behaviors rated on a continuum, and provides descriptive examples of behaviors to assist the rater. An overall score is obtained by totaling the subscales, and results fall into classifications of "not autistic" (15–29.5), "mild to moderately autistic" (30–36.5), and "severely autistic" (37 and over).

The Autistic Diagnostic Observation Schedule (ADOS; Lord et al., 1989) has been used clinically and in research, and measures social functioning, communication, play, and interest by presenting the child with structured and unstructured tasks designed to elicit certain skills. Behaviors are rated based on direct observation.

TABLE 2.5. Selected Measures for Assessing Pervasive Developmental Disorder

Instrument	Ages	Comments
Child Autism Rating Scale (CARS; Schopler et al., 1986)	2 years and older	Consists of 15 subscales completed based on direct observation. Total score classifications include "not autistic," "mild to moderately autistic," and "severely autistic."
Autistic Diagnostic Observation Schedule (ADOS; Lord et al., 1989)	5–12 years	Child is presented with structured and unstructured tasks and then rated based on direct observation.
Autistic Diagnostic Interview (ADI; LeCouteur et al., 1989)	4 years–early adulthood	Interview format with primary caregiver. Behavior is coded based on delays, impairment, and deviance.
Repetitive Behavior Scale—Revised (Lam & Aman, 2007)	3 years and older	Assesses restricted repetitive behaviors.

The Autistic Diagnostic Interview (ADI; LeCouteur et al., 1989) can be used for children from age 4 years to early adulthood, including individuals with a mental age of 2 years and above. The ADI is administered in an interview format with primary caregivers, and then involves coding behaviors based on descriptions that consider not just delays but also qualitative impairments and deviance (Marcus & Schopler, 1993).

The Repetitive Behavior Scale—Revised is useful in assessing restricted repetitive behaviors, a core symptom in children with PDD (Lam & Aman, 2007). This measure is clinically valuable, as repetitive and ritualistic behaviors impact many areas of the child's functioning, including interfering with social interactions, learning tasks, and attention. The measures for assessing PDDs are summarized in Table 2.5.

Eating Disorders

Garner and Parker (1993) point out that assessing for eating disorders can be a complex and dynamic task and may include clinical interviews, semistructured interviews, behavioral observations, self-report measures, symptom checklists, clinical rating scales, self-monitoring procedures, and standardized test measures. Assessment measures are helpful in identifying the diagnosis-specific symptoms, measuring the individual's attitudes and behaviors characteristic of eating disorders, and measuring overall functioning (Garner & Parker, 1993). Garner and Parker recommend beginning with a detailed clinical interview, and they outline key content areas that should be addressed. Semistructured interviews assist the clinician in obtaining the needed history and information to make an accurate diagnosis and assist with treatment planning. Suggestions for these and other instruments for assessing eating disorders are listed in Table 2.6.

The Eating Disorder Examination (EDE) is a clinical interview that assesses symptoms of anorexia nervosa and bulimia nervosa (Cooper & Fairburn, 1987; Fairburn & Cooper, 1996; Wilson & Smith, 1989). The EDE contains two behavioral scales (overeating and methods of weight control), as well as four subscales (restraint, eating concerns, shape concerns, and weight concerns). The psychometrics are extremely strong and make the EDE a highly recommended tool (Anderson, Lundgren, Shapiro, & Paulosky, 2004).

The Clinical Eating Disorder Rating Instrument (CEDRI; Palmer, Christie, Condle, Davies, & Kenwick, 1987) also measures behavior and attitudes, but additionally taps other common symptoms found with eating disorders, such as depression and self-esteem.

Several child-report measures have also been developed for assessing eating disorder symptoms. The Eating Disorder Inventory–2 (EDI-2; Garner, 1991) is a child self-report of psychological and behavioral traits of eating disorders. Items are rated by the child on a 6-point scale, and eight basic subscale scores are obtained based on the first 64 items. Additionally, three provisional subscales are derived from the final 27 items of the measure (asceticism, impulse regulation, and social insecurity).

Another child-report measure is the Eating Attitudes Test (EAT; Garner & Garfinkel, 1979), which provides clinicians with a total score and three subscale scores (dieting, bulimia/food preoccupation, and oral control). The child rates each item on a 1–6 scale, and a total score is obtained, with a cutoff score of 30 used to identify concerns typical of patients with anorexia (Garner & Garfinkel, 1979). More recently, the EAT has been modified for younger children and for grade 3 and older (Children's Eating Attitudes Test [Maloney, McGuire, & Daniels, 1988]; Adapted Eating Attitude Test [Vacc & Rhyne, 1987]), but they have been criticized for their content (Candy & Fee, 1998).

The Eating Behaviors and Body Image Test (EBBIT; Candy & Fee, 1998) may be more useful with preadolescent girls in grades 4 and up. This 38-item measure assesses body image dissatisfaction, restricted eating behaviors, and binge eating behaviors. The EBBIT yields two subscales, body image dissatisfaction/restrictive eating and binge eating.

TABLE 2.6. Selected Measures for Assessing Eating Disorders

Instrument	Ages	Comments
Eating Disorder Examination (EDE; Cooper & Fairburn, 1987)	12 years and older	Assesses symptoms of anorexia nervosa and bulimia nervosa.
Clinical Eating Disorder Rating Instrument (CEDRI; Palmer et al., 1987)	13 years and older	Measures behaviors and attitudes related to eating disorders, as well as other common symptoms found with eating disorders (depression and self-esteem).
Eating Disorder Inventory–2 (EDI-2; Garner, 1991)	12 years and older	Child self-report of psychological and behavioral traits of eating disorders. Yields eight basic and three provisional subscales.
Eating Attitudes Test (EAT; Garner & Garfinkel, 1979)	13 years and older	Child report measure yielding a total score and three subscale scores (Dieting, Bulimia/Food Preoccupation, and Oral Control). Modifications for younger children have been criticized for content.
Eating Behaviors and Body Image Test (EBBIT; Candy & Fee, 1998)	11 years and older	38-item measure of body image dissatisfaction, restricted eating behaviors, and binge eating behaviors.
Body Attitude Test (BAT; Probst et al., 1995)	13 years and older	20-item self-report measure. Assesses dissatisfaction with body size, shape, and appearance.

The Body Attitude Test (BAT; Probst, Vandereycken, Van Coppenolle, & Vander-linden, 1995) consists of 20 items. This self-report measure assesses the youth's dissatisfaction with body size, shape, and appearance. The following subscales have been identified: negative appreciation of body size, lack of familiarity with one's own body, and general body dissatisfaction (Kronenberger & Meyer, 2001). The BAT can distinguish individuals with eating disorders from nonreferred individuals; patients with bulimia tend to score highest. Overall, the BAT is useful for clinicians assessing body image issues.

Specific Cognitive-Content Measures

CBT is based on an information-processing model (A. T. Beck & Clark, 1988; Dozois & Dobson, 2001; Ingram & Kendall, 1986). Cognitive products, structures, operations, and content are elements in this model. Automatic thoughts (ATs) represent cognitive products. Cognitive distortions are the processes inherent in cognitive operations. Cognitive structure and content are reflected in schemas. The specific cognitive content measures allow you to identify particular ATs and their underlying schemas. (Specific cognitive content measures are listed in Table 2.7.)

AUTOMATIC THOUGHTS

ATs are well known to all cognitive behaviorally oriented psychotherapists and most other psychotherapists. ATs are stream-of-consciousness thoughts, judgments, appraisals, conclusions, evaluations, interpretations, and/or images from any time perspective (past, present, future; Padesky, 1988). ATs are a youngster's situationally specific inner voice. They are provoked by triggers linked to emotional experiences. ATs are usually directly accessible and easily linked to children's symptoms and problems. Assessing these products with the measures described below allows you to clearly pinpoint children's distressing thoughts. Treatment can then target these specific thoughts. You can readminister these measures to evaluate progress. Different emotional states are characterized by specific cognitions (content-specificity hypothesis; A. T. Beck & Clark, 1988; D. M. Clark, Beck, & Alford, 1999; Jolly, 1993; Jolly & Dykman, 1994; Jolly & Kramer, 1994; Laurent & Stark, 1993).

Childhood and adolescent depression are characterized by the negative cognitive triad (A. T. Beck et al., 1979). Depressed youngsters explain their experiences through a negative view of themselves, a negative view of others/their own experiences, and a negative view of the future. Overall, anxious children overestimate the probability of danger, overestimate the magnitude of danger, neglect rescue factors, and ignore their own coping skills (Kendall et al., 1992). More specifically, socially anxious patients fear negative evaluation (Albano, Chorpita, & Barlow, 2003). Anxious children often attribute bodily symptoms to something being catastrophically wrong with them and then believe they might die (Mattis & Ollendick, 1997; Ollendick, 1998). Adolescents with panic disorder catastrophically misinterpret normal bodily changes (Mattis & Ollendick, 1997).

Angry and aggressive youngsters have very different automatic thoughts (Coie & Dodge, 1998; Crick & Dodge, 1996). A hostile attribution bias characterizes angry moods and aggressive behaviors (Dodge, 1985). Simply, these youngsters see the world

TABLE 2.7. Selected Measures for Assessing Cognitive Content

Instrument	Ages	Comments
Automatic thoughts		
Children's Negative Cognitive Error Questionnaire (CNCEQ; Leitenberg et al., 1986)	8–12 years	Measures cognitive distortions; discriminates between clinical and nonclinical populations. It can be used as a way to initially target specific cognitive errors and then repeatedly administered to evaluate progress.
Cognitive Triad Inventory for Children (CTIC; Kaslow et al., 1992)	9–12 years	36-item scale measuring negative cognitive triad for depression.
Children's Attributional Style Questionnaire (CASQ; Kaslow et al., 1978; Seligman et al., 1984)	8–13 years	48-item measuring of children's explanatory style (internal, stable, and global factors) associated with depression.
Children's Automatic Thoughts (CATS; Schniering & Rapee, 2002)	7–16 years	40-item broad-band measure addressing negative self-statements. Good option for treatment planning and evaluating treatment response.
Negative Affect Self-Statement Questionnaire (NASSQ; Ronan et al., 1994)	8–15 years	Assesses more cognitive content/self-statements associated with depression and anxiety.
Schemas		
Beck Self-Concept Inventory (J. S. Beck et al., 2001)	7–14 years	Reflects enduring perceptions of competency, agency, and self-worth.
Schema Questionnaire for Children (SQC; Stallard & Rayner, 2005)	11–16 years	12 items rated on a 1–10 point scale by the children. The SQC has been shown to discriminate between community and clinical samples (Stallard, 2007).
Schema Questionnaire—Short Form (SQ-SF; Young, 1998)	16–18 years	75 items assessing emotional deprivation, abandonment, mistrust/abuse, social alienation, defectiveness, subjugation, self-sacrifice, emotional inhibition, unrelenting standards, entitlement, and insufficient self-control.

through a lens that commonly confuses what is deliberate with what is accidental. Because these youngsters see ambiguous or neutral events as deliberate provocations, they are quick to attack. Additionally, anger is associated with a fundamental perception of unfairness, a violation of personal rules (imperatives, shoulds), and a labeling of other people. In depression, critical attention is directed toward oneself, whereas in anger, negative attention is targeted toward another person or the environment.

The Children's Negative Cognitive Error Questionnaire (CNCEQ; Leitenberg, Yost, & Carroll-Wilson, 1986) measures cognitive distortions of overgeneralization, catastrophizing, inaccurately assuming too much responsibility for negative outcomes, and disproportionate attention being directed to negative aspects of an event. The measure is appropriate for fourth through eighth grade. The CNCEQ discriminates between clinical and nonclinical populations. It can be used as a way to initially identify specific cognitive errors and then repeatedly administered to evaluate progress.

The Cognitive Triad Inventory for Children (CTIC; Kaslow, Stark, Printz, Livingston, & Tsai, 1992) is a 36-item scale for children ages 9 through 12 years, which simultaneously measures all three aspects of Beck's negative cognitive triad for depression. Each item offers three response options (yes, maybe, no). Kaslow et al. reported mean scores for depressed children as 39.5 (total), 13.8 (negative view of self), 12.6 (negative view of the world), and 13.1 (negative view of the future).

The Children's Attributional Style Questionnaire (CASQ; Kaslow, Tanenbaum, & Seligman, 1978; Seligman et al., 1984) offers 48 items measuring children's explanatory style associated with depression. Simply, the CASQ is based on the finding that depressed children explain negative outcomes through internal (e.g., "The bad thing happened because of me."), stable (e.g., "It's going to last forever."), and global (e.g., "It's going to effect everything I do.") factors. The CASQ yields a total depressive attribution score as well as scores on the internal, stable, and global factors.

The Children's Automatic Thoughts Scale (CATS; Schniering & Rapee, 2002) is a broad-band measure addressing negative self-statements in children ages 7–16 years. It consists of 40 items covering four factors, including physical threat, social threat, personal failure, and hostility. Children indicate their endorsement by circling one of five response options (0, not at all–4, all the time). The CATS is a good option for treatment planning and evaluating treatment response.

The Negative Affect Self-Statement Questionnaire (NASSQ; Ronan, Kendall, & Rowe, 1994; Lerner et al., 1999) is somewhat of a more cognitive content measure for children ages 7–15 years. The NASSQ assesses self-statements associated with depression and anxiety. There are 57 anxious or depressive stems (e.g., "I am going to make a fool of myself.") and 13 positive self-statements. Patients report their endorsement of various cognitions by selecting one of five options (1, not at all–5, all the time). A cutoff score of 49 is recommended for anxiety-related cognitions (Snood & Kendall, 2007).

SCHEMAS

Schemas are core meaning structures that represent a child's central philosophy or worldview (Mash & Dozois, 2003). Schemas filter individual experiences into general templates and guide behavior (Kendall & MacDonald, 1993). Markus (1990, p. 242) wrote that "schemas provide categories by which to render experience meaningful." Schemas are core beliefs that reflect deep cognitive structures tied to intense emotional experience (Padesky, 1994). Prolonged exposure to ongoing negative or detrimental experiences may lead to negative self-views (Guidano & Liotti, 1983, 1985). Eder (1994, p. 180) noted that since schemas are covert, they are "often experienced but rarely articulated."

Schemas may be most salient, powerful, and pivotal for adolescents (Hammen & Zupan, 1984). However, the vulnerabilities associated with maladaptive schemas may also be operating in elementary school children (Taylor & Ingram, 1999). Taylor and Ingram (1999) astutely commented:

> Each time a negative mood state is encountered, high-risk children may be developing, accumulating, strengthening, and consolidating the reservoir of information in the dysfunc-

tional self-referent structures that guide their views of themselves and how information is processed when adverse events evoke these structures in the future. (p. 208)

With few exceptions, research on schemas in children and adolescents is limited (Cooper, Rose, & Turner, 2005; Stallard, 2002, 2007; Stallard & Rayner, 2005).

The Beck Self-Concept Inventory (J. S. Beck et al., 2001) reflects enduring perceptions of competency, agency, and self-worth. Like the other scales in the Beck Youth Inventories, it consists of 20 items. Raw scores are converted into *T*-scores for standardized comparisons.

The Schema Questionnaire for Children (SQC; Stallard & Rayner, 2005) consists of a single question reflecting early maladaptive schemas (EMS). The SQC's 12 items are rated on a scale of 1–10 by the children indicating to what extent the item applies to them. Higher scores reflect stronger endorsement. The SQC was able to discriminate between community and clinical samples (Stallard, 2007).

The Schema Questionnaire—Short Form (SQ-SF; Young, 1998) assesses emotional deprivation, abandonment, mistrust/abuse, social alienation, defectiveness, subjugation, self-sacrifice, emotional inhibition, unrelenting standards, entitlement, and insufficient self-control (Young, 1998; Wellburn, Coristine, Dagg, Pontefract, & Jordan, 2002). It consists of 75 items scored on a 6-point scale. Higher scores reflect stronger endorsement of the particular schema content. The SQ-SF is appropriate for older adolescents (16–18 years).

The psychometrics for the SQ-SF are acceptable (Wellburn et al., 2002). Wellburn et al. found that females scored higher on self-sacrifice, enmeshment, failure, abandonment, and defectiveness schemas.

IDIOGRAPHIC SELF-MONITORING TECHNIQUES

Self-monitoring is the basic building block of goal-directed, intentional behavior (Bandura, 1977a, 1977b, 1986). Unless youngsters first attend to their thoughts, feelings, and behaviors, change will be difficult for them (Bandura, 1977a, 1977b). Self-monitoring provides essential feedback regarding what needs to be changed and how well the change process is going (Brewin, 1988). Additionally, self-monitoring is often a first-change strategy. Observing a behavior changes it (Bateson, 1972). More specifically, positive behavior increases and negative behavior decreases when monitored (Ciminero & Drabman, 1977). Self-monitoring may reveal either too much critical attention directed to the self or others, or insufficient attention given to problematic behaviors or impulses that contribute to problems in self-control (A. T. Beck, 1976). Table 2.8 lists idiographic self-monitoring methods discussed in the remainder of the chapter.

Emotional Self-Monitoring

Self-monitoring is a way for children and adolescents to mind their moods. There are a variety of nonverbal and verbal ways for youngsters to track their feelings. For identifying feelings, *Feeling Faces* is a simple and commonly used procedure. In its most basic application, a copy of four blank or expressionless faces is given to the child. The child

TABLE 2.8. **Idiographic Self-Monitoring Methods**

Tool	Purpose	Ages
Watch, Warning, Storm!	Emotional self-monitoring	7–11 years
Feeling Compass	Emotional self-monitoring	7–16 years
Behavioral Chart	Behavioral self-monitoring	Any
Keepin' My Stats	Behavioral self-monitoring	8–15 years
File My Fears Away	Hierarchy construction	Any
Up, Up, and Away	Hierarchy construction	Any
What's Buggin' You?	Cognitive self-monitoring	8–11 years
Your Brainstorm	Cognitive self-monitoring	11–16 years
My World	Cognitive, behavioral, and emotional self-monitoring	Any

is then asked to draw happy, sad, mad, and worried faces. These drawings represent the child's emotional code. The child is given the homework assignment to draw the face representing the emotion every time he or she experiences a strong feeling.

Cartoons are often particularly compelling for children and can be used for mood monitoring. Cartoons such as Coping Cats (Kendall et al., 1992), Coping Koalas (Barrett et al., 1996), and PANDY (Friedberg, Friedberg, & Friedberg, 2001), and the illustrations in *Think Good, Feel Good* (Stallard, 2002) provide fun drawings for children. With the advent of clip art, cognitive-behavioral therapists can invent their own cartoons for mood monitoring. Access clip art from your word processing or PowerPoint program, white-out the character's expression, and ask the child to draw expressions for a mood chart. This gives you a nearly limitless number of options you can use with children.

There are a number of commercially produced Feeling Faces charts. While these charts have value, you should use them sensitively. These charts can include many feeling choices that can overwhelm children. The emotional labels used in most charts (e.g., exasperated) are often not part of a young person's vocabulary. While some feeling charts are produced in non-English versions, the faces usually remain male and Caucasian.

Scaling the feeling is another important way to mind moods. It is one step more advanced than feeling identification. Identifying feelings is categorical (either you are happy, sad, worried, mad, or not), whereas scaling rates "how much" of the emotion the patient is experiencing. Scaling adds specificity to the self-monitoring process. Through scaling you can readily see the level of emotional intensity in various circumstances. Further, scaling communicates to young patients that emotions exist on a continuum rather than as an all-or-none phenomena.

Feeling rulers, thermometers, traffic signals, and other measures to gauge emotional intensity are essential in CBT with children. Generally, one end of the scale is high intensity whereas the other is low. The scales typically range from 1–10 or from 1–100. Children simply mark or color in the point that represents the intensity. For example, in the traffic signal scale, red means high intensity, yellow is medium intensity, and green is low intensity.

Occasionally, younger, less sophisticated children do not understand the scaling process. They will need more concrete referents. Friedberg and McClure (2002) suggested the use of different levels of colored water or colored beads in clear cups to represent emotional gradients. Additionally, we frequently use hand gestures paired with verbal descriptors. For instance, we say, "Do you feel sad a little (hands close together), kind of (hands moderately apart), or a lot (hands far apart)?"

WATCH, WARNING, STORM!

Ages: 7–11 years.

Purpose: Scaling technique; monitoring emotional intensities.

Materials Needed:

- Watch, Warning, Storm! Diary (Form 2.1).
- Pencil or pen.

Teaching children to track their feelings at different intensities is a key emotional self-monitoring task. Often, distressed children do not notice their feelings until they are extreme in intensity. Consequently, the feeling gets away from them and impulsive, destructive, and self-injurious behaviors ensue. Through this inattentiveness to minimal cues, they learn to respond only to high emotionality. This commonly teaches others to react to them with high emotion. Since high levels of emotion are more difficult to modulate, children learn that emotions are dangerous and uncontrollable. Tracking emotions' intensity enhances predictability. Feelings no longer seem to come out of the blue. Explosions and meltdowns become more predictable and subsequently more manageable.

Like other scaling techniques, Watch, Warning, Storm! teaches patients to catch their feelings at different intensities. It also prepares them for the cognitive self-monitoring technique What's Your Brainstorm?, presented later in this chapter. Watch, Warning, Storm! is a 3-point scaling technique that uses the language of weather reporters when forecasting storms. "Watch" represents the lowest levels of feeling intensity, "Warning" means the emotional storm is brewing and building in intensity, and "Storm" reflects the highest level of intensity and is usually associated with meltdowns (e.g., tantrums, self-mutilation, aggression to others).

Watch, Warning, Storm! is easy to implement. The first step involves presenting the metaphor and exercise to the child. Next, you begin to fill out the form with the child in the session. The third step is assigning the emotional self-monitoring task for homework. The following transcript illustrates this three-step process.

THERAPIST: Evan, do you ever watch the weather?

EVAN: Sometimes.

THERAPIST: OK, good. You know weather people track snow storms and thunderstorms by first calling a watch, then a warning, and then the real storm arrives.

EVAN: They use radar.

THERAPIST: Exactly. And your strong feelings are like storms. So we can track them using a kind of emotional radar. We can use the same rules the weather people use. An emotional storm watch means the feeling is just in its beginning stages.

EVAN: Like a small or baby amount of feeling.

THERAPIST: Pretty much. Then what is an emotional warning?

EVAN: When the feeling is getting bigger and bigger and is about to blow.

THERAPIST: You've got it. And the arrival of the storm?

EVAN: When the feeling is like an explosion or a tornado or something.

THERAPIST: Let's get started with a homework assignment. What feeling should we track?

EVAN: Frustrated and angry?

THERAPIST: OK, every time you start to feel frustrated or angry, write down the date. To rate whether it is a watch, warning, or storm, just put a check in the column.

The final step is following up with the task in the next session. The following transcript illustrates the follow-up with Evan.

THERAPIST: Let's take a look at your Watch, Warning, Storm! Diary. How many storms did you have?

EVAN: They were all storms.

THERAPIST: What do you make of that?

EVAN: I dunno.

THERAPIST: Well, there are all storms and no warning or watches. No wonder it seems like your meltdowns come out of the blue and you seem out of control. We have to track the beginning of the storms.

EVAN: Why?

THERAPIST: Good question. When a storm comes, you don't want to get caught in it. If we can help you notice the anger storm early, you can learn to deal with the feeling before it gets stronger and floods you. How does this sound?

EVAN: OK, I guess.

THERAPIST: OK. What are the signs that an anger storm is brewing inside you?

In the above transcript, note that the therapist first used the data to empathize with Evan. The therapist then used the diary to provide the rationale for attending to the minimal or early cues of Evan's anger. The therapist's use of "storm" sets the stage for the Brainstorm Diary, which helps children catch their cognitions. Figure 2.1 shows Evan's Watch, Warning, Storm! Diary.

FIGURE 2.1. Evan's Watch, Warning, Storm! Diary.

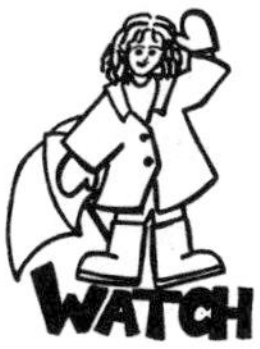

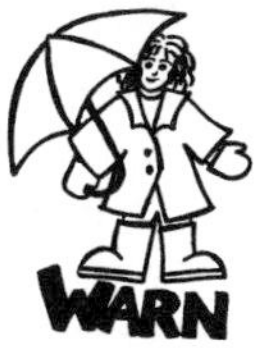

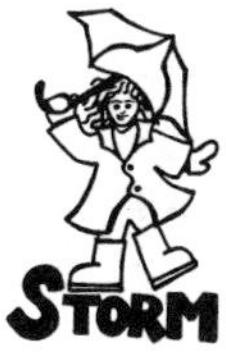

Date (time)	Emotion	Watch	Warning	Storm
2/11	Angry			X
2/12	Angry			X
2/13	Angry			X
2/14	Angry			X
2/15	Angry			X
2/16	Angry			X

FEELING COMPASS

Ages: 7–16 years.

Purpose: Feelings identification and monitoring.

Materials Needed:

- Round sheet of cardboard or stiff paper.
- Arrow of same material.
- Grommet.
- Markers or crayons.

Feeling Compass offers another hands-on approach to the self-monitoring of emotion. This technique serves as a creative self-monitoring and priming intervention and is similar to Thought–Feeling Watch (Friedberg & McClure, 2002). Feeling Compass may be included in the "survival kit" presented in Chapter 4. The compass needle indicates feelings instead of directions and includes a movable arrow. Children can draw the feelings onto the compass and then move the arrow to indicate the feeling they are experiencing. They can change the direction of the arrow as needed to indicate changes in feeling. As additional coping strategies are learned in therapy, the children can apply them and then indicate if the feeling direction changes. When the child changes the direction of the arrow, the therapist should inquire as to what may have led to the change.

Creating the compass in session can be useful in building self-monitoring skills. The following transcript illustrates how to introduce the Feeling Compass with 7-year-old Lucas.

THERAPIST: Do you know what a compass is?

LUCAS: Yeah, we used one at Cub Scouts to know what way we were going.

THERAPIST: That's right, and today we are going to make a Feeling Compass to help us see "what way" your feelings are going. First, we can draw faces [or write the feeling labels] on the four sides of the compass. Which feelings should we use?

LUCAS: We could use the ones from my Feeling Faces paper. I think they were happy, sad, mad, and scared.

THERAPIST: Good idea. Go ahead and draw those.

LUCAS: (*Draws faces.*) (*smiling*) I'm done!

THERAPIST: You worked hard on that! If our arrow was already on the compass, where would it be pointing?

LUCAS: On the happy face. It was cool making the faces.

THERAPIST: Your face looks happy right now, you have a smile on your face (*pointing out nonverbal cues to feeling changes*). Now attach the arrow.

LUCAS: Oh man! My arrow ripped when I tried to stick it on. This stinks!

THERAPIST: It looks like your feeling direction just changed. If the arrow was on the compass, where would it be pointing?

LUCAS: At mad! I don't like this!

THERAPIST: I can tell you feel mad because your face has changed and your voice sounds angry too. What would have to happen to make the direction go back to happy? [The therapist can then work with the child on problem solving, and then identify any change in his feeling.]

As this example illustrates, the process of creating a self-monitoring tool can begin to teach the skills of self-monitoring and set the stage for other interventions. The therapist took a collaborative approach with Lucas, and incorporated his terminology and responses into the technique. In addition, the therapist attended to Lucas's changes in affect during the session, and took the opportunity to acknowledge the feelings. Further, the therapist illustrated how the Feeling Compass could be applied at the point of each shift in mood. The therapist helped Lucas attend to nonverbal expressions of emotion, while also illustrating that feelings can change, not just toward more negative feelings, but also back to positive feelings. This sets the stage for future interventions such as problem solving. Lucas's Feeling Compass and its components are shown in Figure 2.2.

Behavioral Self-Monitoring

BEHAVIORAL CHARTS

Behavioral self-monitoring tasks are relatively simple (Thorpe & Olson, 1997). Parents, teachers, and children keep track of target behaviors. Many of the behavioral interventions in Chapter 4 are set up by the self-monitoring procedures we describe next. Generally, these are paper-and-pencil measures. Stickers or other creative materials may be

FIGURE 2.2. Feeling Compass: What direction am I headed?

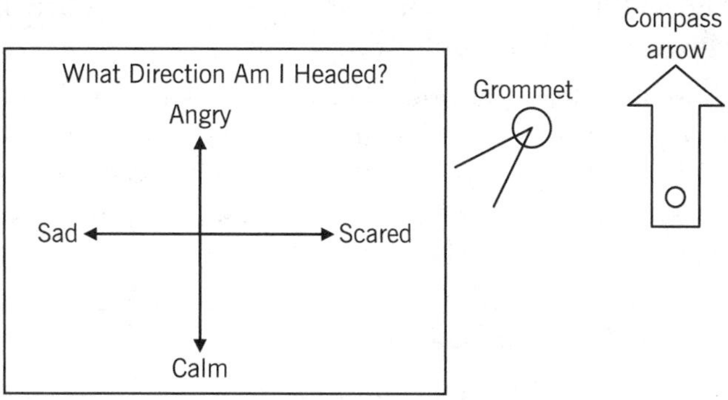

used. It is relatively easy to craft individualized behavioral monitoring forms, but there are excellent resources that are full of ready-made forms for school and home use (Kelley, 1990).

The procedures for behavioral monitoring charts have several common elements. Typically, target behaviors are defined with specifics (e.g., picking up backpack from floor after school by the nth time asked). Contextual factors are also considered in this definition, such as the time and place the behavior occurs. The charts may also include the people who were present and involved in the situation. The frequency (how often), intensity (how much), and duration (how long) of the behavior may also be noted. Finally, the antecedents are recorded. These are the things that come before or cue the behavior, such as commands or transitions. The consequences are also recorded; these are the things that follow the behavior, such as reinforcers and punishers. Form 2.2 provides a sample chart.

Behavioral tracking forms are useful for collecting data and helping patients become more mindful of their behavior. For less frequent habits, a frequency count may be appropriate (e.g., 12 times on Monday). For behaviors that occur at a high rate or for a certain time period (e.g., bit nails for 10 minutes), duration could be recorded instead (e.g., 55 minutes on Wednesday morning). Children may not always be aware that the behavior is occurring, and thus parental and therapist monitoring and cuing may also be appropriate to increase the child's awareness before moving on to the competing response phase of treatment.

In the following example, the therapist is introducing a behavioral chart to track hair pulling to a child and her mother.

THERAPIST: We have discussed your goal of decreasing the frequency and severity of your hair pulling. In order to do this, we first need some information. We need to know how often you are pulling your hair, and when it is most likely to occur. This information will help us make change more quickly, as well as give us a way to check if the hair pulling is lessening. Specifically, after we try some strategies, we will keep track of hair pulling to see if the numbers change. Does that make sense?

KARA AND HER MOTHER: Sure, I guess.

THERAPIST: What questions do you have?

KARA: Well, I guess I don't know who will keep track. And I usually pull the entire time I do homework. How will I record that?

THERAPIST: Those are great questions. Let's take a look at the form and see if that helps. Let's pretend you are sitting in math class and you start to pull your hair. You would write "math class" so we know when the pulling happened, and then you would make a mark in the second column to show you pulled. If it happens again during math that day, you simply put another mark each time.

KARA: OK. That makes sense. But sometimes I don't realize I am pulling right away, especially during homework or on the bus.

THERAPIST: Then instead of the number of times you pulled, you would record the amount of time you spent pulling, just making your best estimate.

KARA: Oh, I see. I usually pull on the bus. So if half-way to school I realize I was pulling, I could write 12 minutes because that is about half the bus ride.

THERAPIST: Exactly, now you've got it! Go ahead and write that on the chart as a reminder.

KARA'S MOTHER: What should I do if I see Kara pulling, like during homework?

THERAPIST: Kara, what would be helpful for you?

KARA: Well, I hate when you start saying "Kara, don't pull!"

THERAPIST: That is frustrating for you. What could your mom do or say that would be more helpful?

KARA: Maybe you could just say "Chart" as a reminder for me to mark my chart and pay attention to what I am doing.

THERAPIST: How does that sound to you?

KARA'S MOTHER: I can do that.

In this example, the behavior chart is explained and Kara gains some experience starting it in session. The parent's and child's questions are addressed, and potential obstacles to success are problem-solved. By including Kara's mother in the plan, as well as giving Kara some input into the cuing approach, the therapist is increasing the chances of follow-through. Kara's chart can be seen in Figure 2.3.

KEEPIN' MY STATS

Ages: 8–15 years.

Purpose: Behavioral self-monitoring.

Materials Needed:

- Paper.
- Pen or pencil.
- Watch or timer if measuring time.

FIGURE 2.3. Example of Kara's behavioral self-monitoring chart for hair pulling.

Date/time period	Count/frequency
Monday —*math class*	IIII
—*lunch*	IЖ III
—*soccer practice*	II
Tuesday—*bus ride to school*	*12 minutes*
—*presentation*	III
—*homework*	*5 minutes*
Wednesday	
Thursday	
Friday	
Saturday	
Sunday	

Keepin' My Stats is a behavioral self-monitoring task inspired through work with a noncompliant boy who loved baseball (Friedberg & Wilt, in press). We presented the task as similar to computing and tracking batting averages. His "stats" were target behaviors and his compliance was the percentage. We augmented the task by putting a digital picture of the child on one side of the chart, and the stats were on the other side, just like a baseball card. When the child's compliance rates increased, he was on the road to the Hall of Fame. Figure 2.4 shows an example of Keepin' My Stats.

BEHAVIORAL HIERARCHIES

Behavioral hierarchies rank situations from least distressing to most distressing, using scaling techniques. Subjective units of distress (SUDS) represent the amount of distress experienced in each hierarchy item. Hierarchies set the stage for systematic desensitization (Chapter 4), cognitive interventions (Chapters 5 and 6), and exposure-based techniques (Chapter 7). The following section describes two hierarchy exercises.

FIGURE 2.4. Keepin' My Stats.

Date	# of parental commands (at bats)	# of compliance (hits)	% (batting average)	# compliance without reminder (home runs)
4/20	20	7	.350	2
4/21	15	3	.200	0
4/22	18	6	.333	3
4/23	9	6	.666	4
4/24	21	7	.333	3

FILE MY FEARS AWAY

Ages: Any age.

Purpose: Hierarchy construction.

Materials Needed:

- Index cards.
- Pen or pencil.
- File folder, envelope, or small box to organize cards (optional).
- File My Fears Away form (Form 2.3).

The File My Fears Away technique involves identifying various distressing items or tasks and writing or drawing a representation of each on an index card (see Figure 2.5). The therapist then helps the child to arrange or "file" the cards by degree of distress into a hierarchy. The cards allow for flexibility in modifying the hierarchy as the child adds items between previously identified steps or scenes. For example, a 13-year-old boy with OCD and social anxiety used File My Fears Away to develop and confront hierarchical steps. He initially recorded fear of calling a friend on a card. The therapist assisted the child in scaling the degree of fear and then identifying less fearful tasks that could precede calling a friend. Younger children can draw the fear, cut out pictures from magazines, or use photographs, while older children and adolescents may opt to write a verbal description. For some youngsters, having the therapist write the items as they verbalize their fears is a nice collaborative activity. You may help identify items with prompts such as "What level would your anxiety be if ... ?" and "What would be a level 4?" Once the cards have been made and placed in order, a small box or envelope can be used to keep them organized or "filed." The 13-year-old in the above example initially colored in his predicted level of anxiety for the various tasks. Three steps have been selected to illustrate a portion of his hierarchy (Figure 2.5a–c).

As the exposures to each item are occurring, the patient circles, colors, or simply points to his or her anxiety level on the cards. This visual cue regarding anxiety strength will alert children and the therapist to any changes in feeling intensity. Laminating the cards after the scenes have been written, and then using a dry erase marker for rating, is helpful when the same cards are repeatedly used during each exposure in cases when

FIGURE 2.5 a–c. Example of File My Fears Away.

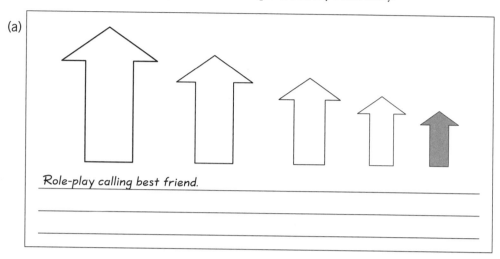

(a)

Role-play calling best friend.

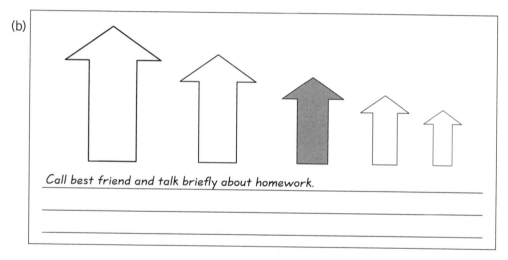

(b)

Call best friend and talk briefly about homework.

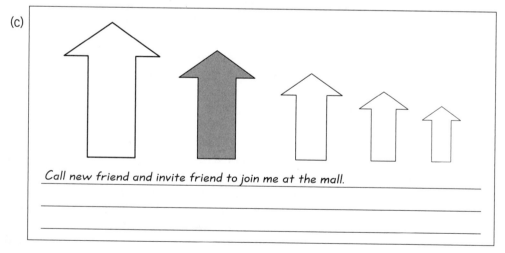

(c)

Call new friend and invite friend to join me at the mall.

scenes have to be presented multiple times. Alternatively, different colored pens/markers can be used for the rankings so the child can visually see the changes in his or her fear intensity.

Figure 2.6 demonstrates the use of File My Fears Away with a younger child. Six-year-old Alexa was so scared of getting in the swimming pool that she refused to swim even in shallow water. Her fear was starting to generalize to the bathtub, and her mother began giving her sponge baths since Alexa refused to get in even shallow bath water. Alexa drew pictures on her cards. The least fearful card pictured her looking at shallow water. The next pictured her putting her toe in the water. In the most feared, she drew herself standing in the water.

UP, UP, AND AWAY

Ages: Any age.

Purpose: Hierarchy construction.

Materials Needed:

- Index cards.
- Yarn or string (such as shoe strings).
- Hole punch.
- Markers/crayons for drawing.
- Optional: Game piece or token/coin to use to mark location on hierarchy.

Some children may enjoy or require a more active approach to self-monitoring and creating/completing hierarchies. Up, Up, and Away takes the basic components of hierarchy construction and applies them in a game-like fashion. This approach is ideal for a more active child, such as one with comorbid ADHD, or a child that requires higher levels of distraction or stimulation to engage in therapy tasks. This technique adds in a reinforcer for completion of hierarchical steps. The Up, Up, and Away technique utilizes index cards, such as those found in the File My Fears Away technique, and makes an active game out of systematic desensitization to help children make their fears "go away."

As hierarchical items are identified, they are drawn or written on cards. Then the cards are strung in hierarchical order onto the string. The string is laid on the ground so that each item can be seen, like steps up a ladder (see Figure 2.7). At the top of the string, a reinforcer for completion can be added to increase motivation and follow-through. This item should be selected collaboratively with the child to ensure it is a true motivator. The child then stands or sits at the first card as the exposure or visualization is occurring. When the hierarchical item is completed, the child physically moves to the next item. Alternatively, a game piece can be used to mark the spot on the hierarchy. Reinforcers can be added to various parts of the hierarchy if needed.

For example, 9-year-old Tony had a severe fear of storms. The sound of thunder often caused him to run to the basement at home, cover his ears, and cry. His fear had grown so intense that even the threat of rain or dark clouds kept Tony from his normal

FIGURE 2.6. Example of Alexa's File My Fears Away.

(a)

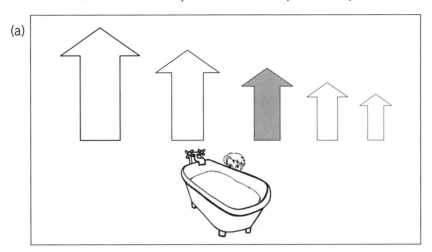

(b)

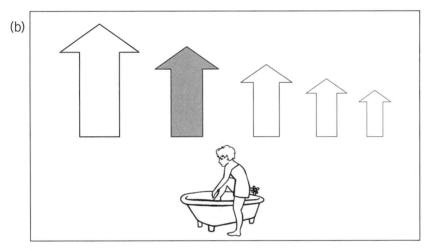

(c)

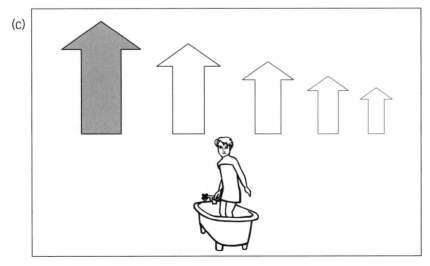

FIGURE 2.7. Up, Up, and Away.

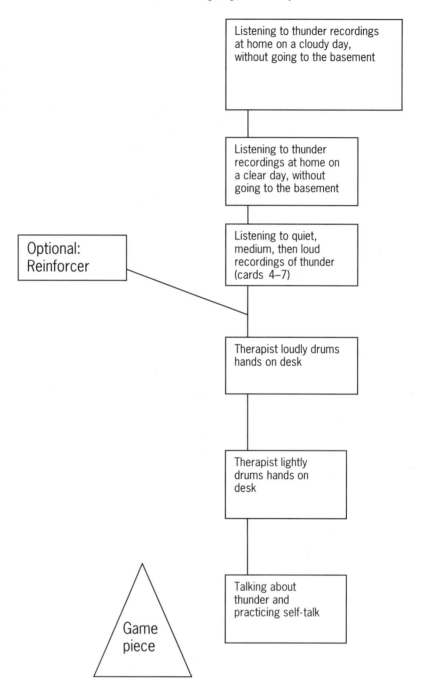

daily activities. A hierarchy was created in session. It started with Tony's least distressing items. Tony ranked talking about thunder and practicing self-talk as the least distressing step; this item was recorded on the first card. Listening to the therapist lightly drum her hands on the desk in a repetitive manner was written on the second card, followed by louder drumming recorded on the third card. The fourth through seventh cards involved listening to recordings of thunder at various volumes, starting with very soft (card/item 4) up to loud volumes (card/item 7). The final two cards included listening to the thunder recordings at home, without going into the basement, first on a clear day and finally during a cloudy day. Tony chose his own reinforcers, which his mother agreed to, and they were inserted in the flow of cards. After completion of the fifth card, Tony would be permitted to invite a friend over to play, and after the last card, Tony would be able to go to his favorite restaurant. Once the hierarchy was created, the cards were strung together with a shoe string. Tony marked his spot on the hierarchy with a sticky note, allowing him to easily move his spot as items were successfully completed and self-monitoring occurred. After two therapy sessions, and several exposures at home, Tony had completed the hierarchy and was proud of his success. He could easily see how far he had "climbed" to overcome his fears when looking at the string of cards that he had completed.

Cognitive Self-Monitoring

Cognitive self-monitoring typically involves thought diaries that are used to identify children's "hot" thoughts. These diaries connect the cognitions to their situational contexts and unite thoughts with their accompanying feelings. There are many types of thought diaries for adolescents (J. S. Beck, 1995; Friedberg, Mason, & Fidaleo, 1992; Greenberger & Padesky, 1995). Thought diaries for children generally use cartoons and thought bubbles. The Coping Cat (Kendall et al., 1992), PANDY (Friedberg et al., 2001), and human figure cartoons in Stallard (2002) are excellent examples of child-friendly thought records. For very young children, thought flower gardens are good options (Bernard & Joyce, 1984).

Despite the many variations, thought diaries have several common elements. First, activating events or situations are listed. Second, the children note their feelings/emotions and scale them in intensity. Last, they catch hot thoughts by responding to the question "What is running through your head?" or its variants, such as "What is going through your mind?" or "What are you saying to yourself?"

While this procedure is relatively straightforward, there are several important points to remember to make the most of thought catching. First, make sure the child and you identify the specific situation. Vague descriptions (e.g., "Had a bad day at school.") should be clarified into operationalized ones (e.g., "Two kids picked on me in the hall."). Second, you should check that the situations are objectively described (e.g., "Jimmy did not say hi to me in the hall.") and are free from automatic thoughts (e.g., "Jimmy rejected me."). Third, be sure that feelings are not confused with thoughts. Friedberg et al. (1992) offered a good decision rule: thoughts are conclusions, evaluations, judgments, and interpretations and therefore are always open to question. You should remain mindful that the cognitions should correspond to the content-specificity hypothesis described earlier in this chapter.

WHAT'S BUGGIN' YOU?

Ages: 8–11 years.

Purpose: Self-monitoring of negative automatic thoughts.

Materials Needed:

- What's Buggin' You? Diary (Form 2.4).
- Pen or pencil.

What's Buggin' You? is a way to present and apply thought records to children. Negative automatic thoughts are irritating and annoying, like bugs that swarm around in young patients' heads. In fact, child behavior therapists refer to capturing cognitions as "catching NATS" (negative automatic thoughts; Shirk, 2001, p. 157). What's Buggin' You? is a way to make use of this metaphor to help children capture the thoughts that buzz around in their heads when they are distressed. It also flows nicely into the self-instructional technique Swat the Bug presented in Chapter 5.

What's Buggin' You? includes components of a traditional thought diary. Children record the date, situation, and the thought that "bugged them." A bug cartoon on the diary form illustrates the nagging aversive nature of irritating cognitions. The following transcript with Regina shows its use.

THERAPIST: Regina, have you ever had a bug buzz around you?

REGINA: Yeah, it's annoying mainly when I am eating ice cream.

THERAPIST: I'm sure it gets on your nerves.

REGINA: My last nerve!

THERAPIST: Well, that is like the things that run through your mind when you are sad, mad, and worried.

REGINA: I'd like to swat them.

THERAPIST: We'll get to that. Before you swat them you have to catch them, right?

REGINA: Right.

THERAPIST: So look at this diary. It has a place for the date, situation, and your feeling. And look at this bug. This is the thought bug. Here is where you write the thought that is bugging you. Can you read the question by the bug?

REGINA: What bug buzzed through your mind?

THERAPIST: Great. Let's try one. What's the date today?

REGINA: October 10th.

THERAPIST: What happened that made you feel sad today?

REGINA: When my parents got mad at me for punching my little sister.

THERAPIST: What buzzed through your head?

REGINA: They love her more than me.

THERAPIST: You caught the bug.

FIGURE 2.8. Regina's What's Buggin' You? Diary.

Date	Situation	Feeling	What bug buzzed through your head?
10/10	Parents got mad at me for punching my sister	Sad	They love her more than me.

The dialogue illustrates the gradual way the diary is introduced. The therapist systematically stepped Regina through the thought-catching process. Once Regina caught the thought, the therapist reinforced her. Figure 2.8 shows Regina's diary as filled in during the session. Regina's mention of swatting the bug will lead naturally to the Swat the Bug procedure (see Chapter 5).

YOUR BRAINSTORM

Ages: 11–16 years.

Purpose: Self-monitoring negative automatic thoughts.

Materials Needed:

- Your Brainstorm Diary (Form 2.5).
- Pen or pencil.

Your Brainstorm is another variation of a thought record. It is similar to What's Buggin' You? but may be more appropriate for older children. Your Brainstorm naturally follows from Watch, Warning, Storm! It precedes and forms the basis for the simple rational analysis procedure, Whether Report (Chapter 6), which is a child-friendly test of evidence. Your Brainstorm is based on the metaphor that negative automatic thoughts and images are "storms" that disrupt the young patient's emotional climate. There may be a variety of storms including anger, sadness, anxiety, and/or shame. The youth's task is to be an emotional weathercaster or meteorologist. He or she has to describe the brainstorm in the emotional weather report.

Your Brainstorm is easy to complete. The date is recorded along with the feeling, its intensity, and cognitive components. Figure 2.9 illustrates a completed Your Brainstorm Diary. The task can be augmented by having the child make a TV weather report. The report could be videotaped or used in group or family work, where children present their brainstorm to the viewing audience. The following example shows a therapist introducing the technique to 10-year-old Terrance. Terrance's Your Brainstorm Diary can be seen in Figure 2.9.

FIGURE 2.9. Terrance's Your Brainstorm Diary.

Situation	Feeling	How strong (1–10)	Brainstorm
In therapy	Angry	9	This is bullshit. I hate this lame shit. I wish my mom would not make me come to this lame shit.

THERAPIST: Terrance, remember when you did such a great job on your Watch, Warning, Storm! Diary?

TERRANCE: I guess.

THERAPIST: I have another diary for you.

TERRANCE: Lucky me.

THERAPIST: I am sensing you are not too excited about this.

TERRANCE: Wow! Did you graduate from college to figure that out? This is boring.

THERAPIST: How are you feeling right now?

TERRANCE: A little pissed.

THERAPIST: (*Writes in the diary.*) OK. Now I bet you are having a brainstorm.

TERRANCE: What?

THERAPIST: A brainstorm. ... Something that goes through your head when you are having strong feelings. You see, we have to help you continue to be an emotional weatherman.

TERRANCE: This is bullshit. I hate this shit. I wish my mom would not make me come to this lame shit.

THERAPIST: (*Writes in the diary.*) This makes a lot of sense. I understand how pissed you would be if you saw this stuff as lame. You are good at catching brainstorms. (*Shows diary to Terrance.*) Let's talk about how lame this stuff is and see if you have any more brainstorms and we'll write them down.

The dialogue illustrates the experiential nature of self-monitoring. The therapist used Terrance's annoyance in the session to fuel the Your Brainstorm Diary. By applying the brainstorm to his spontaneous expression, the therapist taught Terrance how to easily complete the diary. Additionally, the diary was completed in a quick, nonthreatening manner, which led to a further discussion of Terrance's frustration. Consequently, Terrance learned that the diary is useful in promoting communication, understanding, and problem solving.

MY WORLD

Ages: Any age.

Purpose: Self-monitoring of cognitions, behaviors, and emotions.

Materials Needed:

- Poster board.
- Color markers.
- Game pieces.
- Blank cards.
- Dice.

My World is a self-monitoring technique based on a game concept. It was particularly useful with a very avoidant 8-year-old with severe OCD. Kortni, her mother, father, and the therapist developed the game board, pieces, and game cards based on her danger and safe zones. A large piece of poster board was divided up into spaces much like the Monopoly game board. Safe zones (bed) were placed on the board and colored green. Danger zones (closet floor, swing set) were similarly drawn, but colored red. The board was started in session and completed as a homework assignment.

Once the board was drawn, the game play began. The idea was for everyone to get a sense of what it was like to live in Kortni's world. When players landed on a space, they asked themselves: "What is it like to live in Kortni's world? What goes through her mind? How does it feel?" Naturally, when mother and father landed on her spaces, they were clueless. At this point Kortni often corrected their misperceptions, which gave her a much needed sense of control and efficacy. More importantly, through the game, Kortni's thoughts and feelings contained in different situations could be better clarified. Kortni felt very understood and experienced less shame about her symptoms due to the game play.

CONCLUSION

In this chapter, we outlined numerous formal measures and informal techniques for self-monitoring. These serve as data collectors as well as interventions. The data help clarify the case formulation and test hypotheses. This approach is also collaborative and keeps the treatment focused on treatment goals. Symptoms are monitored to determine changes and antecedents to change, and therefore help guide treatment and relapse prevention. Self-monitoring and assessment should occur throughout treatment, and continually be addressed as agenda items during sessions in order to communicate the importance of the information to the family, as well as to make full use of the data that is being collected. Thus, the data guide treatment planning decisions regarding the frequency of sessions, termination/discharge, and referrals for medication.

Watch, Warning, Storm! Diary

Date (time)	Emotion	Watch	Warning	Storm

Behavioral Chart

Date/ time	Behavior	Frequency count	Duration	Place	People	Cues	Consequences

File My Fears Away

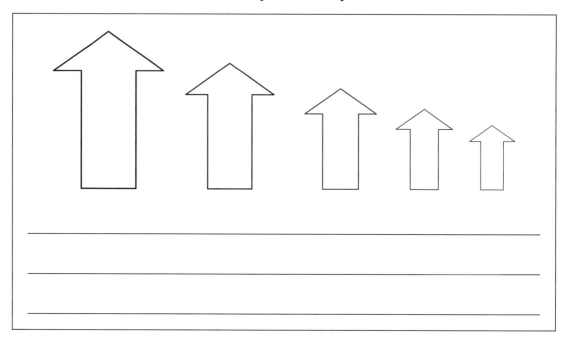

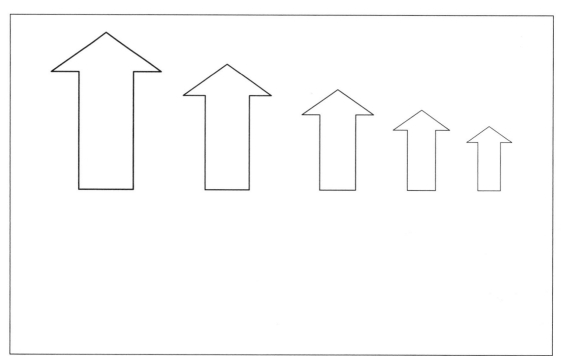

What's Buggin' You? Diary

Date	Situation	Feeling	What bug buzzed through your head?

53

FORM 2.5

Your Brainstorm Diary

Situation	Feeling	How strong (1–10)	Brainstorm

CHAPTER 3

Psychoeducation

Psychoeducation serves a central role in cognitive therapy. It orients children, youth, and families to CBT. Its purpose includes communicating information to the family to increase their understanding of symptoms, treatment, and diagnoses and thus to facilitate the change process. We want patients to be informed and educated partners in the psychotherapeutic enterprise. As Goldfried and Davila (2005) have said, psychoeducational methods and books may instill hope in patients. Necessary information needs to be presented in an easily accessible, understandable, and engaging manner and it should avoid jargon (Piacentini & Bergman, 2001). Piacentini and Bergman have also suggested the use of stories, anecdotes, and metaphors to concisely illustrate information.

In this chapter, we offer different metaphors and creative worksheets to help the psychoeducation portion of treatment be meaningful, memorable, and effective. This chapter also outlines multiple resources (e.g., books, websites), allowing therapists to choose those that fit the learning styles and presenting problems of the families with whom they are working.

INFORMATION FOR PARENTS

Psychoeducation is not a passive process. Therapists must treat the patient as an active consumer rather than as a mere recipient of information. In this way, psychoeducation becomes a dynamic ingredient in the therapeutic mix. For instance, printed material should not merely be handed out and never again revisited in therapy. Instead, the materials should be provided, processed, and repeatedly referenced (e.g., "What parts apply to you?"; "What parts don't seem to apply to you?"; "What parts do you agree with?"; "Which parts do you disagree with?").

This processing sends a variety of overarching messages to patients. First, psychoeducation is a collaborative rather than a prescriptive endeavor. Second, the patient's

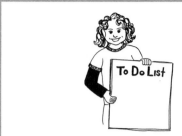

BOX 3.1. Tips for Psychoeducation

- Psychoeducation is an active process.
- Materials should be relevant, developmentally and culturally appropriate, and engaging.
- Concrete metaphors are useful.
- Keep the case conceptualization in mind.

task includes reading and personalizing the information, rather than simply adopting it. You want patients to *mindfully* think over material rather than *mindlessly* swallow it. Finally, by asking patients what parts they agree and disagree with, you are teaching them to decrease their absolute thinking.

When you give out psychoeducational material, it also communicates several messages that help to enhance the therapeutic relationship at a time that is critical in the early phases of treatment. Sharing this information tells the patient you have his or her best interests at heart. Patients can literally "take away" these tools from therapy and they concretely learn they "get something from therapy." In addition, they learn that therapy takes place outside the 50-minute hour and continues outside the office.

As a suggestion, an initial psychoeducational homework assignment might involve the patient and family being given reading material and a highlighter. They are then asked to underscore all the material that they see applying to them. In the subsequent session, the therapist discusses the highlighted material, as well as any pertinent information that is not highlighted.

Disorder-Specific Information for Parents

Developing a library of patient education materials is a handy idea. Fortunately, there are many resources to rely upon. Table 3.1 lists key online resources where disorder-specific information can be found. New York University's Child Study Center website, *about-ourkids.org,* is particularly valuable. It contains a multitude of parent-friendly materials on disorders and treatment options. Websites maintained by the National Institute of Mental Health and the Substance Abuse and Mental Health Services Administration offer information on disorders and treatment, as well as child-friendly coloring books, stickers, and activities that can be ordered or downloaded free of charge. Division 53 (Clinical Child Psychology) of the American Psychological Association offers an array of information on disorders and empirically based treatment. The American Academy

TABLE 3.1. Selected Websites with Parent Education Materials

Source	Location	Topic
New York University Child Study Center	*www.aboutourkids.org*	Disorders, development, parenting, medications, CBT
American Academy of Child and Adolescent Psychiatry	*www.aacap.org*	Disorders, development, medications, parenting
National Institute of Mental Health	*www.nimh.org*	Disorders, treatments
Academy of Cognitive Therapy	*www.academyofct.org*	Cognitive therapy, disorders
American Psychological Association Division 53	*www.clinicalchildpsychology.org*	Disorders, treatments
Association for Behavioral and Cognitive Therapies	*www.abct.org*	Disorders, treatments
Substance Abuse and Mental Health Services Administration	*www.samsha.gov*	Disorders, treatments, parenting information
Anxiety Disorders Association of America	*www.adaa.org*	Disorders, treatment
Worrywise Kids	*www.worrywise.org*	Disorders, treatment, parenting information
Autism Speaks	*www.autismspeaks.org*	Parenting information and treatment

of Child and Adolescent Psychiatry operates useful websites where information on medications, disorders, and treatment options can be downloaded. The Academy of Cognitive Therapy and the Association for Behavioral and Cognitive Therapies websites are the authoritative sites for CBT. The Anxiety Disorders Association of America is a rich resource for information on childhood anxiety and treatment. Similarly, Worrywise Kids is a comprehensive site for parenting material for parents of anxious children. Autism Speaks is an authoritative site for parenting information on autism and PDD. Finally, each of these core sites contain valuable links to other sites.

These above resources offer several advantages for clinicians. For the most part, the material is free. Second, the information is up-to-date and based on recent research. Third, the patient information is very readable and the children's material is fun. The availability and minimal cost of this information allows you to give this material to patients to carry home.

Parent Training and Education

Parent training is obviously often a difficult business. Most parents enter treatment timidly, worried they have "screwed up" their children. Recommending parent education and training procedures will likely trigger parents' self-critical cognitions ("The doctor thinks it's all my fault.") and, at times, avoidant/defensive behavior ("Why do I have to change?"). These thoughts, feelings, and behaviors need to be addressed. For instance, instead of just assigning some material to parents, the alert therapist should collaborate and inquire, "What went through your mind when I suggested that you read this chapter on parenting?" or "How did you interpret my suggestion?"

THERAPIST: I am going to recommend this book called *SOS: Help for Parents*. (*Parents sigh and look down.*) What goes through your mind when we talk about a parenting book?

FATHER: I don't know. Do you think we are bad parents?

MOTHER: Shouldn't we know all this? Are we doing wrong things?

THERAPIST: I can see you really want to do well for your child. So much so that sometimes a recommendation seems like a criticism. Is there any other way to look at learning new techniques?

MOTHER: I just feel bad.

THERAPIST: I understand. It's difficult, but what might be a way to look at parent education other than as you did something wrong?

FATHER: We're stupid or slow learners.

THERAPIST: Wow. That's a lot of pressure. Do you think you could be a good parent and still make mistakes and learn new things?

MOTHER: (*Pause.*) I always thought I had to be perfect.

THERAPIST: Then when things go badly, you see yourself as ...

MOTHER: A bad mother.

THERAPIST: So your equation is imperfect mothering equals bad mothering.

FATHER: I am the same way.

THERAPIST: I see. How possible is it for you to see parenting as a process that includes trial and error, change, and flexibility?

MOTHER: That's different. I guess it is possible.

FATHER: Yeah, it's new.

THERAPIST: So if your parenting is trial and error and a learning process, would learning new techniques from a book be a way to work toward better parenting?

MOTHER: Let's give it a try.

This transcript illustrates several important parts of the psychoeducational process. First, empathy and understanding were communicated. Second, automatic thoughts regarding parents' perceptions of implied criticisms were elicited. Third, the therapist conducted a Socratic dialogue to test the parents' assumptions.

In the initial stages of parent education, we often use a sports fan metaphor. Sports fans follow and root for their teams despite their losses, slumps, and poor seasons. A fan readily recognizes that a rare team goes undefeated and players rarely compete perfectly. Nonetheless, a genuine fan's interest and loyalty does not wane despite disappointments. Teams sometimes cause fans heartbreaks but they remain hopeful and optimistic (e.g., "There's always next year.").

This metaphor is especially apt for parenting. No child is perfect and undefeated. Children inevitably will do something that disappoints or even infuriates their parents. Nevertheless, parents ultimately remain their children's fans, cheer their successes, and soulfully absorb their setbacks without giving up on them. The following transcript illustrates the use of the metaphor.

THERAPIST: Mr. and Mrs. Freed, I remember that both of you are New York Giants fans.

MR. FREED: We *love* the Giants. You?

THERAPIST: I happen to be a big fan. You know they went through many lean years.

MRS. FREED: We were there for all of them. We suffered.

MR. FREED: It was a rocky road for awhile.

THERAPIST: How come you stayed with them for all those years?

MR. FREED: We're not fair-weather fans. We are *true* fans. We don't jump from the bandwagon.

MRS. FREED: I guess our loyalty never wavered.

THERAPIST: Even when they stunk and were awful?

MR. AND MRS. FREED: (*Laugh.*) Yes.

THERAPIST: Well, you know Jennifer is having a "rough season" now. How can you stick with her through this?

MRS. FREED: Hmm, we should really have more faith in her.

THERAPIST: Yeah, kids and sports teams disappoint you and sometimes even break your heart.

MR. FREED: Like Jennifer skipping school and having sex with her boyfriend.

THERAPIST: I know that hurts you, but can you not give up on her like you stayed with the Giants through those hard times?

MRS. FREED: I never thought about it that way.

MR. FREED: I guess when I scream at her it's like I am booing her off the field.

The dialogue with Jennifer's parents helps them shift their perspective. The metaphor allowed for the parents to see they were communicating a loss of faith in their child. Finally, the sports team metaphor limited the parents' defensiveness.

Parenting training is not an abstract exercise. In most cases, educational material alone does not create much change. Parents need to acquire and practice different strategies. They need to receive corrective feedback from therapists. We have found that *in vivo* practice is very effective. We describe some parenting strategies in the behavioral interventions and exposure/experiential chapters. Therefore, the psychoeducation module helps parents acquire skills, but actual practice with corrective feedback facilitates skill acquisition and change.

Developmental and disorder-specific information help parents set realistic and attainable goals for their family. As the literature has shown us, the environment in which children grow up is obviously linked to some of their symptoms. Through psychoeducation, parents can become aware of how to reinforce positive behaviors and how to avoid reinforcing maladaptive patterns. Books for parents are also helpful aids. Many parents find comfort in knowing they are not alone in their struggles. In addition, books with research backing can help to validate the work you are doing in therapy. For some, getting information from books is more palatable, and they avoid having to spend several sessions with a therapist reviewing particular issues. When using parenting books, the therapist must keep in mind that the books must be processed in sessions to communicate importance and to follow up on comprehension and application of skills. The following transcript illustrates how to address parenting books in session.

> THERAPIST: So, Mrs. Barker, how is it going with the parenting book I recommended last session?
>
> MRS. BARKER: Well, I felt kind of embarrassed buying it last week. Like the cashier was going to think I was a bad parent. But then I thought, they must sell a lot of these books since there was an entire section for them at the bookstore! I just started reading it a few days ago.
>
> THERAPIST: What has been the most interesting thing you have read?
>
> MRS. BARKER: It was interesting how the examples seem so true to life. It was like the author knew Tommy and was writing about his behavior and struggles.
>
> THERAPIST: How did you feel when you read that?
>
> MRS. BARKER: I felt relieved. If there are enough kids out there like Tommy that they actually have books about it, there must be hope for helping him. It also helped me not blame myself so much. I know there are things I can do differently, but I also see that part of this is who Tommy is and finding a parenting style that is appropriate for him.
>
> THERAPIST: It sounds like you are really using the book as a way to learn new things and to reflect on how you are parenting Tommy.
>
> MRS. BARKER: Definitely. Now I see what you meant at the start of treatment, about how my husband and I have to be a part of Tommy's treatment and not just "drop him off" once a week to be "fixed."
>
> THERAPIST: So, what things have you used at home so far?

This transcript illustrates how the therapist can use the parent's experience with the book to capture some of her thoughts and feelings, as well as to assess how the family is applying the information in the home environment. By spending some time talking with Mrs. Barker about the book, the therapist communicates that the information she is reading is important and will be incorporated into treatment. Doing so may also motivate her to continue to read and apply the strategies, knowing they will be discussed at upcoming sessions.

Table 3.2 outlines a range of resources for families. *Parents Are Teachers* (Becker, 1971) and *Living with Children* (Patterson, 1976) are classic parenting texts that present behavioral concepts and techniques. They include plentiful examples and sample forms. *SOS: Help for Parents* (L. Clark, 2005) offers parents basic child management strategies in a very readable and cartoon-rich format.

TABLE 3.2. Recommended Parenting Book Resources

Book (author and year)	Application
SOS: Help for Parents, Third Edition (L. Clark, 2005)	Simple behavioral strategies for parents
Parents Are Teachers (Becker, 1971)	Behavioral child management strategies for parents presented in a simple programmed learning format
Living with Children (Patterson, 1976)	Behavioral child management strategies for parents presented in a simple programmed learning format
Your Defiant Child (Barkley & Benton, 1998)	Parenting information, behavior management techniques, and communication skills for parents with oppositional and defiant children
Your Defiant Teen (Barkley, Robin, & Benton, 2008)	Parenting information, behavior management techniques, and communication skills for parents with oppositional and defiant children
Taking Charge of ADHD (Barkley, 1995)	Strategies for parenting children with ADHD
Parents and Adolescents (Patterson & Forgatch, 1987)	Strategies for managing defiance, noncompliance, and oppositionality in adolescents
Parenting Your Out of Control Child (Kapalka, 2007)	Strategies for managing tantrums, noncompliance, oppositionality, defiance, and aggression
The Explosive Child (Greene, 2001)	Parenting strategies for children with angry, rebellious, noncompliant, oppositional, and defiant behavior
What Childhood Is All About (Vernon & Al-Mabuk, 1995)	Information on normal development and parenting strategies
First Feelings (Greenspan & Greenspan, 1985)	Enhancing parent and young children relationships (especially useful with children with PDD spectrum disorders)
The Essential Partnership (Greenspan & Greenspan, 1989)	Enhancing parent and children (ages infancy to 4) relationships (especially useful for children with PDD spectrum disorders)
The Hurried Child (Elkind, 1981)	Information on normal development, strategies to reduce unrealistic parental expectations and pressure
All Grown Up and No Place to Go (Elkind, 1984)	Information on normal development, strategies to reduce children's pressures regarding rushing into adulthood
Stressed-Out Girls (Cohen-Sandler, 2005)	Expectations, pressure, teenage girls
Helping Your Child with Autism Spectrum Disorder (Lockshin, Gillis, & Romanczyk, 2005)	Guide for parents with autistic children
If Your Adolescent Has Depression or Bipolar Disorder (Evans & Andrews, 2005)	Parenting bipolar children
Raising a Moody Child (Fristad & Goldberg-Arnold, 2004)	Parenting bipolar children

(cont.)

TABLE 3.2. *(cont.)*

Book (author and year)	Application
The Optimistic Child (Seligman, Reivich, Jaycox, & Gillham, 1995)	Parenting information and skills to teach children how to cope with distressing situations
Help for Worried Kids (Last, 2006)	Parenting strategies for children with anxiety and worries
Helping Your Child with Selective Mutism (McHolm, Cunningham, & Vanier, 2005)	Tips for parents of children with selective mutism
Freeing Your Child from Obsessive–Compulsive Disorder (Chansky, 2000)	Tips for parents of children with OCD
Talking Back to OCD (March, 2007)	Tips for parents of children with OCD
If Your Adolescent Has an Anxiety Disorder (Foa & Andrews, 2006)	Tips for parents of children with anxiety disorders
Getting Your Child to Say "Yes" to School (Kearney, 2007)	Parenting strategies for school avoidance and refusal
Helping Your Child Overcome Separation Anxiety or School Refusal (Eisen & Engler, 2006)	Parenting strategies for separation anxiety and school refusal
If Your Adolescent Has an Eating Disorder (Walsh & Cameron, 2005)	Parenting information for eating disorders
Help Your Teenager Beat an Eating Disorder (Lock & le Grange, 2005)	Parenting strategies for eating disorders
Playground Politics (Greenspan, 1993)	Parenting strategies to deal with interpersonal struggles in elementary school

First Feelings (Greenspan & Greenspan, 1985), *The Essential Partnership* (Greenspan & Greenspan, 1989), and *Playground Politics* (Greenspan, 1993) are very helpful for parents of younger children. Although these books are grounded in psychodynamic theory, they can have a place in cognitive-behavioral psychotherapy. They offer an excellent adjunct to behavioral management and give parents a fresh perspective on their children's developmental, emotional, and interpersonal lives. We have also found them to be helpful with parents challenged by their children's PDD.

Table 3.2 also includes a number of disorder-specific parenting books. Depression, OCD, anxiety disorders, eating disorders, disruptive behavior disorders, and PDD are all represented. Each of these resources includes both developmental information, background knowledge on the disorder, and handy tips. *Stressed-Out Girls, The Hurried Child,* and *All Grown Up and No Place to Go* deal with developmental struggles children experience. These resources allow parents to place the child's behavior in a developmental context.

Parenting books can serve several helpful roles in the treatment of children and adolescents. First, recommending and then discussing parenting books communicates to parents that they serve an important role in treatment. It sets up a collaborative stance, as the parents' role as cotherapist is directly addressed. In addition, information is empowering to parents. The information they read in the parenting manuals can increase parents' confidence and engagement in treatment. It communicates the active role parents must take in their child's treatment, rather than being a passive observer.

DISORDER-SPECIFIC MATERIALS FOR CHILDREN
AND ADOLESCENTS

Storybooks

There are a variety of children's storybooks available addressing a range of disorders and coping skills. Stories hold a number of advantages for socializing patients and their families to CBT (Friedberg & McClure, 2002). Stories are woven into the fabric of childhood and most children are familiar with reading and being read to. Otto (2000) concluded that stories are less likely than direct instruction to elicit defensiveness and avoidance. Cook, Taylor, and Silverman (2004) noted that stories promote motivation and vicarious learning. Additionally, stories may even enhance the working alliance (Blenkiron, 2005). There are many specific storybooks that teach children and their families about various disorders and treatments. Some of these resources are explicitly CBT in focus (Shaw & Barzvi, 2005; Wagner, 2000; Waters, 1979, 1980).

Table 3.3 lists a number of these storybooks that present complex information in simple ways. We invite children to color the characters while reading the stories. Additionally, we frequently pause on each page and ask the child salient questions to augment the experience (e.g., "How do you think _____ is feeling?"; "What is going through his mind?"; "What do you think will happen next?").

Finally, to increase identification with the characteristics and facilitate internalization of the information, we pose different questions (e.g., "When do you feel the same way as _____?"; "What goes through your mind when _____ happens?"; "What do you do when _____ happens?").

Adolescents' Personal Accounts

There is a very interesting series of firsthand accounts of various adolescent mental health disorders, published by Oxford University Press. The series, Adolescent Mental Health Initiative, contains teenagers' accounts of eating disorders (Arnold & Walsh, 2007), depression (Irwin, Evans, & Andrews, 2007), schizophrenia (Snyder, Gur, & Andrews, 2007), social anxiety (Ford, Liebowitz, & Andrews, 2007), obsessive–compulsive disorder (Kant, Franklin, & Andrews, 2008), bipolar disorder (Jamieson, 2006), suicide (Lezine & Brent, 2008), and substance use (Keegan, 2008). These books may speak to adolescents' subjective experiences of their disorders. Moreover, they are concrete reminders that young patients are not alone in their distress—they communicate universality. Finally, each of these books offers handy coping skills that can easily be integrated into a cognitive-behavioral package. These valuable books are listed in Table 3.4.

Games

There are many games that are extremely helpful in the psychoeducational process. We find the cognitive-behavioral games pioneered by Berg (1986, 1989, 1990a, 1990b, 1990c, 1992a, 1992b, 1992c) particularly helpful. The games come with game board, pieces, dice, chips, and domain-specific cards. Each card represents an opportunity for teaching the connection between thoughts and feelings, problem solving, the cognitive model of change, and communicating that problems are universal. Table 3.5 lists our recommendations.

TABLE 3.3. Storybooks for Psychoeducation

Book (author and year)	Application
Rational Stories for Children (Waters, 1980)	Common distortions
Color Us Rational (Waters, 1979)	Common cognitive distortions
Who Invented Lemonade? (Shaw & Barzvi, 2005)	Pessimism, catastrophizing
Up and Down the Worry Hill (Wagner, 2000)	OCD (ages 8–14 years)
What to Do When Your Brain Gets Stuck (Huebner, 2007b)	OCD (ages 6–12 years)
What to Do When You Grumble Too Much (Huebner, 2007a)	GAD (ages 6–12 years)
Worry Wart Wes (Thompson, 2003)	Worry
When Fuzzy Was Afraid of Losing His Mother (Maier, 2005b)	Separation anxiety (ages 3–7 years)
Catchin Cooties Consuelo (Thompson, 2004a)	Hypochondria, worries about getting sick
Mookey the Monkey Gets over Being Teased (Lonczak, 2007)	Coping with teasing (ages 4–8 years)
Mind over Basketball (Weierbach & Phillips-Hershey, 2008)	Worry and stress (ages 8–12 years)
Too Nice (Pellegrino, 2002)	Lack of assertiveness (ages 8–12 years)
What to Do When You Worry Too Much (Huebner, 2006)	GAD (ages 6–12 years)
The Lion Who Lost His Roar (Nass, 2000)	CBT for fearfulness (ages 6–10 years)
The Koala Who Wouldn't Cooperate (Shapiro, 2006b)	CBT for noncompliance (ages 4–9 years)
The Bear Who Lost His Sleep (Lamb-Shapiro, 2000)	CBT for worrying (ages 4–9 years)
Loud Lips Lucy (Thompson, 2002)	Self-control
Busy Body Bonita (Thompson, 2007)	ADHD
When Fuzzy Was Afraid of Big and Loud Things (Maier, 2005a)	Sensitivity to loud things and unexpected sounds (ages 3–7 years)
The Rabbit Who Lost His Hop (Nass, 2004)	CBT for self-control (ages 4–8 years)
The Penguin Who Lost Her Cool (Sobel, 2000)	Anger management (ages 6–10 years)
The Chimp Who Lost Her Chatter (Shapiro, 2004)	Shyness (ages 4–8 years)
The Horse Who Lost Her Herd (Shapiro, 2006a)	Social skills (ages 4–8 years)
What to Do When Your Temper Flares (Huebner, 2008)	Anger management (ages 6–12 years)
Full Mouse, Empty Mouse (Zeckhausen, 2008)	Disordered eating (ages 7–12 years)
The Hyena Who Lost Her Laugh (Lamb-Shapiro, 2001)	Negative thinking, perfectionism (ages 6–10 years)
When Lizzy Was Afraid of Trying New Things (Maier, 2005c)	Perfectionism (ages 3–7 years)
Blue Cheese Breath and Stinky Feet (DePino, 2004)	Bullying (ages 6–12 years)
The Putting on the Brakes Activity Book for Young People with ADHD (Quinn & Stern, 1993)	ADHD (ages 8–13 years)
Annie's Plan (Kraus, 2006)	Completing homework (ages 6–11 years)
Clouds and Clocks (Galvin, 1989)	Encopresis (ages 4–8 years)
It Hurts When I Poop (Bennett, 2007)	Encopresis (ages 3–6 years)
Feeling Better (Raskin, 2005)	Description of psychotherapy (ages 8–14 years)
In Grown Tyrone (Thompson, 2004b)	Coping with teasing

TABLE 3.4. Adolescents' Personal Accounts from the Oxford University Press Adolescent Mental Health Initiative Series

Book (author and year)	Application
Mind Race (Jamieson, 2006)	Bipolar spectrum disorder
Eight Stories Up (Lezine & Brent, 2008)	Suicide
Monochrome Days (Irwin, Evans, & Andrews, 2007)	Depression
What You Must Think of Me (Ford, Liebowitz, & Andrews, 2007)	Social anxiety
The Thought That Counts (Kant, Franklin, & Andrews, 2008)	OCD
Next to Nothing (Arnold & Walsh, 2007)	Eating disorder
Chasing the High (Keegan, 2008)	Substance abuse

Games offer a number of advantages (Friedberg, 1996). First, they are familiar and nonthreatening to most children. Thus, they are "ecologically valid" or, to put it more simply, they are the stuff of childhood. Second, they do not overly rely on traditional "talk" methods. Games involve action and interaction. Finally, information from games is easily communicated. Typically, children are given the homework assignment to create their own cards that reflect their own individual realities.

AFFECTIVE EDUCATION

Affective education is a key psychoeducational component. Children with a variety of disorders and presenting complaints require affective education. Many children with psychological difficulties are less skilled in emotional understanding (Suveg, Kendall, Comer, & Robin, 2006). Affective education teaches children about different feelings, demonstrates that negative emotions are part of the human experience, and promotes emotional expression (Deblinger, Behl, & Glickman, 2006). Children's identification

TABLE 3.5. Cognitive-Behavioral Games

Game	Ages	Application
Assertiveness Game (Berg, 1986)	8–13 years	Social skills, assertiveness
Feelings Game (Berg, 1992b)	8–13 years	Learning the connection between thoughts and feelings
Anger Control Game (Berg, 1989)	8–13 years	Identification of anger-producing triggers, anger management, problem solving
Anxiety Management Game (Berg, 1990a)	8–13 years	Identify negative cognitions, learn self-instruction
Self-Control Game (Berg, 1990c)	8–13 years	Learning about symptoms of ADHD and how to deal with them
Conduct Management Game (Berg, 1992a)	8–13 years	Psychoeducational material for behavior problems
Self-Concept Game (Berg, 1992c)	8–13 years	Decreasing negative views of self

and recognition of feelings are initial cues for cognitive skills and skill application (Friedberg & McClure, 2002). Suveg et al. (2006) noted that identification of emotions is a pivotal precursor to emotional regulation.

Books, Movies, Television, and Music

Children may use a variety of methods to learn about emotions. Books, movies, television shows, songs, plays, or any other media are great stimuli. These media have the added advantage of flexibility. Material can be selected based on the children's developmental and ethnocultural context. Cartledge and Milburn (1996) offer a large number of culturally responsive resources.

Movies and television shows offer compelling educational advantages (Davis & Pickard, 2008; Finamore, 2008; Gallo-Lopez, 2008; Hesley & Hesley, 2001; Robertie, Weidenbenner, Barrett, & Poole, 2008; Wedding & Niemiec, 2003). Films help young people identify emotion and communicate the universality of emotional experience. Table 3.6 offers listings of several books, movies, television shows, and song lyrics we find useful. Hesley and Hesley (2001) offer a very helpful summary of many movies and their psychological content. However, we strongly recommend getting the parents' consent before showing or playing a movie, TV show, or song.

The movie version of *The Wizard of Oz* (Fleming, 1939) is a personal favorite for both affective education and cognitive experiences with children (Friedberg & McClure, 2002). The characters display readily recognizable emotions in a simple manner. The child watches the movie with the therapist, then the film is paused at emotionally salient moments, and the therapist helps the child identify feelings.

Adolescents may be more responsive to song lyrics than to movies. Popular songs and rap are typically filled with emotionally loaded material. The recent Broadway rock musical *Spring Awakening* (Slater & Sheik, 2006) deals with various provocative aspects of adolescents' experiences, such as teen angst, suicide, runaways, dating, teen pregnancy, and sexual abuse. "My Junk Is You" contains various emotionally touching lyrics and is excellent for affective education.

The following transcript illustrates the use of affective education using song lyrics with a 17-year-old girl named Tasha. She reluctantly entered therapy after the breakup of a long-term relationship, which led to depressive symptoms. She did not know what to expect from therapy and was quite distant from her emotional and cognitive experiences.

> THERAPIST: I know you are upset about the breakup with your boyfriend. It's hard to talk about the thoughts and feelings you have about it. Let's try something different. I'd like to play a song that kind of speaks about the things you may be experiencing. Would that be OK?
>
> TASHA: OK. What's the song?
>
> THERAPIST: It's called "My Junk Is You" from a show called *Spring Awakening*. It's about many of the struggles teenagers encounter. (*Plays the song.*) What did you think?
>
> TASHA: I liked it. It makes me sad, though.
>
> THERAPIST: This is a good first step. What touched you?

TABLE 3.6. Movies, Plays, Television Shows, and Books for Affective Education

Source	Focus
Feeling Scared (Berry, 1995) (book)	Identifying scared, anxious feelings
Feeling Sad (Berry, 1996) (book)	Identifying sad feelings
Alexander and the Terrible, Horrible, No Good, Very Bad Day (Viorst, 1972) (book)	Frustration tolerance
Smoky Night (Bunting, 1994) (book)	Anxiety, trauma, children of color
Amazing Grace (Hoffman, 1991) (book)	Identifying feelings, African American girls
The Feelings Book (Madison, 2002) (book)	Identifying feelings, girls
The Meanest Thing to Say (Cosby, 1997) (book)	Teasing, peer relationships, African American boys
Searching for Bobby Fischer (Zaillian, 1993) (movie)	Pressure, performance anxiety, giftedness
Stand and Deliver (Menendez, 1988) (movie)	Academic achievement, gangs, Latino/Latina children
Little Man Tate (Foster, 1991) (movie)	Giftedness, peer rejection
The Breakfast Club (Hughes, 1985) (movie)	Teen issues, identity
Good Will Hunting (Van Sant, 1997) (movie)	Identity
Crooklyn (Lee, 1994) (movie)	Loss, coping, African American family
Fly Away Home (Ballard, 1996) (movie)	Family conflict
Antwone Fisher (Washington, 2002) (movie)	Child abuse, identity, African American males
This Boy's Life (Caton-Jones, 1993) (movie)	Child abuse, conduct disorders
Finding Forrester (Van Sant, 2000) (movie)	Identity issues, African American males
Half Nelson (Fleck, 2006) (movie)	Substance abuse
Stand by Me (Reiner, 1986) (movie)	Friendship, identity
Beauty and the Beast (Trousdale & Wise, 1991) (movie)	Self-efficacy, separation, independence
The Lion King (Allers & Minkoff, 1994) (movie)	Fearfulness, loss, identity
Mulan (Bancroft & Cook, 1998) (movie)	Self-efficacy, separation, independence
Alladin (Clements & Musker, 1992) (movie)	Self-efficacy, separation, independence
Little Mermaid (Clements & Musker, 1989) (movie)	Self-efficacy, separation, independence
Father of the Bride (Shyer, 1991) (movie)	Independence, letting go
Penelope (Palansky, 2008) (movie)	Self-acceptance, body image, teenage issues, relationships
Juno (Reitman, 2007) (movie)	Teen pregnancy, depression, relationships
Thirteen (Hardwicke, 2003) (movie)	Adolescence, drugs, sexuality, acting out, conduct problems, family conflict
Akeelah and the Bee (Atchison, 2006) (movie)	Coping with stressors, family life, achievement, African Americans
Little Miss Sunshine (Dayton & Faris, 2006) (movie)	Dealing with negative circumstances, family relationships, loss
The Incredibles (Bird, 2004) (movie)	Family life
Mi Familia, My Family (Nava, 1995) (movie)	Latino family life, teen issues
Quinceanera (Glatzer & Westmoreland, 2006) (movie)	Teen issues, teen pregnancy, family conflict
Everybody Hates Chris (LeRoi & Rock, 2005) (television show)	Middle school issues, African American youth
Joan of Arcadia (Hall, 2003) (television show)	Teen issues, family life
American Family (Nava, 2002) (television show)	Latinos, family life
Spring Awakening (Slater & Sheik, 2006) (musical)	Teenage issues, sexuality, depression, relationships, family conflict, sexual abuse

TASHA: The words and music. It is kinda how I feel.

THERAPIST: (*Takes the lyric sheet and hands it to Tasha.*) Which part of the song seems to speak most to your thoughts and feelings?

TASHA: The part where it talks about being nothing without a relationship. How relationships make you into something.

THERAPIST: You looked like you had some tears.

TASHA: I did. It puts my feelings into words.

THERAPIST: It is touching. Which parts?

TASHA: The parts where she sounds hooked on the boy.

THERAPIST: Hooked?

TASHA: Like she is addicted. I feel like I was hooked on Andre. Like I am nothing and worthless without him. Small. Like they said, my life is a mess.

THERAPIST: When these things run through your head, how do you feel?

TASHA: Alone. Hopeless. Sad. Afraid. Frustrated (*teary*).

THERAPIST: Although it is hard and painful, you are taking the first steps toward feeling better. You are putting words to your thoughts and feelings.

The dialogue with Tasha illustrates several important points. First, the use of the song allowed the therapist to tap thoughts and feelings in a nonthreatening way. More-over, the choice of the song likely enhanced the therapeutic alliance by communicating that the therapist understood how important romantic relationships are to young people. The music was also a mini-mood induction and contributed to hot thoughts and feelings boiling up to the surface. The lyrics communicated that these distressing thoughts and feelings are universal. Finally, Tasha learned that sharing unpleasant thoughts and feelings are part of psychotherapy.

VOLCANO

Ages: 6–18 years.

Purpose: Affective education.

Materials Needed:

• Volcano science kit.

Or

• Plastic cone.
• Baking soda.
• Vinegar.

We also use a volcano metaphor to talk about inhibition and explosion of emotional expression. Like a volcano, unexpressed and neglected levels of emotion may simmer, bubble, and boil beneath the surface before they erupt and spill out uncontrollably.

An elementary science project involving a volcano, familiar to most children, nicely demonstrates this concept. Together, the therapist and the patient can build a volcano or volcano science kits can be purchased in most novelty, craft, or educational supply stores. The therapist equates the baking soda to the child's thoughts and feelings. The vinegar or stressor associated with the inhibition is then added to the baking soda which is hiding peacefully within the volcano. Naturally, the "laws of science" demonstrate that these feelings will overflow unless properly monitored, expressed, and modulated. The following transcript illustrates the process.

> THERAPIST: Do you know what a volcano is?
>
> MULIK: Sure. It is a mountain that blows up.
>
> THERAPIST: Want to make one?
>
> MULIK: Sure. I did one in science class.
>
> *(Therapist and patient get the materials and pour the baking soda into the volcano.)*
>
> THERAPIST: What do you guess will happen if we pour in the vinegar?
>
> MULIK: It will blow up.
>
> THERAPIST: What do you mean?
>
> MULIK: The lava will flow out.
>
> THERAPIST: Let's see. *(Pours in vinegar.)*
>
> MULIK: Cool.
>
> THERAPIST: You know, this volcano is kind of like you.
>
> MULIK: What do you mean?
>
> THERAPIST: Well, you hold in too many things for too long and they blow up.
>
> MULIK: Like my anger.
>
> THERAPIST: Just like your anger.
>
> MULIK: It kind of makes a mess.

Through this exercise, Mulik gained a concrete appreciation of the negative consequences of psychological inhibition. The volcano held his interest and graphically represented the "mess" pent-up feelings can cause when they erupt. The therapist was sure to personalize the metaphor ("You know, this volcano is kind of like you.").

NAMING THE ENEMY

Ages: 8–18 years.

Purpose: Affective education.

Materials needed:

- Paper.
- Pencil or pen.

Naming the Enemy is a psychoeducational procedure developed by Fristad and her colleagues (Fristad & Goldberg-Arnold, 2003; Goldberg-Arnold & Fristad, 2003). It is simple, yet engaging and enlightening for many families. Children divide a sheet of paper by drawing a line down the middle of the paper on both the front and back of the sheet. The right-hand column on the front of the paper is labeled "Things I like about me." The paper is then turned over and the right-hand column is labeled "My symptoms." Patients list all their symptoms. Next, they turn the paper over and list all their positive qualities or strengths. In the last step, they fold the paper so that the symptom column effectively hides or covers the strengths. Now, patients and their families have a referent for the way symptoms obscure strengths.

EDUCATION ABOUT THE COGNITIVE MODEL

Introducing the cognitive model is a standard component of psychoeducation in CBT. Learning about the cognitive model helps familiarize young patients to treatment and demystifies the process. CBT's simple commonsense language makes complex problems understandable to young people. By recognizing that there is a basic template from which to view their symptoms, patients are better able to describe their problem and set collaborative goals. The key points to illustrate are:

1. Physical, emotional, cognitive, and behavioral symptoms are all causally related so that changes in one contribute to changes in the other three.
2. Making sense of the world is a natural human process.
3. Sometimes these processes are problematic and inaccurate.
4. When the conclusions are accurate, we will problem-solve together.
5. When the conclusions are inaccurate, we will teach you to form better conclusions.
6. Behavioral experiments ("adventures") will be used to test conclusions.

There are various means for introducing the model, including the traditional CBT paradigm (J. S. Beck, 1995; Greenberger & Padesky, 1995), the telephone metaphor (Friedberg & McClure, 2002), and Diamond Connections (Friedberg et al., 2001). The basic cognitive model suggests that four connected factors contribute to psychological difficulties. The separate variables are emotional functioning, physiology/biology, behavior, and cognition. Each individual factor influences and in turn is shaped by the others in a causally interactive manner.

Diamond Connections breaks this complex paradigm into a fun baseball metaphor. Each factor is illustrated by a base on a baseball diamond. The importance of each variable is captured by the notion that a baseball diamond must have four bases. Children note their symptoms on the appropriate base (e.g., writing feelings on second base, which is labeled "Feelings").

The telephone metaphor utilizes three columns labeled situation, feelings, and thoughts. Under the situation, the therapist writes "telephone rings." Together, the therapist and the teenager write different potential feelings associated with getting a phone call (e.g., excited, worried, mad). Then they hypothesize about who is calling (e.g., boyfriend, mother, probation officer, principal). Feelings and thoughts are connected (e.g., "If you thought it was your probation officer, how would you feel?"). The notion of interpretations rather than events determining emotional reactions is also illustrated via a Socratic dialogue (e.g., "How many thoughts are there?"; "How many feelings?"; "How many situations?"; "If situations solely determined feelings, how can one situation produce so many feelings?"). Last, you help the adolescent see what might happen if she falsely predicted it was the probation officer and it was really her boyfriend (e.g., become needlessly distressed). You also hammer home the idea that the only way to know who is on the phone is to answer the phone or check the caller ID (i.e., gather data). The following procedures listed in this section are intended to augment these traditional interventions.

Kendall (2006) offers a humorous story augmented by a cartoon about stepping in dog poop to illustrate thought–feeling connections. These can evoke a variety of thoughts, conclusions, and interpretations. Some youngsters will be self-critical ("I'm a klutz. I should have seen the dog poop there.") and feel sad. Others may feel embarrassed, anxious, and dread negative evaluation ("What if my mom saw me and yells at me?"). Still other youngsters may feel angry ("Damn! What idiots didn't pick up the dog shit? They must have done this on purpose."). Many young patients will find this example amusing and readily be able to see that the way you interpret situations powerfully shapes emotions and behavior.

The use of alarms is a good metaphor to teach patients about anxiety disorders (A. T. Beck, Emery, & Greenberg, 1985; Friedberg et al., 2001; Piacentini, Langley, & Roblek, 2007a, 2007b; Piacentini, March, & Franklin, 2006; Shenk, 1993). A. T. Beck et al. (1985) noted that in anxiety, the alarm is often worse than the fire itself. This is particularly true if patients are plagued by false alarms—alarms that do not accurately predict true dangers. Piacentini et al. (2006, pp. 309–310) explained:

> A false alarm. What happens? That's right. Even though there is no fire, the loud noise makes everyone nervous as if there was a fire, and they want to leave the building. People think they are in a dangerous situation even when they aren't.
>
> OCD is just like a false fire alarm. When you start to worry about germs, it's like a fire alarm going off—you feel nervous and think something bad is going to happen. However, just like the false alarm, nothing bad is going to happen. In treatment, you will learn that your OCD fears are false alarms and that if you ignore them they will go away and nothing bad will happen.

IT'S IN THE BAG

Ages: 6–18 years.

Purpose: Teaching the cognitive model.

Materials Needed:

- Magic wand.
- Two brown paper sandwich bags.
- Can of soda.

It's in the Bag is a psychoeducational procedure based on a humorous carnival trick. The task teaches children that to discover truths behind tricks, data must be collected. It's in the Bag involves pretending you are a magician (a bad one at that!!). You try to move a can of soda from one bag to another by the mere waving of your magic wand. The way the audience is convinced is by not seeing the evidence that the bag has not actually moved. The "illusion" is founded on blind faith, just like the negative beliefs most children faithfully hold. You need two brown bags, a can of soda, and a magic wand. You may introduce the procedure in the following way:

> "Did you know I can do magic? Here is what I am going to do. I am going to make this one can of soda move from this bag and then back again. All we need is magic words. Do you have any magic words?"

In the next stage, you augment the process just like a real magician would. You say:

> "I need some more help. First check out this can of soda. [Hand it to the patient.] Is there anything unusual about it? Now, inspect the bag. [Give the bag to the patient.] Anything unusual about it?"

After the patient has examined the bag, you perform the trick.

> "Watch me do the trick. Abracadabra. The can moved from one bag to the other bag [Don't let the child check!]. Now, I'm going to wave my magic wand so it moves back. Abracadabra. [Wave wand.] Look, it moved!"

Children readily recognize the trick and point out that the can did not move. You then ask, "How did you know the can did not move?" and "What did you have to do to prove my trick was wrong?" The children learn they should check out data to verify assumptions. This "trick" will set up a discussion about negative beliefs and collecting data. It is memorable for the child and primes him or her for later interventions.

A DOZEN DIRTY TRICKS YOUR MIND PLAYS ON YOU

Ages: 8–15 years.

Purpose: Education on cognitive distortions.

Materials Needed:

• A Dozen Dirty Tricks Your Mind Plays on You (Form 3.1).

Techniques for naming cognitive distortions are traditional psychoeducational interventions (Burns, 1980; Persons, 1989). Although teaching children to discover the errors in their thinking is an important step in psychoeducation, both the terminology and the process can be tough for youngsters to grasp. Adolescents generally can be given a list of cognitive errors or distortions found in many cognitive therapy texts (J. S. Beck, 1995;

Burns, 1980) and workbooks (Friedberg et al., 1992; Greenberger & Padesky, 1995). The Blurry Thinking Diary (Friedberg et al., 1992) is a naming the distortion intervention for adolescents. Younger children may profit from a more fun and metaphorical approach. We recommend presenting the distortions as tricks children's minds play on them. We have simplified the naming of the distortion procedure as A Dozen Dirty Tricks Your Mind Plays on You and the accompanying Spot the Dirty Trick Diary.

A Dozen Dirty Tricks Your Mind Plays on You is a handout you can give to children and their parents to teach them about cognitive errors (Form 3.1). In Chapter 5, the cognitive restructuring procedures Trick or Truth and Clean Up Your Thinking refer to the Dozen Dirty Tricks.

After the children learn the Dozen Dirty Tricks, we invite them to practice identifying the distortions using a fun game. Twelve small bags are labeled with each "dirty trick." Then, the youngster is given a distorted thought on a slip of paper or an index card. Their task is to decide which dirty trick is reflected in the distorted thought. Once they have made their choice, they drop the thought into the proper bag. This exercise teaches the child to examine thoughts for possible dirty tricks and then categorize them into appropriate categories.

Music and television shows can also help adolescents learn about cognitive distortions (Friedberg et al., 1992). After they learn the dirty tricks, teenagers can be instructed to listen to their favorite songs or watch their preferred television shows and note the dirty tricks that are embedded in the lyrics or dialogue. This exercise trains patients to attend to thoughts and discern their accuracy. The assignment also pairs a fun and frequently occurring activity (listening to music, watching TV) with a psychoeducational assignment (learning about cognitive distortions).

SPOT THE DIRTY TRICK DIARY

Ages: 8–15 years.

Purpose: Identifying cognitive distortions.

Materials Needed:

- A Dozen Dirty Tricks Your Mind Plays on You (Form 3.1).
- Spot the Dirty Trick Diary (Form 3.2).

Spot the Dirty Trick Diary is a way for children to name the distortion. It is conceptually similar to the Blurry Thinking Diary (Friedberg et al., 1992). Patients record the date, situation, feeling, and thought in columns 1–4. In column 5, they record the dirty trick. Like the Blurry Thinking Diary, children practice by watching a favorite TV show or listening to a favorite song and then identify the dirty tricks reflected in the dialogue or lyrics. Once they have practiced the naming the distortion technique, they apply the skill to their own automatic thoughts in the Spot the Dirty Trick Diary.

The following dialogue illustrates the Spot the Dirty Trick Diary with Omar, a 13-year-old boy with depression. Omar's filled-out Spot the Dirty Trick Diary can be seen in Figure 3.1. Form 3.2 is a blank diary form.

FIGURE 3.1. Omar's Spot the Dirty Trick Diary.

Date	Situation	Feeling	Thought	Dirty Trick
9/23	Two girls said I was fat	Sad	I'm the ugliest kid. No one will want to go to the dance will me.	Lame Blaming. Too Fast Forward thinking
9/23	Dad said I was too scared of the ball	Sad	He thinks I'm a wimp and doesn't like me.	Tragic Magic and One-Eyed Ogre
9/24	Got nervous talking to Marlena	Bad	I'm uncool.	Prisoner of Feeling

THERAPIST: Omar, let's use the List of Dirty Tricks to spot tricks in your thinking.

OMAR: OK.

THERAPIST: You said that yesterday two girls said you were fat.

OMAR: Yeah, at the pep rally. I felt really sad because I like them.

THERAPIST: What did you say to yourself?

OMAR: I'm the ugliest kid around. No one will want to go to the dance with me.

THERAPIST: Look at your list of dirty tricks. Can you spot one?

OMAR: Umm, lame blaming and too-fast-forward thinking.

THERAPIST: Great. You are good at this. Want to do another one?

OMAR: Sure.

THERAPIST: What happened last night that upset you?

OMAR: My dad said I was too scared of the ball during my baseball game. I felt really sad because I think he doesn't like me and thinks I'm a wimp.

THERAPIST: Can you spot the trick?

OMAR: Tragic-magic and one-eyed-ogre thinking.

THERAPIST: You are getting to be an expert at this. How about what happened today?

OMAR: I was talking to Marlena and I felt nervous and got flustered. I felt bad because I am so uncool. Hey, that's prisoner of feeling thinking!

Omar became increasingly able to spot the dirty trick. By the end of the dialogue, Omar was able to identify the distortion without being prompted by the therapist.

CONCLUSION

Psychoeducation is a necessary beginning step in effective CBT, but does not have to be dry and lectured. The techniques presented in this chapter, summarized in Table 3.7,

TABLE 3.7. **Psychoeducational Techniques**

Technique	Ages	Uses for technique
Storybooks	3–13 years	Socializes families to CBT, increases motivation, promotes learning
Books with adolescent personal accounts	13–18 years	Introduces teenagers to the nature of their disorders and self-help skills
Games	8–13 years	Builds rapport while teaching skills
Volcano	8–18 years	Affective education
Naming the Enemy	8–18 years	Provides concrete illustration for the way symptoms obscure strengths
Movies, plays, television shows, music (see Table 3.6)	All	Affective education
Diamond Connections	8–13 years	Teaches cognitive model
Telephone Example	13–18 years	Teaches cognitive model
It's in the Bag magic trick	6–18 years	Teaches cognitive model
A Dozen Dirty Tricks Your Mind Plays on You	8–15 years	Naming-the-distortion techniques
Spot the Dirty Trick Diary	8–15 years	Used after skills in naming the distortion have been developed, provides practice in identifying their own automatic thoughts

provide interactive and fun strategies for accomplishing psychoeducation in a manner the child or adolescent will remember, and therefore be more likely to apply in future treatment sessions. These techniques provide patients with the building blocks necessary to make future therapy interventions effective. Therapists have to keep in mind the case conceptualization, even during the psychoeducation phase of treatment. Doing so will help you choose appropriate psychoeducation strategies, apply them in a flexible manner, and modify them when needed.

A Dozen Dirty Tricks Your Mind Plays on You

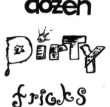

ONE-EYED OGRE: Seeing things from only one side and ignoring all other sides.

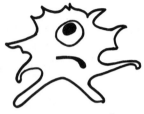

PRISONER OF FEELING: Using your feelings as the main guide for your actions and thoughts.

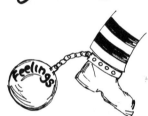

DISASTER FORECASTER: Falsely believing something awful will happen with very little to back up your ideas.

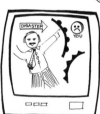

MAXI-ME THINKING: Falsely believing all the bad things that happen to you or other people are all your fault.

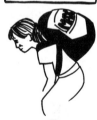

LAME BLAMING: Using a label for yourself ("I'm bad") or others ("She's a witch. It's all her fault.").

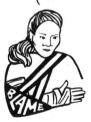

(continued)

MULES RULES: Stubbornly insisting that your ideas about how you, other people, and the world should act are the only ones that are right.

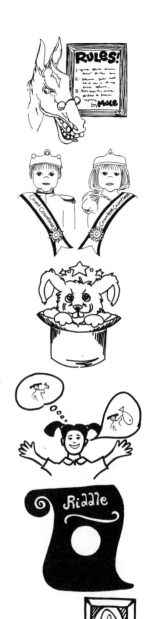

COUNTLESS THINKING: Convincing yourself that strengths, successes, and good experiences do not count.

TRAGIC MAGIC THINKING: Incorrectly believing you know exactly what is going through someone else's mind without checking it out or asking him or her.

TALL-TALE THINKING: Believing something despite there being little to back up the ideas.

NO MIDDLE RIDDLE: Seeing things in only two ways, like you are perfect or you are a total loser.

CIRCUS MIRROR THINKING: When you look at yourself, other people, or what happens to you, you shrink the positive (+) or supersize the negative (−).

TOO FAST FORWARD: Jumping to big conclusions by using small bits of information. Not waiting to get all the results or information you need.

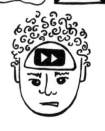

Spot the Dirty Trick Diary

Date	Situation	Feeling	Thought	Dirty Trick

CHAPTER 4

Behavioral Interventions

There are good reasons to start with behavioral interventions in the treatment of most childhood problems. Many children in treatment lack skills in self-regulation and will therefore gain a tremendous initial benefit by learning how to calm their feelings and control their behaviors. When children are overwhelmingly anxious or angry they generally cannot attend to cognitions and will therefore struggle with the more sophisticated cognitive interventions. In addition, introducing behavioral approaches in the beginning phase of treatment builds rapport, increases the child's motivation and engagement in treatment, expands coping repertoires, and primes youngsters for subsequent interventions. Behavioral interventions often produce quicker changes and facilitate follow-through with treatment. Behavioral techniques are also beneficial for assisting parents in modifying behaviors outside of the therapy sessions, which facilitates generalization.

Behavioral techniques decrease the frequency and severity of undesirable behaviors, as well as increase the frequency of desirable behaviors. In addition, changes in the child's attitude, emotion, and cognition may follow changes in behavior, and thus lead to an overall improvement in functioning. Behavioral interventions involve direct instruction in skills and parent training, as well as in-session practice of skill application (Friedberg & McClure, 2002). Since behavioral techniques are more concrete, they can be used quickly and easily with many different populations and presenting problems.

In this chapter, we present a variety of effective behavioral techniques. We briefly describe the techniques and a rationale for their use. We then present numerous applications. We designed the descriptions to try to make implementation easy for the therapist. Handouts should be helpful in presenting the techniques to clients. Charts can be found at the end of each section to guide therapists in choosing the approaches that are most appropriate for various presenting problems. Finally, the end of the chapter offers helpful descriptors of techniques to assist parents and teachers wanting to prompt or reinforce the child's use of the techniques. The handouts assist therapists in bridging the gap between sessions and daily life.

RELAXATION TECHNIQUES

Without skills in self-regulation and self-calming, children may be unable to follow through with therapy interventions in the face of high levels of emotion (Goldfried & Davison, 1976). Therefore, relaxation is a basic behavioral technique that cannot be overlooked. Relaxation strategies allow enough reduction in symptoms so that additional techniques can be successful. These strategies are also often fun for young patients. Thus, in addition to improving emotional functioning, these techniques strengthen the therapeutic alliance.

Progressive Muscle Relaxation

Progressive muscle relaxation (PMR; Jacobson, 1938) is a traditional relaxation strategy used to treat various symptoms by teaching clients to tense and relax muscle groups. Children are first taught to tense various muscle groups; then, after about 5–8 seconds, the child is instructed to completely release the tension and relax the muscles. Often the muscle groups are targeted one at a time, going from one end of the body to the other. Children will often require more specific instructions, demonstrations by the therapist (Goldfried & Davison, 1976), visualization, and/or metaphors (Koeppen, 1974) to assist with this process. Demonstration can be helpful, as can descriptors, such as "Your arm should feel loose and limp like spaghetti" to convey the change the child may feel. Telling the child to envision squeezing a lemon and trying to squeeze all the juice out (Koeppen, 1974) is a good example of how to assist younger children with the tensing process. Repeated practice is generally needed when building this skill; thus, both in-session and home-based practice sessions are utilized.

Deep breathing exercises are often paired with PMR to assist with the relaxation. Deep breathing has been introduced to children in creative ways to increase motivation and compliance with the breathing exercises. For example, Wexler's (1991) Ten Candles approach has the child imagine 10 candles in a row and then blow them out one by one. Instructing the youth to actually blow bubbles with a commercial bubble solution and wand can also teach deep breathing (Warfield, 1999). Both are fun ways to encourage younger children to slow their breathing and breathe more deeply. By combining visualization (e.g., with the Ten Candles approach) or actual visual cues (e.g, bubbles) with the deep breathing, therapists are more likely to engage the youth. In addition, visual cues can help reinforce children's efforts, as well as provide a means for youth to monitor their breathing. For example, children can observe the flow of the bubbles to monitor their rate of breathing. If the bubbles are not smoothly flowing from the wand, children can practice decreasing the force and rate of the breath to a slower and softer exhale. An added benefit is that the bubbles serve as a nice distraction for many youngsters.

If bubbles are not an option, some children enjoy using a straw to blow a cotton ball across a table or the floor. The movement resulting from the breaths serves as a visual cue and reinforcer, as well as a nice distraction, further relaxing the child. When teaching relaxation to older children, it is important to adapt some strategies for use in social environments (e.g., school). Children will not likely do deep breathing or other exercises if they believe their peers might notice and tease them.

We encourage youth to be creative and find ways to apply skills in their daily lives. In the following transcript, one anxious youngster adapted the deep breathing technique by "whistling" when frustrated.

SARAH: The bubbles are fun and make my body calm down at home, but I can't blow bubbles at school. Even during recess, I would get in trouble 'cause we can't bring stuff like that to school.

THERAPIST: What *could* you do during recess?

SARAH: I don't know. If I just pretend to blow bubbles like I do in the car with my mom, I would probably look stupid and the other kids would tease me more.

THERAPIST: I like that you are trying to think of other ideas. What else might work?

SARAH: I know! I could whistle. It would be like blowing out air, and no one else would know what I was doing.

THERAPIST: Wow, Sarah, what a creative idea! Why don't you try that this week, and see how it works.

In the above example, the therapist validates Sarah's concerns by supporting the problem-solving process. The therapist reinforces her efforts, and then begins to set up behavioral experimentation to increase follow-through and to provide data to determine if the technique is helpful for her.

Other Relaxation Techniques

The balance of this section outlines several more relaxation techniques for youth. Table 4.1 is a guide to choosing appropriate techniques for specific children. Since all of the

TABLE 4.1. Choosing Relaxation Techniques

Technique	Ages	Use	Appropriate problems/ diagnoses	Format
Calming-down kits/Survival kits	4–10 years—use pictures and items; 9 years and older—can add in text-based items	Relaxation Self-monitoring Self-regulation	Anger Anxiety Impulsivity Sensory integration dysfunction Irritability/depression	Individual Family Group
Progressive muscle relaxation	4 years and older	Relaxation Self-regulation	Anger Anxiety Impulsivity	Individual Family Group
Cue cards	4 years and older (pictures for younger children, and written words for older youth)	Nonverbal cues for use of relaxation strategies; increases independent use of techniques and helps with generalization of skills	Anger Anxiety Impulsivity Sensory integration dysfunction Irritability/depression	Individual Family Group
Scripts for relaxation	4–10 years	Provide opportunities for memorization of self-talk and coping statements	Anger Anxiety Impulsivity Sensory integration dysfunction Irritability/depression	Individual Family Group

techniques listed generally teach the same skill set, therapists are encouraged to choose the options that best match the child's developmental level and interests.

RELAXATION SCRIPTS

Ages: All ages.

Purpose: Relaxation.

Materials Needed:

• Prewritten script.

While relaxation is a relatively straightforward procedure, many children will experience difficulty with straightforward instructions (e.g., "Tense up your jaw, then let go and relax."). Therefore, concrete and developmentally friendly instructions can help in the coaching process. There are a number of excellent relaxation scripts for children and adolescents (Geddie, 1992; Kendall et al., 1992; Ollendick & Cerny, 1981).

Meaningful relaxation scripts for youth include clear visual images. They make use of objects and situations that are within the child's experience. Demonstrations by the therapist are also useful. Koeppen (1974) taught muscle tensing in the hands and arms by having the child pretend to squeeze a lemon. The image of a stretching cat was used to target the arms and shoulders, and a turtle pulling its head into the shell was used to teach tensing of the neck and shoulders. Further descriptive examples included chewing a big piece of gum (for jaw tensing) and a fly on the nose for face/nose tensing. Kendall et al. (1992) offer detailed step-by-step relaxation training scripts. The scripts can be read by the therapist or parent. The child is taken through the process of tensing and relaxing each targeted muscle group. Choosing an appropriate script is similar to choosing other appropriate techniques for youth. That is, the therapist needs to be cognizant of the conceptualization so that the specific script chosen will be engaging and meaningful for that particular child.

The dinosaur script (Geddie, 1992) is a very engaging and inviting relaxation script. Children pretend they are dinosaurs and relaxation procedures are specific and understandable. For example, to tense forehead muscles, the script suggests, "As you begin to move slowly through the trees with sweet leaves on them, you think you also see some juicy berries. But because you are walking into the sun, you have to squint hard to see the berries." The instruction for arm tension is: "When you get to the waterhole, you see it is covered with rocks. You have to lift the rocks out of the way with your arms. Bend your big dinosaur arms up at the elbows and lift the rocks out of the way with your arms."

CALMING-DOWN KITS

Ages: All ages.

Purpose: Relaxation, self-monitoring, self-regulation.

Materials needed:

- Shoe box or bag (such as a paper lunch bag).
- One or more from the following: bubbles, candle (e.g., birthday candle), straw, and cotton ball.
- Squeeze ball/Koosh ball.
- Small pillow or stuffed animal.
- Paper, scissors, and crayons or markers.

Many children in our practices have benefited from creating a portable calming-down kit. This kit can take various forms, depending on the child's age, interests, and clinical symptoms. Relaxation skills are taught to the child, then the child practices the techniques, assembles a kit, adds his or her own creative "calming" idea, and decorates the kit. A bag or shoebox then can be used in session during role plays and exposures. Sometimes separate kits are created for home and school. Depending on the child's interests, the kit can take the form of a purse, survival kit, tool box, backpack, or treasure chest. Table 4.2 provides ideas for content in each kit. Additional strategies for distraction items can be added to individualize the kit for each youth.

A survival kit is a popular method. The kit may include camping items that can be used as cues for traditional relaxation techniques. A candle serves as a symbol for deep breathing, and children can pretend to blow out the candle "flame." A small pillow may be squeezed to cue tensing and relaxing muscles. The Feeling Compass for self-monitoring, presented in Chapter 2, can be added to the kit. When the child detects a change in feelings and indicates it on the Feeling Compass, that may serve as a prompt to use other items in the kit to target relaxation.

The materials may seem overwhelming at first, but many items can be ordered through companies such as SmileMaker. Fun bubbles, colorful squeeze balls, and small stuffed animals come in multipacks. Candles, cotton balls, and straws are easy to find and store. These hands-on items are more engaging and fun for the youth than simply teaching PMR and breathing on their own. In addition, the items are visual reminders for each of the techniques, assisting in use of the strategies outside of the session. The actual process of creating the kit in session (e.g., decorating the box, assembling the kit) also serves as a rapport-building activity.

TABLE 4.2. Contents for Calming Kits

Item	Deep breathing	Muscle relaxation	Feeling identification/ rating	Distraction
Bubbles	X			X
Candle	X			X
Straw and cotton ball	X			X
Koosh or squeeze ball		X		X
Pillow/stuffed animal		X		X
Cue cards	X	X	X	X
Feeling Compass			X	X

CALMING CUE CARDS

Ages: All ages.

Purpose: Relaxation, self-regulation.

Materials Needed:

- Cards.
- Cue pictures.
- Markers, crayons, or pen.

Some children and teens may not be interested in completing an actual kit. For those youth, the "kit" can take the form of cue cards that are created, laminated, and connected by punching a hole in the card and stringing or clipping the cards together. For younger children, picture cues are fun prompts, while older youth may prefer word cues. Examples for cue cards may include pictures of a bottle of bubbles, a squeeze ball, calming images or pictures, stuffed animals, and speech bubbles with self-talk statements. These cards can easily be kept in a backpack, a purse, or even a pocket. A teen may have a mini-book of cue cards with reminders of self-talk statements and relaxation techniques, and the teen can glance at these cards to help prompt use of the strategies throughout the day. Children are encouraged to come up with their own ideas for how to make the cue cards most useful for them. For example, one child with anxiety chose to attach the cue cards to her water bottle during soccer games to review and prompt herself during the games. Figure 4.1 illustrates some examples of cue cards.

Implementing Calming Kits and Cue Cards Techniques

Once the "kit" is created, regardless of its form, it is beneficial to teach families how to use the kit at home to assist with generalization. We recommend teaching families to prompt the child to use the kit, and to reinforce the use of the kit. This prompting/reinforcing should first occur during role plays (modeled first by the therapist, and then with parents), and then generalized to real-life situations at home.

Consider the following example, in which 8-year-old Tara is learning to apply relaxation strategies when her younger brother bothers her. First, the therapist demonstrates the use of role plays for the family, and then prompts the family to complete a role play. A plan for generalization to home is then made.

THERAPIST: Let's pretend you just got a new art tablet for your birthday, and your brother drew all over it with markers. You walk into the kitchen and discover the book is ruined. You are very angry and feel your muscles tighten and your face turn red. Show me how you could use your calming kit.

TARA: I could pretend to blow bubbles and squeeze my squishy ball.

THERAPIST: Great job remembering your tools! Show me how you would blow the bubbles and squeeze the ball. (*Tara uses the items from the calming kit.*) Wow, Tara, you are really getting good at relaxing your muscles and calming your breathing! Now, I want you and Mom to practice. What is something else that might happen that would make you angry at your brother?

FIGURE 4.1. Examples of Calming Cue Cards

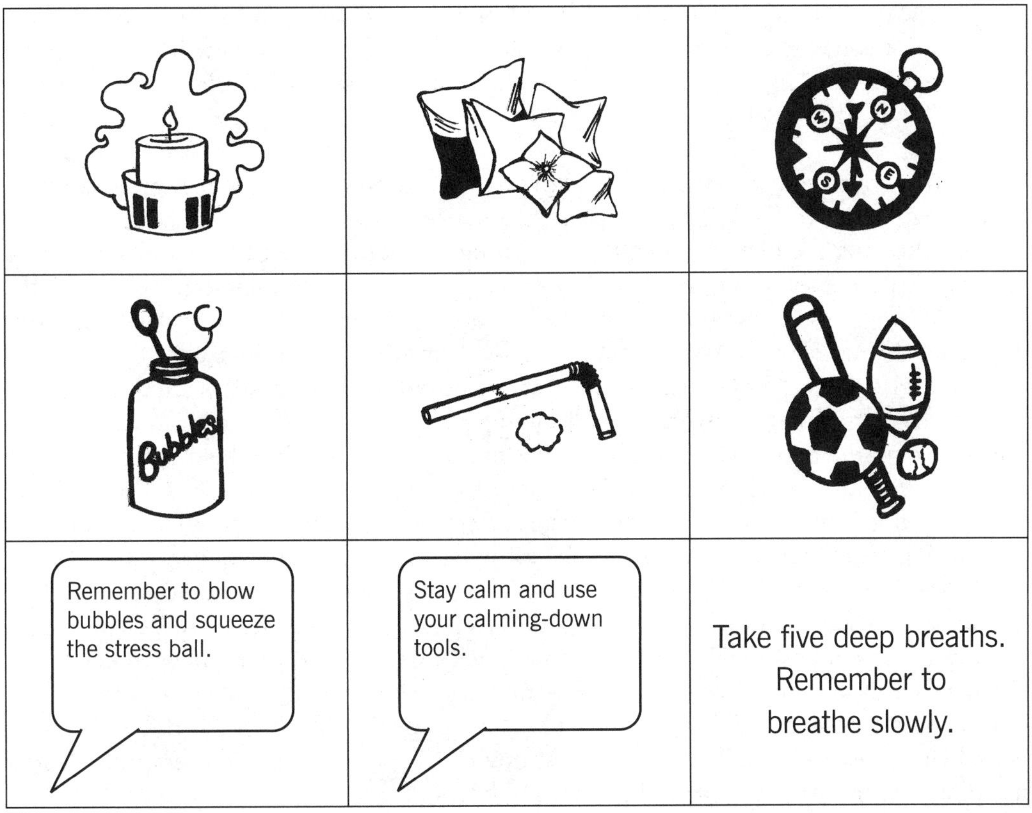

Remember to blow bubbles and squeeze the stress ball.

Stay calm and use your calming-down tools.

Take five deep breaths. Remember to breathe slowly.

TARA: I get really mad when he comes into my room.

MOTHER: That is true! That often leads to a big fight or tantrum.

THERAPIST: OK, I want the two of you to practice a role play about that.

MOTHER: Alright—let's see ... Tara, pretend you are on your bed reading a book, and your brother throws open your door and walks right in.

TARA: I would really be mad. He is supposed to knock first and he always comes right in without asking.

THERAPIST: OK, and remember before you can solve the problem, you have to be calm.

MOTHER: Yes. So, Tara, show me what you could use from your calming kit to stay in control.

TARA: (*Picks up kit and pulls out small stuffed animal.*) I would squeeze a stuffed animal since there would probably be one on my bed!

THERAPIST: (*Quietly prompts mom.*) Praise and prompt.

MOTHER: That's a good one to start with! What could you do next?

TARA: I could use this card. It says, "Stay calm and you won't get in trouble!" and then I would go get you.

MOTHER: Great thinking, and then I would help you solve the problem!

THERAPIST: Nice job with the role play! Now, it will be important for you to practice some role plays at home. What would be a good homework assignment?
[The therapist and family then collaboratively establish a plan for practice at
home that week.]

In this transcript, the reader sees how to help families practice using the calming
kit during role plays. By having the parents practice in session with the child, the therapist is increasing the likelihood of follow-through at home. The therapist observed and
shaped the parent's and the child's behavior as needed during the session. Consequently,
the child was successful and generalization occurred. In addition, the collaborative
approach to a homework assignment can help identify potential obstacles to success.

To assist in skill building, the scenarios initially include mild to moderately distressing triggers, and then work up to more upsetting triggers drawn from the presenting problem and examples provided by the family. The role plays help children create
a script for dealing with common situations at home. Having a concrete "kit" to take
home prompts families to use the strategies. Parents and children should be cautioned
that initially it may be difficult to use the kit when emotions are strong.

Consider Tara again. If she is on her bed reading, her mother could point out, "This
is kind of like we practiced in therapy today. What if your brother came in your room
right now, without asking?" Then later in the week if Tara's brother comes in her room,
she may be more likely to use calming strategies. Also, her mother could prompt her
"in the moment" (e.g., "Tara, you look like you are getting upset. What did we practice
earlier this week that might help you right now?"). Tara's mom could then praise Tara's
use of any of the strategies from her calming kit.

Practicing techniques and predicting times for use is crucial when building skills.
The Guessing Game Worksheet described later in this chapter can be used to prompt
youth to guess the outcome of using the kit, and then assess actual usefulness. This
approach is also a useful way to test the evidence when a child is skeptical about using
the techniques. A completed Guessing Game Worksheet will also assist you in assessing
follow-through by the family and identifying obstacles for success.

MODELING

The power of modeling in developing new behaviors is strong. Children learn from
observing their environment. By providing appropriate models, therapists and caregivers can increase the success of techniques. Modeling can be done by caregivers and
therapists, can occur in play with puppets or dolls, or can be illustrated by characters
and story lines in books. Media images, drawn from movies or TV shows, can also
be powerful modeling agents. For example, if relaxation is being taught, the therapist
may use scenes from movies or television shows that illustrate various forms of feeling
expression and self-regulation (or lack of self-regulation). Children can view the scenes
and pick out triggers for changes in emotion, as well as look for strategies the characters
are using or could be using for self-regulation (e.g., deep breathing, clenching fists, verbally expressing their feelings). The child can practice identifying verbal and nonverbal

cues of how the character is feeling and when changes in feeling intensity are occurring. In addition, the child can be asked to assess what self-regulation/relaxation techniques are being used or could be used in the given scene. Children's books can also be used in a similar manner. Children also enjoy stories and puppet shows acting out everyday struggles where characters use therapy techniques to cope. Adults modeling coping strategies and self-talk is also a very powerful teaching tool. Therapist self-disclosure is another modeling technique (Gosch et al., 2006). The therapist can coach parents to verbalize some struggles or problem solving at home in front of the child to illustrate the use of various techniques.

For example, a parent might spill something while making dinner. The parent may then state, "Oh no, I spilled the potatoes all over the floor. Wait, this is not a big problem. Let me just take a breath and think. I know there is always a way to solve the problem. I can get out some more potatoes and just wipe up the ones on the floor."

SYSTEMATIC DESENSITIZATION

Since its 1958 introduction by Joseph Wolpe, systematic desensitization has become an important aspect of anxiety treatment. This counterconditioning procedure involves the use of relaxation strategies while confronting anxiety-producing stimuli. Systematic desensitization works by pairing anxiety-producing stimuli with a counterconditioning "agent," such as deep breathing, PMR, or even humor. Thus, the importance of training the child in counterconditioning agents (CCAs) prior to beginning systematic desensitization is clear.

After relaxation or other CCAs have been taught to the child, an anxiety hierarchy is created. As mentioned in Chapter 2, the anxiety hierarchy consists of descriptions of situations that evoke anxiety in the client. The descriptions must be detailed, and the situations ordered in a hierarchy based on the level of anxiety the client associates with each one.

Systematic desensitization starts by targeting the lowest item on the hierarchy and remaining at that item until the youth can encounter that thought, image, or situation without feeling significant anxiety. Relaxation as a competing response is used during these encounters with anxiety-producing stimuli. Thus, having calming kits and/or cue cards on hand is beneficial. The child stays at each item until he or she is able to produce a relaxed state consistently when faced with that item. Once the child has shown the ability to maintain a relaxed state with the targeted item, he or she moves on to the next item on the hierarchy. After each item on the hierarchy is mastered, the child progresses up the hierarchy until all items have been completed. With each item, relaxation (rather than fear) is paired with the identified source of anxiety. As a result, a classical conditioning response is created. Thus, the link between anxiety and fear-producing stimuli is disconnected and a fresh connection between the fear-producing stimuli and relaxation is established. In effect, a new response to the stimuli (relaxation) is being substituted for the previous, maladaptive response (fear). Since relaxation competes with or inhibits the anxiety, the anxiety decreases. This approach often takes several sessions in combination with home-based practices.

The following transcript demonstrates the systematic desensitization process with Tony.

THERAPIST: Tony, you said you want to get rid of your worries about dogs.

TONY: That's right. I want to be able to go to friends' houses who have dogs, or play outside with my friends without being embarrassed because I am scared of the dogs that are out there.

THERAPIST: OK. Let's work on that today with a tool called Up, Up, and Away. We are going to figure out what things would make you a little nervous, medium nervous, and a lot nervous about dogs. Then we are going to use your calming-down kit to stay calm while thinking about the different situations we talked about.

TONY: But I will get really scared if we start talking about this.

THERAPIST: I know it seems hard to think about these things, but remember we will start with the easier things and use calming strategies until you are ready to go to the next step.

TONY: So I won't have to do the really hard ones right away? I guess that sounds OK.

THERAPIST: We can use these note cards to write down the ideas we have. Remember when we worked on rating how strong your feelings were? We are going to use that and write it on the cards, too.

TONY: OK, let me get my feeling thermometer out of my folder.

THERAPIST: Tony, it is great that you are using your tools! Now, what is a situation that would make you a little nervous?

TONY: Probably if I just thought of a dog in my head. That would be a 1 on my feeling thermometer.

THERAPIST: What would the dog look like?

TONY: Well, it would have to be a kind of friendly dog, like my Auntie's dog—not like Ricky's dog—that would be like a 6!

THERAPIST: OK, let's start with picturing your Auntie's dog. Do you want to write or draw that on this note card?

TONY: I will write it. (*Writes down the description and rating.*)

THERAPIST: OK, what other situations can you think of?

In this example, the therapist helps Tony create a hierarchy to desensitize him to dog-related stimuli that are causing fear. The feared stimuli (dogs) will be paired with relaxation. The therapist helps Tony outline mildly distressing items first, so as not to overwhelm him and risk strengthening his fear. When Tony identifies visualization of a dog as his first hierarchy item, the therapist inquires more to make sure the item is accurately placed. This helps Tony differentiate which dog he will visualize, and also helps identify an item for later on the hierarchy. Each item will be recorded on a separate card. As Tony moves up the hierarchy, he will be able to see how far he "climbed" to overcome his fears by looking at the string of cards that he had completed.

There are a few tips to remember when conducting systematic desensitization (Morris & Kratochwill, 1998). When the first scene is presented, the distressing image should be held for 5–10 seconds if the patient reports no initial anxiety. Subsequent items should be held for 10–20 seconds. The relaxation or other CCA should persist for at least 15–20 seconds between the introduction of the scenes, or until relaxation is achieved. Generally, three to four scenes at most are introduced in a single session.

SOCIAL SKILLS TRAINING

Social skills are critical for children experiencing interpersonal difficulties, isolation, exclusion, and rejection (Erdlen & Rickrode, 2007). Social skills training is used to address a range of presenting problems, including disruptive behavior disorders, anxiety, depression, and pervasive developmental disorders. Although children with these disorders may present with very different behaviors, their deficits in social skills can generally be categorized into the areas of acquisition, performance, or fluency (Erdlen & Rickrode, 2007). Therapists must identify the area(s) needing intervention, and build the youths' skills accordingly. Beidel and Turner (2006) point out the importance of skill building through instruction, modeling, behavioral rehearsal, feedback, and positive reinforcement. Instruction is the direct teaching of the skill, and is accompanied by the rationale for the skills. Modeling by the therapist should be exaggerated, and should include appropriate and inappropriate models for the youth to observe and distinguish between. Modeling can also be accomplished through peers, puppets, books, and media (Cartledge & Milburn, 1996). Beidel and Turner (2006) recommend that the majority of treatment time be spent on behavioral rehearsal and providing repeated practicing of skill sets. Group settings are helpful for this process. Corrective feedback and positive reinforcement also assist with skill improvement. Generalization of skills occurs through specific homework assignments tailored to the individual child (Beidel & Turner, 2006).

Social skills training is a natural match for children and adolescents with PDD. Because of their social and emotional symptoms, and often their secondary affective disorders, children with PDD need training in social functioning that includes affective education and cognitive restructuring (Attwood, 2004). Attwood (2003) points out that children with PDD need assistance with various stages of social development. He emphasizes affective education utilizing strategies such as likening the face to an information center for emotions. Therapists use various activities to train the child to "spot the message." Then they identify various possible meanings of the same nonverbal cue. Attwood (2003) uses the example of a furrowed brow as a sign of anger, bewilderment, or aging skin. In addition, cognitive restructuring is particularly important when conducting social skills training with a population with PDD due to the social deficits that lead to literal interpretations and misinterpretations of social stimuli (Attwood, 2003).

Attwood describes several difficulties these children experience, including differentiating between intentions that are accidental and those that are deliberate. Additionally, children with PDD attend to the act itself and the consequences, without paying attention to the circumstances. Attwood offers a creative approach to improving such skills using visual cues of actual tools to represent therapy techniques. For example, a paintbrush represents relaxation techniques, while a two-handle saw stands for social activities or represents individuals who can help the child with dealing with negative feelings (Attwood, 2003).

We next offer several useful strategies to assist therapists in using social skills training with youth. Making a Book is a flexible technique that can be modified and applied in countless situations. The basic procedure for creating the book is outlined and remains the same across various situations, but the content and level of complexity varies with each patient. Instant Message Role Plays make use of a common technique (role plays), but apply it in a familiar context for youth. Many youth are comfortable using computers and communicate through computers regularly. Applying what they are comfortable with to new interactions can help build social skills in a fun and engaging manner. Etch A Sketch is also presented in this section as a creative social skills training exercise that lends itself well to group treatment settings. Finally, Password is another interactive task that can be used to build skills in perspective taking in a fun and active manner. The following sections outline these interventions in more detail.

MAKING A BOOK

Ages: 4–10 years.

Purpose: Social skills training.

Materials Needed:

- Paper.
- Stapler to attach book pages.
- Markers/crayons for writing/drawing.
- Scissors, glue, and magazine pictures.

For younger children, creating a book about a particular skill can be fun, engaging, and effective. In this Making a Book activity, the action of creating the book is part of the intervention, and the examples used in the book can be specifically tailored to the individual child to make it more meaningful and applicable. The technique begins with the therapist guiding the child in creating the text, while the child illustrates the pictures. The text of the book offers an avenue for direct instruction, while the book provides opportunities for repetitive review, both in session and at home. The child can independently review the text, or do so with parents, to assist with generalization of skills. This technique involves identifying a specific skill to work on, such as dealing with teasing. The skill is discussed in session, then a book is started detailing the skill being targeted. Specifically, the therapist begins the sentence and then the child fills in the remainder of the text. The example below illustrates how to create a book with an 8-year-old girl named Jenna, who is being teased at school.

> THERAPIST: Jenna, I see that the next thing on our list today is to talk about the teasing that has been going on at school [identifying agenda item]. You are such a great artist, why don't we make a book about how to solve this problem.
>
> JENNA: And I can draw the pictures? Can I take it home when we're done?
>
> THERAPIST: Yes. We can write about the problem and how to solve it, then you can draw the pictures, and then you can read the book to practice remembering the tools for making things better at school.

JENNA: OK, but what should we write?

THERAPIST: Let's start with this: "Every day at school we go out to recess. During recess, I enjoy _____." What should we add in there?

JENNA: I really like playing on the swings, walking around, and sometimes talking to other kids.

THERAPIST: Great, let's write that on the first page. Now, what would you like to draw?

In the above dialogue, the therapist introduces the Making a Book technique to address the agenda item of dealing with teasing and building Jenna's social skills. The therapist uses an interest and talent of Jenna's (drawing) to motivate and engage her. By participating in creating the book, Jenna is more likely to take ownership of it and will be more likely to follow through with using the techniques outside the session. Below is an example of what could be included in the remainder of the book. The underlined portion represents the text the child fills in.

- "Every day at school we go out to recess. During recess, I enjoy <u>playing on the swings, walking around, and sometimes talking to other kids</u>."
- "Sometimes when I am swinging, <u>Jared and his friends stand in front of the swing</u>."
- "<u>Jared calls me names, like stupid and fat. I feel sad and mad when that happens</u>."
- "When I see Jared walking toward me, I can <u>get up and walk over to a teacher or friend. Tonya and her friends are usually nice, so I could ask to play with them</u>."
- "If that doesn't work, I will <u>tell Jared to leave me alone. I can use the broken record tool, and just calmly say the same thing over and over</u>."
- "If Jared is still bugging me, <u>I can ask a teacher for help</u>."
- "I will remember to <u>use my calming tools on the playground so that I can stay calm and handle things</u>."
- "I don't like being teased, but <u>I feel better knowing what to do when it happens</u>."

Some children want to improve their social interactions with peers and may be motivated to participate in social skills training. For example, an anxious child may express an interest in making more friends, and may be eager to learn skills necessary to do so. However, children with externalizing disorders, such as oppositional defiant disorder, often lack the motivation to try out some of the social skills problem-solving strategies, and may require further therapeutic interventions to increase motivation. Cognitive restructuring may be beneficial, as well as contingency management. The key is to identify the reason for reluctance to using the strategies, and then intervene accordingly. By keeping the approach collaborative, the therapist should be able to identify the child's perspective on the task, and therefore design effective ways to motivate the child.

The following dialogue shows how to identify the sources of avoidance in an 11-year-old patient named Brady.

THERAPIST: Last week we agreed that you would start a conversation with the guys you sit with at lunch and we role-played ways to do so. So, how did it go?

BRADY: I never really got around to it.

THERAPIST: What got in the way?

BRADY: It was just a busy week. I had a test in science, and we had a basketball game and I just had a lot to do.

THERAPIST: When you think about doing the assignment, how do you feel?

BRADY: (*Looks down and starts to fidget.*) Just bored, I guess. It just seems like a stupid assignment. What's the point?

THERAPIST: [Rather than focusing on Brady's question, the therapist attends to the change in affect.] I noticed you looked down and seemed to move around in your chair more when I asked how you felt.

BRADY: Geeez! Let it go. Why would I want to waste my time with your stupid homework? Those kids don't like me, no one does!

THERAPIST: Wow! I can understand why you wouldn't want to start a conversation if your thought is, "Those kids don't like me, no one does." It would be hard to talk to someone with that thought in your head.

BRADY: (*Calming down.*) Yeah.

THERAPIST: What feeling do you have when you say that to yourself?

BRADY: Really alone and down.

By exploring Brady's avoidance of implementing the social skills techniques they had been addressing in session, the therapist is able to help Brady identify an automatic thought that is getting in the way. Although Brady's initial obstacle was a lack of skills in initiating and sustaining conversation, it became clear that even when the skills were taught, a challenge remained. By addressing the shift in affect during the session, the therapist was able to help Brady catch the automatic thought. Cognitive techniques can then be applied to overcome this obstacle, and to increase the chances of homework compliance in the future.

INSTANT MESSAGE ROLE PLAYS

Ages: 10 years and older.

Purpose: Social skills training.

Materials Needed:

- Cell phones.
- Instant Messaging Social Skills Worksheet (Form 4.1).

Role plays are an excellent way for children with many presenting problems to practice and master self-talk and social skills. In the age of IM-ing, older children and teens can have fun by using an instant messaging approach to role-play various social responses and skills. Vignettes can be presented for the youth to respond to in an appropriate manner. Form 4.1 provides examples that are helpful for in-session practice or for homework assignments. Examples are provided to tap skills in initiating social interactions, as well as responding to initiations by others. Therapists are encouraged to tailor additional IM vignettes to address targeted areas with the individual child. This engaging and effective approach can be graduated based on the youth's current skill level, and adapted to address specific skill areas. It can be difficult to connect with some teens, and adolescents may view therapy interventions as boring and "uncool." By using metaphors that include interests and communication styles familiar to teens, the working relationship may be more effective, and the teen may be more motivated and engaged in the tasks. Therefore, the interventions will increase in effectiveness.

The following transcript illustrates the use of the Instant Messaging Social Skills Worksheet with an anxious and skeptical teenager named Sarina.

THERAPIST: We have been talking about ways to respond to your classmates at school, and you are getting really good at it.

SARINA: I still feel like I don't know what to do or say.

THERAPIST: Well, I have a fun way for you to practice. I know you said you like to chat online a lot.

SARINA: Too much, if you ask my mom!

THERAPIST: I have an Instant Messaging Worksheet that gives you situations that might come up at school. I want you to think of how you could respond, and IM it back to me. (*Smiles.*)

SARINA: But it is so much harder to actually do it—I never know what to say.

THERAPIST: This worksheet will help you practice figuring out what to say more quickly, and we can rate your anxiety before and after to test if it works.

SARINA: All right, I am at a 7 now—I can't believe I am this nervous!

THERAPIST: Let's give it a try. The first one says, "You are walking down the hall at school and a new student smiles at you." Now, write in your IM response.

SARINA: (*Writes "How's it goin'?" :) or nod my head.*) Look, I wrote the smile with an IM smile. (*Laughs.*)

THERAPIST: I notice you are smiling and joking. How is your anxiety?

SARINA: Down to a 3. This wasn't as bad as I thought!

THERAPIST: OK, try the next one.

In this example Sarina has already been taught basic social skills. When it comes time to practice the skills, the therapist chooses this creative approach to keep Sarina engaged and motivated. When Sarina expresses anxiety, the therapist proceeds with the technique, communicating confidence that Sarina is capable of completing the technique. Feeling rating is used to collect data on how Sarina feels before and after using the technique.

After the child or adolescent has practiced social responses on paper and in role plays with the Instant Messaging approach, he or she will be better prepared to try the skills in real-life situations. Thus, the worksheet and in-session role plays offer a graduated step in skill development and application. By using examples from the youth's life, the therapist can assist in the generalization to the youth's life. The youngster can try out rehearsed social responses, and then report back as to how the exposures went. Reinforcement and feedback can be provided accordingly by the therapist.

ETCH A SKETCH

Ages: 6–18 years.

Purpose: Teaching social skills.

Materials Needed:

- Etch A Sketch toy.
- Designs to be copied.

The children's toy Etch A Sketch lends itself nicely to social skills training. Ginsburg, Grover, Cord, and Ialongo (2006) used the task to study overcontrol and criticism in parent–children dyads. However, the toy can also be easily applied to peer dyads. The task is structured so it is a cooperative exercise that requires teamwork for success. As Ginsburg et al. (2006) recommended, a two-child team is given one Etch A Sketch toy and instructed to copy designs. One team member controls the left knob and the other controls the right knob. Thus, success is achieved only by working together. A time limit and an evaluation component may be added to increase anxiety.

The therapist processes the task with the team members. He or she provides positive feedback for appropriate behavior (e.g., "Nice going. You two are working together."), helps them monitor their problematic thoughts, feelings, and behaviors ("What's going wrong here? How are you feeling? What is going through your mind when you aren't working together?"), and guides them toward more appropriate self-talk when they are feeling frustrated or anxious. Additionally, the therapist fosters behavioral flexibility (e.g., "Let's see what the two of you could do. What about if you take turns giving directions?") and corrects inappropriate behavior (e.g., preventing them reaching for the other knob). Finally, the therapist helps the patients cement the experience by writing out a summary (e.g., "Write down on a card what you learned from this.").

The following transcript illustrates the procedure with a brother and sister named Ethan and Malea, who have control battles.

THERAPIST: This next activity is for Ethan and Malea to do together. Here's an Etch A Sketch and I want the two of you to work together to make this shape. (*Shows shape.*) But here's the catch: each of you can only work one knob.

ETHAN: This will be easy.

MALEA: Yeah, easy.

THERAPIST: Go ahead and try it.

[*They begin the task. Ethan gets frustrated and starts to use Malea's knob.*]

ETHAN: Do it this way! Here, I will show you!

MALEA: Keep your hands off it!

THERAPIST: OK, stop. Ethan, what is going through your mind?

ETHAN: She's stupid and ignorant. I have to do it for her.

MALEA: I'm not stupid. You are! I'll smack you if you do it again!

THERAPIST: All right, calm down. I see how hard it is for you to work together. How can you finish this without arguing or smacking?

ETHAN: She needs to do what I say!

MALEA: Why? Who died and left you boss?

ETHAN: Shut up, you brat.

THERAPIST: Let's try something different. What do you need to do to work together?

ETHAN: (*Pause.*) Maybe we can tell each other what direction we are going.

MALEA: And stop calling names!

THERAPIST: Sounds like a plan.

Malea and Ethan began to talk their way through the activity and accomplish the cooperative task. As shown above, the activity revealed the thoughts, feelings, and behaviors associated with their control battles. The experiential task facilitated productive behaviors such as communication and perspective taking, which led to success.

PASSWORD

Ages: 8–18 years.

Purpose: Social skills training.

Materials Needed:

- Password board game.
- Index cards.
- Pen or pencil.

Password is a board game that decreases egocentricity and self-absorption. Password requires that one member of the team provides a one-word clue so the teammate can guess the secret word. Vocabulary words can be selected to match the children's expressive and receptive vocabulary levels. In order to be successful, players have to be skillful in appreciating another person's perspectives. Players who give non sequitors or clues based on idiosyncratic logic will not do well. For this reason, we often use this activity with children who have high-functioning autism spectrum diagnoses.

Each round can be processed and these youngsters can be given concrete positive and constructive feedback on their performance. The feedback can be recorded on index cards (e.g., "Try to see things like Mom does"). Constructive feedback can be given by the partner ("I didn't understand when you said 'Banana ranger.' Maybe you could use a word we both know.") The partner can also model productive perspective taking ("I tried to give you clues you would know. Like I thought about your interests in *Battlestar Galactica* and used the word *Cylon* to see if you would say 'robot.' ").

PLEASANT ACTIVITY SCHEDULING

Pleasant activity scheduling (PAS) involves setting up positive activities during the week, with the purpose of increasing reinforcement in the child's life, while also assisting the child in attending to the pleasant activities (A. T. Beck et al., 1979; Greenberger & Padesky, 1995). Youth are typically asked to rate their mood prior to and following the activity to highlight improvements. PAS can decrease depression and increase motivation and activity in the otherwise uninvolved child. It provides external structure and rewards for engaging in tasks, which is helpful when internal motivation is lacking.

Depressed youth often have difficulty generating ideas for PAS independently; angry or anxious youth may resist doing so as well. By developing lists of options, youth are more likely to choose from the list than come up with something on the spot. Below are some creative ways for developing lists of activities and engaging the youth in scheduling and completing activities.

MY PLAYLIST OF PLEASANT EVENTS

Ages: 10 years and older.

Purpose: Increasing positive mood, providing reinforcement.

Materials Needed:

• Activity Scheduling iPod Playlist (Form 4.2).

Or

• Paper and pencil.

Listening to music is a popular pastime for adolescents, and creating lists of activities in an iPod "playlist" format can be engaging and fun. Creative youngsters may even wish to make up song titles to reflect the activities they will complete. This playlist metaphor helps the therapist connect with adolescents, and allows teens to apply interventions with familiar language. For anxious children and adolescents, familiarity may increase comfort with the intervention tasks, and consequently increase compliance. In addition, arranging the events in playlists helps with organization and comprehension of the task. Figure 4.2 gives examples of playlists, and Form 4.2 can be used as a worksheet on which the youth can develop his or her own playlist. The following transcript provides an example for activity scheduling using Form 4.2.

THERAPIST: Do you listen to much music?

NICHOLAS: I love music. I take my iPod everywhere—in the car, on the bus, even in the waiting room here. (*Smiles.*)

FIGURE 4.2. Example of Completed Activity Scheduling iPod Playlist.

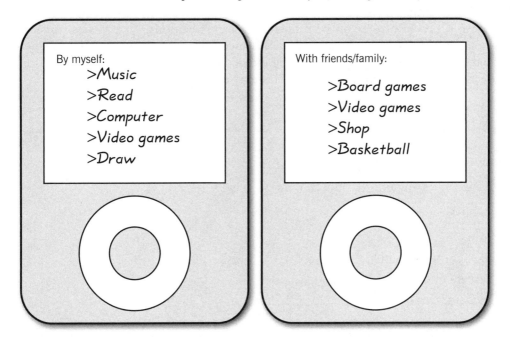

THERAPIST: What are your favorite songs on your iPod? (*Spends a few moments with Nicholas discussing his favorite music.*)

THERAPIST: What if we made a playlist of activities instead of songs?

NICHOLAS: What do you mean?

THERAPIST: Well, it seems that listening to your music makes you feel good. But there might be other things that could help with your depression that we could list. Then you could try those things to see if they change your mood at all.

NICHOLAS: (*Jokes and smiles.*) I get it, another one of your "experiments."

THERAPIST: You're really getting the hang of this! Remember when we talked about the connection between feelings, actions, thoughts, and body? (*Nicholas nods.*) Well, we are going to focus on actions and how those actions might effect your feelings.

NICHOLAS: So this will help me not feel so depressed?

THERAPIST: That is the goal. We will have to pay attention to your feeling ratings to see which things help change your feelings the most. So, let's make a playlist of things you can try when you are by yourself.

NICHOLAS: Well, I like listening to music as long as it is nothing too depressing. Reading my sci-fi books sometimes makes me forget about whatever I am down about. Oh, comedy shows can usually make me laugh.

THERAPIST: Great, let's put those on the first playlist. Now we need to decide when you will choose something from the list.

In this transcript, the therapist demonstrates a genuine interest in Nicholas's music. By paying attention to what is important to Nicholas, the therapist is able to talk with him on his level and come up with meaningful interventions. Nicholas can then refer to the playlist for ideas for behavioral activation, and items can be added or deleted as needed. For example, if the feeling rating indicates that a particular item is consistently ineffective in changing his mood, Nicholas may decide to delete it from the list.

ACTIVITY SCHEDULING GRAB-BAG

Ages: 6 years and older.

Purpose: Increasing positive mood, reinforcement.

Materials Needed:

- Brown lunch bag.
- Index cards or small pieces of paper.
- Markers or crayons for writing/drawing.
- Magazines, scissors, and glue for pictures.

For younger children, a grab-bag with pictures of activities is often fun and helpful. The activity scheduling grab-bag involves children generating a list of events/activities that they predict may be enjoyable. Each item is then written or drawn on a card. Alternatively, the child cuts pictures out of magazines and glues the pictures on individual cards. The cards are placed in a small bag, such as a brown lunch bag, which is decorated by the child. The child is instructed to pick an item or card out of the bag, and then rate the results in the traditional pleasant activities schedule format. There can be a place on the back of each card to record the date and rating of the event. Then the cards can be reviewed to determine the usefulness of each activity in improving the child's mood. Figure 4.3 provides examples of cards that could be created and put in a grab-bag.

GUESSING GAME

Ages: 6 years and older.

Purpose: Scheduling and rating pleasant activities.

Materials Needed:

- Guessing Game Worksheet (Form 4.3).

Visual and concrete methods for tracking and rating pleasant activities are often needed, and are a natural follow-up to activity scheduling (J. S. Beck, 1995; Persons, 1989). As discussed in Friedberg and McClure (2002), children make inaccurate predictions of various kinds. Depressed youth often underestimate the amount of fun they will have, while anxious youth overestimate anticipated distress. However, once the event is

FIGURE 4.3. Grab-bag items for scheduling pleasant activities.

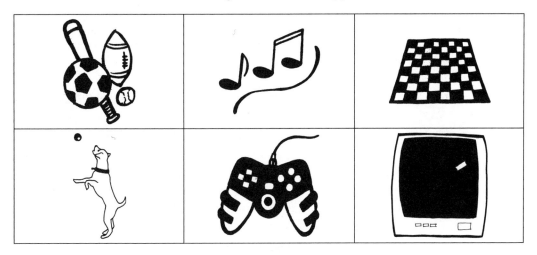

Back of grab-bag cards:

Date: _____	Rating: _____
Date: _____	Rating: _____
Date: _____	Rating: _____
Date: _____	Rating: _____
Date: _____	Rating: _____

over, youth rarely reflect on their own predictions, and thus do not independently assess the accuracy of their predictions. As a result, these patients do not learn from their inaccurate predictions, and they continue to make the same errors over and over again. By assisting children to examine their predictions and outcomes more closely, as well as to look for patterns in the accuracy of their predictions, you set the stage for future cognitive techniques. Youth are primed to start assessing evidence for their thoughts. Setting up predictions visually allows patients to track their predictions easily as well as provides a written record for future references.

The Guessing Game provides a format for scheduling and rating pleasant activities in a fun and engaging manner. For children who are sometimes reluctant to make the schedule, "scheduling pleasant activities" can be the first item on the Guessing Game Worksheet. In the far left column, children draw or write the event or activity (e.g., birthday party, swim lessons, playing a board game). Children then mark the level of fun they guess they will have during the event in the middle column. After the event is completed, children mark the level of fun they actually experienced. This worksheet then provides a visual record of predicted and actual feelings to assist with modifying future guesses and increasing willingness to engage in activities.

The Guessing Game can also be helpful when completing systematic desensitization. Rather than ranking pleasant activities, children could rate anxiety regarding various items on the fear hierarchy. After each exposure, they record the anxiety level.

When the rating has decreased, the child is done with the item and can move to the next item on the hierarchy.

Below is an example of 10-year-old Tina, who is pessimistic about upcoming events. The therapist introduces the Guessing Game to help test out her predictions about the scheduled events.

TINA: I don't want to do anything. I know it will be boring and I just don't feel like it.

THERAPIST: It seems like you don't even feel like doing things that used to be fun for you.

TINA: I used to love going to my dance class, but I just don't feel like it now. And my cousin and I used to play "American Idol" all the time, but now I don't even want to go to her birthday party this weekend. I just know I won't have any fun.

THERAPIST: Sounds like you have already made some guesses about how things will go.

TINA: Yeah. Not good!

THERAPIST: Would you like to play a little game? You make a guess about how something will go, then you try it out and we see if your guess was right.

TINA: Well, I guess that is OK. My mom said I am going to my cousin's party no matter what, so I don't really have a choice!

THERAPIST: So, what is your guess? From 1–10, how much fun do you think you will have at the party?

TINA: Maybe a 2. (*Fills in the worksheet [Figure 4.4].*)

FIGURE 4.4. Tina's Guessing Game Worksheet.

THE GUESSING GAME

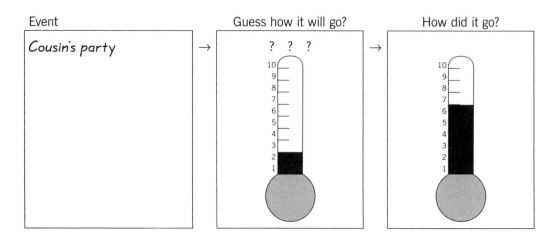

THERAPIST: OK. After the party, do you think you can fill in the number for how much fun it actually is?

TINA: Sure, that sounds easy enough.

The Guessing Game will help Tina test her prediction, while creating a visual record of the predictions and outcomes. This data can be used to detect and point out patterns in underestimating positive or overestimating negative outcomes.

HABIT REVERSAL

Repetitive behaviors, such as tics or nervous habits, lead to social and physical problems (Miltenberger, Fuqua, & Woods, 1998). A child struggling with these issues may become emotionally distressed and unsure of how to cope. Patients become increasingly self-conscious about the appearance of the behaviors, and the behaviors themselves may be distracting during school or interfere with social or extracurricular activities. For these reasons, behavioral interventions are often used to reduce the frequency of tics in individuals with tic disorders, compulsions, or other repetitive behaviors (e.g., trichotillomania, stuttering, nail biting and other nervous habits, self-stimulatory behaviors that occur with PDD). Habit reversal has been shown to be an effective treatment for tics, stuttering, and nervous habits (Woods & Miltenberger, 1995).

Habit reversal involves having the individual practice actions that are the "reverse" or opposite of the habit that is being treated (Azrin & Nunn, 1973). Thus, someone who is repeatedly biting her nails may be taught to hold onto an object rather than biting the nails. In addition to imposing a "reverse" behavior, Azrin and Nunn recommended several other steps in the habit reversal treatment. Specifically, patients were taught to record the frequency of the habits. Increasing patient awareness of the habit is an important step in this treatment, and may involve having patients watch themselves in a mirror and give detailed descriptions of the habit. Azrin and Nunn also recommended teaching patients to identify and detect early signs of the habit.

Once the youth is aware the behavior is occurring, he or she is instructed to engage in some competing response. This is a behavior that cannot be completed at the same time as the habit, and is done in place of the habit. By practicing the competing behavior in therapy and/or in front of a mirror, the child may become more used to using it. For example, if children demonstrate repeated throat clearing, deep breathing exercises and sipping water from a water bottle may be used. If the behavior is found to increase with certain stressors, the relaxation strategies reviewed earlier in this chapter can be helpful for stress management. Finally, positive reinforcement can be provided for the patients' efforts and successes (Azrin & Nunn, 1973). Visual and verbal cues for using the technique can be provided, and differential reinforcement of the alternative behavior can be given, both verbally and through a contingency management program if needed (see the Contingency Management section later in this chapter). Continuing to measure the frequency or duration of the habit is helpful for self-monitoring and tracking progress. A visual graph or chart can illustrate changes in the frequency of the habit, and further motivate the child to continue with the approach.

Stemberger, McCombs-Thomas, MacGlashan, and Mansueto (2000) recommended some simple behavioral interventions to compete with tic and habit behaviors. Many of these strategies can also be used with perseverative and self-stimulating behaviors experienced by patients with autism spectrum disorders. For hair pulling or putting fingers in one's mouth, finger bandages or rubber gloves may be used. Clenching fists or squeezing a Koosh ball or other toy may be useful to occupy hands and fingers. Wetting and brushing hair or fiddling with dental floss, nylon fishing lines, fuzz on a tennis ball, or anything that feels like hair are competing responses. Drinking water or deep breathing may effectively compete with vocal grunts and tics (Miltenberger, Fuqua, & Woods, 1998; Woods & Miltenberger, 1995). Woods and Luiselli (2007) suggested slow soothing verbal statements as a competing response to vocal tics. Additionally, they used rhythmic controlled blinking on a 2-second schedule to treat eye muscle tics. Neck stretching exercises can also compete with head jerking.

Mansueto, Golomb, Thomas, and Stemberger (1999) offered many specific behavioral strategies for treating trichotillomania. They recommended using scents on wrists and fingers as well as wearing an elastic elbow brace to increase motoric and sensory feedback. Wearing glasses and/or sunglasses, pulling hair back, dying hair, and keeping fingernails closely trimmed can facilitate response prevention. Mansueto et al. also suggested competing response training with fist clenching; squeezing Play Doh, worry beads, or Silly Putty; knitting; bead work; and needlepoint. If reinforcement is gained from sensory stimulation, brushing the area or rubbing it with a textured sponge may be useful. Additionally, if the patient bites or eats the hair, Mansueto et al. employed "crunchy foods" such as celery, carrots, or candy with fleshy textures.

BACK UP!

Ages: 6–10 years.

Purpose: Habit reversal.

Materials Needed:

- Back-Up! map.
- Markers, crayons, pencil, or pen.
- Small toy car or paper on which to draw and cut out car.

The Back Up! technique uses the metaphor of a car driving down a road to help the child understand the purpose of habit reversal. Using a map like the one in Figure 4.5, the therapist explains to the child that if someone was driving along and missed the road he or she was supposed to take, the driver might "back up" by reversing the car until he or she could continue down the correct route. The main road represents the path to more desirable behaviors, and decreased tics or habits. The "wrong turns" represent use of the habit. The therapy technique helps the child back up and get on the "right track." The child can draw a car or truck to cut out and push along the road. A small toy car also works well and is fun for the youth. Along the road are signs, and the child is instructed to write in coping strategies such as relaxation techniques, competing responses, and self-instructional statements that may help him or her with the habit

FIGURE 4.5. Example of a back-up map.

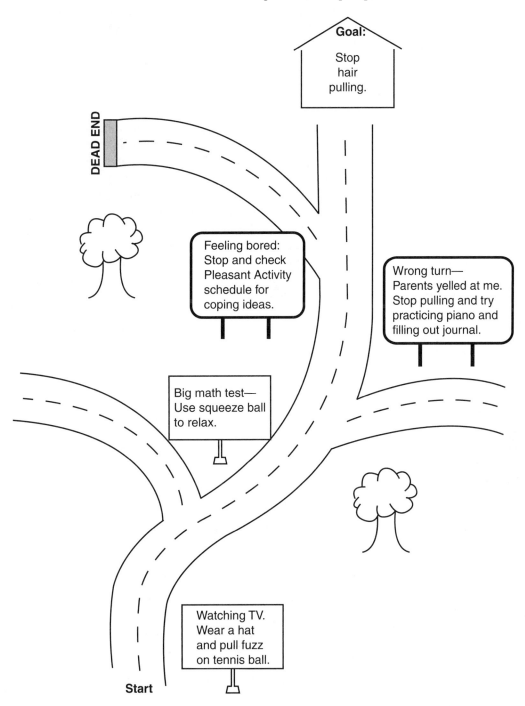

reversal. The "destination" is the elimination or reduction of the habit, with the specific goal filled in by the child. The car is stopped at various intersections along the way, representing stressors and triggers for the habit. The child then practices the intervention skills and continues on the desired path.

BEHAVIORAL DISTRESS TOLERANCE SKILLS

Distress tolerance skills help children and adolescents accept and manage emotional discomfort. Emotional intolerance contributes to impulsivity, vulnerability, and poor self-regulation (Corstorphine, Mountford, Tomlinson, Waller, & Meyer, 2007). Linehan (1993a, 1993b) pioneered teaching patients ways to change their emotional, behavioral, and sensory sets through various techniques. Linehan (1993a) defines *distress tolerance* as the capacity to accept and endure negative affect so productive problem solving can occur. While distress tolerance skills are useful for many patients, they may be especially useful for children with PDD who have distressing sensory sensitivities. Additionally, eating disorders are characterized by low distress tolerance (Corstorphine et al., 2007).

The basic idea is to develop sensory experiences that compete with the patients' distress. Items might be placed in a kit like the calming techniques described earlier in the chapter. Sze and Wood (2007) also suggested the use of coping skills housed in a "museum box" for a young child with Asperger syndrome. The boxes and kits could be decorated with drawings, stickers, beads, and play jewels. Figure 4.6 lists a number of skills drawn from Linehan's work as well as from our own clinical experiences.

CONTINGENCY CONTRACTING

Contingency management is essentially setting up a contract for rewards and consequences to be applied in response to specific behaviors. Contingency management is beneficial for increasing and shaping desirable behaviors (Kazdin, 2001). The contract provides incentives (reinforcements) to increase motivation and structure to aid follow-through with goals, both for the child and the caregiver. A first step in contingency management is to establish a specific and realistic behavioral goal (Barkley, 1997; Sha-

FIGURE 4.6. Examples of distress tolerance skills.

- Painting fingernails/ toenails.
- Listening to favorite music.
- Putting on hand lotion.
- Blowing bubbles.
- Using a hand fan.
- Putting on favorite cologne, perfume, and/or body splash.
- Sucking on a lemon or orange.
- Chewing flavorful gum (e.g., sour cherry, hot cinnamon).
- Taking a bubble bath.
- Petting cat/dog.
- Holding ice.
- Brushing or braiding hair.
- Rubbing silk, fur, ribbon, or favorite fabric.
- Putting cold compress on forehead.
- Smelling a scented candle.
- Smelling spices (garlic, cinnamon).
- Sucking an atomic fire ball candy or very sour hard candy.
- Working puzzles.
- Massaging scalp.
- Squeezing a toy or Koosh ball.

piro, Friedberg, & Bardenstein, 2005). Once the goal is established, it is broken down into steps or time periods. For example, if the behavioral goal is to increase independent completion of the get-ready-for-school morning routine, the contract would outline each step of the child's morning routine and provide reinforcement for completion of each step. If the behavioral goal is to reduce aggression, then the day may be broken down into time periods and the child is rewarded for exhibiting nonaggressive behaviors during each of the time periods.

In addition to identification of specific target behaviors, the consequences of completing or not completing the target behavior must be clearly defined (Spiegler & Guevremont, 1998). This includes not only what the behavior is, but also when or how often the behavior will occur and who will be responsible for various aspects of the target behavior (Spiegler & Guevremont, 1998). For example, a goal of improving compliance with brushing teeth may state, "If Joey brushes his teeth within 10 minutes of finishing breakfast Monday through Friday, his mother will drive him to BlockBuster where he can pick a game to rent for the weekend." This example clearly outlines the target behavior (brushing teeth), when it will occur (within 10 minutes of completing breakfast), the responsibilities of various participants (mother will take him to the store, Joey will choose the game), and the consequence/reward (renting a game for the weekend).

Spiegler and Guevremont (1998) point out the various benefits of using contingency contracts. Specifically, the contracts decrease conflict by clearly defining expectations. Having families take an active role in developing the contracts and signing the contracts can increase their commitment to the plan. Moreover, they benefit the parent–child relationship by encouraging positive interactions and cooperation. Further, contracts help parents follow through with consistent consequences for desirable behaviors and undesirable behaviors, and also decrease multiple warnings (the contract should specify "completes task the first time child is told").

PUZZLE PIECES

Ages: 4–10 years.

Purpose: Making contingency contracts meaningful.

Materials Needed:

- Cardboard or stiff paper.
- Velcro.
- Scissors or box cutter.
- Markers.
- Puzzle pieces.

Puzzle Pieces offers visual and tactile interventions to help contingency contracting become meaningful for even young children. By using this approach, the child may better understand the goal as well as the rewards that may not be immediately available. The biggest challenge to a successful contingency management plan for young children is often making the plan concrete and immediate enough for the child to understand the system and be motivated by it.

Puzzle Pieces is a visual way to reinforce the child immediately, while still working toward longer-term rewards. Using the Puzzle Pieces approach, a reward or generic symbol for a reward is created and cut into puzzle pieces. Velcro can be placed on the back of the pieces and on a piece of cardboard used to assemble the puzzle. The child earns a piece of the puzzle for previously determined behaviors, and then earns the designated reward when the puzzle is complete. The target behaviors are placed on the back of the pieces, and when the puzzle is complete the child reviews the pieces to know what behaviors were reinforced. For example, "unloaded dishwasher," "fed dog," "took bath the first time I was told," and "cleared the table" may be written on the backs of the pieces. When each item is completed, the child adds that puzzle piece to the puzzle. For youngsters who enjoy working for a surprise, the parents could create the puzzle themselves. Then, as the child earns the pieces, he or she can try to guess what is being earned.

Consider 6-year-old Jeni, who bridled against her bedtime routine. Her mother reported telling Jeni multiple times to complete each task (e.g., to change clothes, wash her face, brush teeth), and Jeni would still refuse or ignore her mother. A contingency contract was set up with the goal of increasing Jeni's compliance with the nighttime routine. The specific steps for compliance were outlined. Jeni loved animals, so trips to visit a pet store were very motivating to her. A puzzle of a bear was made (Figure 4.7), with each piece representing a step in the nighttime routine. To earn the puzzle piece,

FIGURE 4.7. Puzzle Pieces: "build-a-bear" example of contingency management.

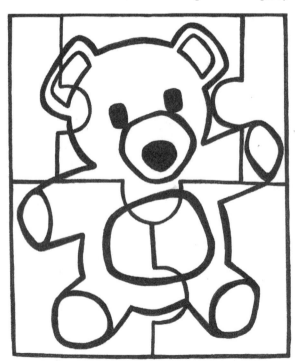

Jeni was required to complete the step with no more than one prompt. Once the puzzle was completed, Jeni's mother took her to the pet store for a visit. After 2 weeks, Jeni was showing more consistent compliance with the nighttime routine. Thus, the system was modified and Jeni began earning one piece for each night that she complied with the nighttime routine. The puzzle had five pieces so if she was compliant all week, she earned a weekend visit.

Reinforcement

Providing positive reinforcement for a behavior is one of the most powerful behavioral interventions. It is a common "first step" in parent training (Barkley et al., 1999; Becker, 1971; Forehand & McMahon, 1981). Positive reinforcement involves providing a positive consequence to a behavior in order to increase the frequency of that behavior. The reinforcer may be something tangible, such as stickers or tokens used during contingency management programs. Reinforcers can also be privileges, such as allowing the child to stay up 15 minutes later following the completion of evening chores in a timely and pleasant manner. Verbal praise from caregivers is also a powerful reinforcer. When praise specifies the desirable behavior, it also teaches appropriate behaviors (e.g., "I like how you are squeezing your calming-down ball and taking deep breaths to help control your feelings.").

Targeted behaviors can also be modified by the use of negative reinforcement. Negative reinforcement works by removing something undesirable or aversive every time a targeted behavior occurs, with the purpose of increasing the frequency of that behavior. For example, a child may be reinforced for sitting at the table nicely during dinner by being excused from cleaning up the dishes. The negative reinforcer is the removal of the dreaded kitchen clean-up chore. The most important point to remember about positive and negative reinforcement is that both types increase the desired behavior.

The terms positive and negative reinforcement can be confusing to caregivers. Plus and minus symbols, (+ and −), can be helpful cues for signifying whether the reinforcement consists of adding something desirable (+, positive reinforcement) or taking away something negative (−, negative reinforcement). Reinforcement can be addressed with parents in a manner such as the one outlined in the following transcript with Ms. Jones.

THERAPIST: So, we have agreed on the goal of increasing Steven's compliance with directions the first time they are given. We are going to use reinforcement to increase the times that Steven complies with your directions the first time.

MS. JONES: (*Smiles.*) Yeah, that sounds great! I just hope it works.

THERAPIST: Well, one thing that is clear to me from watching you and Steven together is that you love each other very much. I can see how much you care about him, and how much he pays attention to how you are responding to him. We want to use that love to improve his behavior.

MS. JONES: But how?

THERAPIST: Well, for one thing, there are things that are very important to Steven, and we will "give" him those things when he follows directions the first time [positive reinforcement]. So, we know your attention is very important to Steven. You will give smiles, high fives, and the praise we talked about before when he follows directions the first time.

MS. JONES: You mean like saying, "I like when you follow directions the first time"?

THERAPIST: Exactly! You are really catching on! Good work.

MS. JONES: Thanks. But I think he likes the computer more than my smiles!

THERAPIST: We will also "give" him access to the computer. So he will have chances to earn computer time and praise from you. We can also take things away that he does not like, and that will be a reward and therefore help him follow directions more often.

MS. JONES: Well, he definitely does not like emptying the garbage.

THERAPIST: Great example. If he meets a certain goal of following directions the first time, he could "earn" not having to take out the garbage. Basically, you will take away something he does not like to reward him for following directions the first time.

MS. JONES: Oh, I get it.

THERAPIST: OK, now let's talk about the specifics of the plan.

In this example, the therapist teaches Ms. Jones about reinforcement through direct instruction, specific examples, and modeling. The therapist includes Ms. Jones in the discussion to increase her attention to the information, to check for understanding, and to obtain meaningful examples from the family's daily life.

Preventing Stimulus Satiation

When talking to parents about implementing a contingency management plan, families often report, "Those things work at first, but always seem to stop working after a few weeks." One of the most common reasons for this occurrence of initial success followed by a regression is stimulus satiation. Stimulus satiation occurs when the reinforcer loses its value for the child, often due to overexposure or too much access to the reinforcer (Barkley, 1997). Children who are rewarded with candy multiple times a day may no longer be motivated to change their behavior for a piece of candy. Likewise, an adolescent who has unlimited access to the television and computer after school (while parents are still at work) may not be as motivated to complete chores in order to earn computer time in the evening. When reinforcers are used more sparingly, or access to reinforcers is limited, the reinforcers are more likely to maintain their value longer. It is often helpful for families to reevaluate and modify the list of reinforcers being used on a regular basis.

Consider 5-year-old Ryan whose parents initially found the use of special treats (e.g., candy, snacks, gum) to be a useful reinforcer in their home behavior plan over the summer. However, after several weeks Ryan's compliance declined despite good follow-through with rewards by the parents. Upon further investigation, Ryan's parents discovered that Ryan was being provided highly desirable snacks after kindergarten by his babysitter. Since that gave him daily access to these previously rare treats, Ryan was not motivated to complete tasks at home to earn the treats. Once Ryan's parents clearly communicated with the sitter about what were acceptable afterschool snacks, and which items could only be given as part of the behavior plan, the rewards regained their value and again became motivating for Ryan, and thus Ryan's behavior improved.

Time-Out

"We've tried time-out and it didn't work" is a common reaction of parents when discussing this behavioral technique. Time-out is a widely used technique that is quite effective when used appropriately, and quite frustrating when it is not! First, parents should agree on the targeted behavior or behaviors that will be disciplined with the use of time-out. Time-out should be used to target one or two specific behaviors, such as aggression, cursing, or noncompliance. If a compliance issue is being targeted, the child is given a command. If the child does not comply, a warning may be used: "You need to _____ [direction from parent] or you will go to time-out." If the child still does not comply, an immediate time-out should be issued. For other behaviors, such as aggression, the child is told ahead of time that the behavior will always result in a time-out. So, when the child is aggressive, no warning is needed and the child is immediately sent to time-out. Parents need to stay calm and in control, using a neutral voice during these interactions. Frustration and yelling on the part of the parent inadvertently reinforces the child's negative behavior, as well as triggers additional negative behaviors and leads to additional family conflict.

When time-out is issued, some children try to comply with the initial demand or to apologize for the inappropriate behavior. The apology or behavior can be praised, but time-out is still completed. The parent may need to escort the child to time-out. For children who cannot be safely escorted to time-out, an additional punishment that would be considered more aversive than time-out can be used. Thus, if the child does not go to time-out when told to do so, that child receives another punishment that is considered less desirable than time-out. The goal is that the child will choose to comply with time-out to avoid the alternative (e.g., "You either need to go to time-out now or you will not be able to go skating this afternoon."). As with all behavioral interventions, follow-through is key. Parents must only state punishments they are willing and able to enforce or else they will be ineffective.

Much has been written about the details of setting up effective time-out interventions (Barkley, 1997). Choosing an unstimulating and safe location, having the child sit for a short period of time (typically, approximately 1 minute per year of age), and avoiding any attention or reinforcement of the child while he or she is in time-out are guidelines. Parents often lecture or attend too much to the child in time-out, which can lead to further acting-out behaviors and decreased effectiveness of this strategy.

In the following example, the therapist has just suggested the use of time-out to Mr. Skeptic.

MR. SKEPTIC: That time-out stuff is crap! It doesn't work.

THERAPIST: You have tried it before?

MR. SKEPTIC: Yeah! But it always just ends up in a disaster.

THERAPIST: How frustrating! Tell me about what happens.

MR. SKEPTIC: Well, first he never goes when I tell him to, so we end up arguing about it. Then, once he's there he just plays in his room and can't even remember why he got in trouble to begin with.

THERAPIST: I see. What if I could show you a different way to use time-out that would solve those problems you just described? Would you be willing to try this different approach?

In this example, the father is immediately turned off by the idea of using time-out. Rather than arguing with him or trying to convince him that time-out will be helpful, the therapist first acknowledges the father's experience and feelings. The therapist then elicits additional information so that the time-out intervention can be presented in an effective and meaningful way. In doing so, common problems are identified and can later be addressed by the therapist. In taking this approach, the therapist is working collaboratively with the father to establish a plan, rather than simply trying to convince him to use time-out.

Response Cost

Whenever discussing contingency management, the issue of response cost is often raised. Response cost involves the removal of a previously earned reward ("cost") in response to an undesirable behavior. For example, a child who has earned 17 tokens for completing her morning chores and getting ready for school on time may later be punished for hitting her sister by losing 10 tokens, leaving her a balance of seven tokens. When beginning a contingency management program, we recommend that rewards not be removed until the behavior program is up and running (Barkley, 1997). After a week or two, caregivers can begin implementing a response cost procedure. Just as behaviors to be rewarded are outlined ahead of time, the behaviors that will be punished should also be clearly designated. When such behaviors occur, a token, chip, or point—whatever currency is being used—is removed. Noncompliance, lack of follow-through, or engaging in certain unacceptable behaviors such as lying, aggression, or cursing may be punished with response cost. If the Puzzle Pieces technique is being used, a piece of the puzzle is taken away.

It is important for caregivers to use the response cost procedure sparingly and for designated behaviors to avoid compromising the effectiveness of the reward system. A child who loses many rewards/points may lose motivation to continue with the program. In addition, if parents do not have clear rules about when and how to remove rewards/points, they may impulsively take away an excessive amount to relieve their own frustration. Barkley (1997) refers to this as the "punishment spiral" which occurs when a child is fined, then reacts negatively to the punishment by exhibiting inappropriate behaviors. Those behaviors are then fined as well, invoking additional misbehavior, thus leading to additional fines and so on. Thus, Barkley recommends fining the child once through the point system. If a negative reaction follows, another form of punishment, such as time-out (see section on time-out earlier in this chapter) should be used.

The following example illustrates what can happen when response cost is not used effectively.

MOTHER: This token system is not working. Toni had a fit yesterday, and I tried taking away chips and it just did not work. Things went down hill, and she doesn't even care about the chips any more.

THERAPIST: Wow, you sound really frustrated. Tell me what happened.

MOTHER: Well, she started yelling at me when I told her to get ready for bed, so I told her she just lost 5 chips.

THERAPIST: That was clearly outlined in your plan with Toni last week. Good job sticking with the contract.

MOTHER: Yah, but it didn't work. She kept yelling, so I took away another 5 chips. Then she got really mad and called me a bitch so I told her she lost 20 chips. She stomped off to the basement and watched TV the rest of the night.

THERAPIST: I see. Let's go back to the plan and see what might have helped this situation go better. What does your behavior plan say about dealing with non-compliance and response cost?

In this example the therapist prompts the mother to share details of the conflict. The therapist acknowledges her frustration, and the problems with the mother's implementation of response cost are revealed (she continued to take away chips and did not stick to the behavior plan to move on to another punishment if needed). The therapist then begins helping the mother solve the problem using a guided discovery approach. This strategy is likely to be more meaningful for the mother in the long run, as she may be more invested in using the plan in the future once she understands for herself what went wrong.

PROMPTS FOR PARENTS/TIPS FOR TEACHERS

One of the challenges for therapists working with children is the generalization of therapy techniques and skills outside of the session. Children often respond well to techniques during sessions, but parents will report the child is not using the techniques at home or at school. Educating caregivers on the purpose and use of certain techniques, as well as ways to prompt and reinforce the child in the home and school environments, will increase the success of generalization. Communication with caregivers is often difficult to arrange, and is time-consuming. By providing caregivers with clear and concise summary sheets that describe the current focus of treatment and the caregiver's role, we are working with these caregivers in a collaborative and realistic manner. Form 4.4 is a user-friendly handout with descriptions of interventions to educate caregivers. Such handouts can be given to parents and sent to the teachers or other caregivers to guide them in working with the child on generalization and use of therapy skills.

CONCLUSION

Behavioral strategies are powerful tools for therapists, parents, and teachers. The benefits of using behavioral techniques outweigh the challenge of implementing them. Spe-

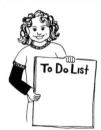

BOX 4.1 Summary Pad for Behavioral Techniques

When to use:

- Often helpful at the start of treatment.
- To produce quicker changes and facilitate follow-through with treatment.
- To assist parents in modifying behaviors outside of the therapy sessions.

For what purpose:

- Builds rapport, increases the child's motivation and engagement in treatment, expands coping repertoires, and primes youngsters for subsequent interventions.
- To decrease the frequency and severity of undesirable behaviors, as well as to increase the frequency of desirable behaviors.
- To make changes in the child's attitude, emotions, and cognitions.

How to use it:

- Through direct instruction in skills and parent training.
- In-session practice of skill application.
- Be creative and collaborative.

cifically, as positive changes in the targeted behaviors occur, parent and teacher satisfaction improves, and often parent–child interactions and relationships improve. It is important for parents and therapists to clearly outline the goals of the behavioral strategies and make sure the goals are communicated to all participants. To make the behavior plan as effective as possible, remember to include the family's input, to employ the child's interests, and to solicit feedback. The therapist's job can often be challenging; you must clearly communicate behavioral principles, keep the strategies "alive" for the child by helping families define goals clearly, establish powerful reinforcers, and follow through consistently with the interventions. The strategies in this chapter offer creative and engaging ways to get started. They are summarized in Table 4.3.

TABLE 4.3. Summary of Behavioral Interventions

Type of behavioral intervention	Specific technique	Ages	Appropriate problems/diagnoses	Format
Relaxation	PMR	4 years	Anger Anxiety Impulsivity	Individual Family Group
	Scripts for relaxation	All ages	Anger Anxiety Impulsivity Sensory integration dysfunction PDD	Individual Family Group
	Feeling Compass	6–9 years	Anger Anxiety Impulsivity Sensory integration dysfunction PDD	Individual Family Group
	Calming Cue Cards	All ages	Anger Anxiety Impulsivity Sensory integration dysfunction PDD	Individual Family Group
Systematic desensitization	Up, Up, and Away	6–9 years	Generalized anxiety OCD Specific phobia Social anxiety	Individual Family Group

(cont.)

TABLE 4.3. (*cont.*)

Type of behavioral intervention	Specific technique	Ages	Appropriate problems/diagnoses	Format
Social skills	Making a Book	4–10 years	PDD Anxiety Impulsivity/ADHD Depression	Individual Family Group
	Instant Message Role Plays	10 years and older	PDD Anxiety Impulsivity/ADHD Depression	Individual Family Group
	Etch A Sketch	4 years and older	Anxiety Anger/frustration tolerance	Individual Family Group
	Password	6 years and older	PDD (high functioning)	Individual Family Group
PAS	My Playlist of Pleasant Events	10 years and older	Depression Anxiety PDD	Individual Family Group
	Grab-bag items for scheduling pleasant events	6 years and older	Depression Anxiety PDD	Individual Family Group
	Guessing Game	6 years and older	Depression Anxiety PDD	Individual Family Group
Habit reversal	Back Up!	6–10 years	Impulse control Anxiety/OCD Tic disorders PDD	Individual Family Group
Contingency management	Puzzle Pieces/Build a Bear	4–10 years	ADHD/Disruptive behaviors ODD Developmental delays Anxiety/depression	Individual Family Group

Instant Messaging Social Skills Worksheet

You are walking down the hall at school and a new student smiles at you.

```
IM response:
```

A student sitting next to you in math class asks if you are going to the football game on Friday.

```
IM response:
```

A boy you have a crush on asks if you are doing the extra credit assignment.

```
IM response:
```

Your teacher announces everyone must find a partner to complete an in-class assignment. You look to the left and the student next to you is looking at you.

```
IM response:
```

There is a dance after the basketball game, and you want to find out if some of your peers are planning to stay for the dance.

```
IM response:
```

Activity Scheduling iPod Playlist

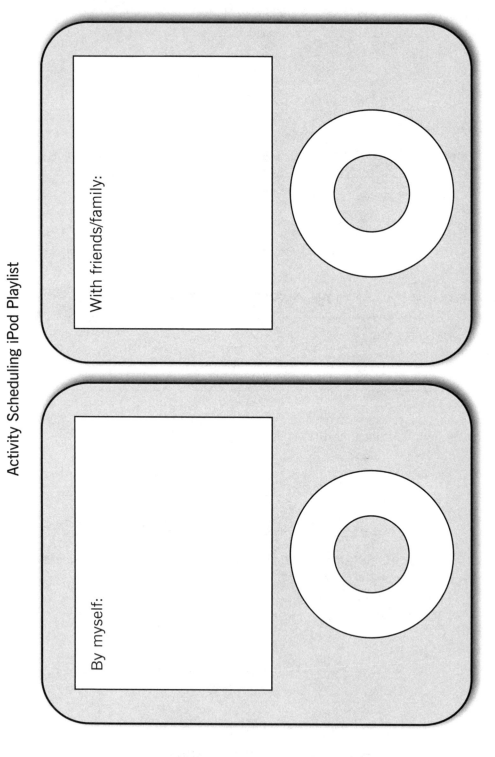

With friends/family:

By myself:

Guessing Game Worksheet

THE GUESSING GAME

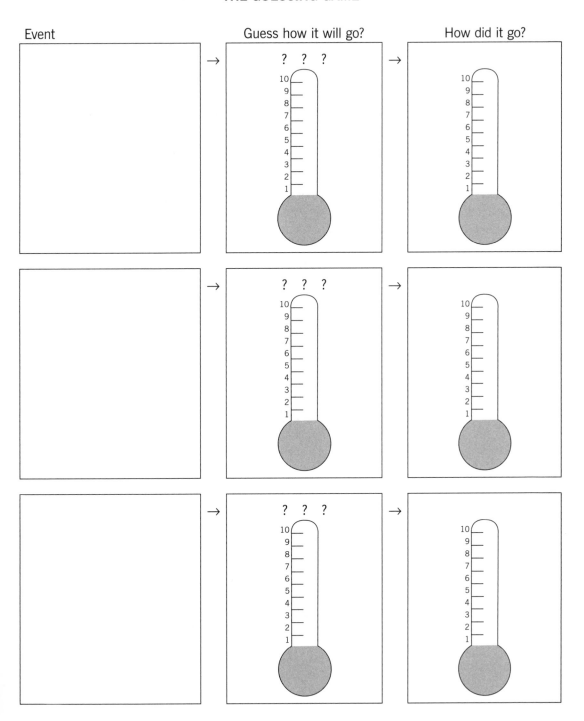

FORM 4.4

Prompts for Parents/Tips for Teachers

Your child/student is building many skills in therapy. Support and encouragement at home and in school are important aspects of success. Currently, we are working on behavior strategies in the checked areas below. Please read these sections for ideas on how to prompt the child's use of skills, as well as to reinforce progress. For all of the checked strategies, the following components are important:

IMPORTANT WAYS YOU CAN HELP

Modeling: You are powerful models for your child/student. Verbalizing your own feelings and responses can be helpful.

Prompting: When you notice your child/student starting to get upset you can prompt his or her use of techniques. Giving choices is also a helpful option. Often children respond better to these optional prompts than to direct instruction.

Reinforcing the Child: Changing habits is hard, especially for kids. If the child makes attempts to use therapy techniques, he or she should be praised for the effort, even if it is not completely successful at first.

Predicting and Problem Solving: When a situation approaches that you predict will be difficult, try preparing your child through hypothetical examples and/or role plays.

Relaxation is being used to teach the child to calm his or her physical reactions and to self-regulate more effectively. Relaxation involves strategies for slowing down the heart rate, relaxing muscles, and using self-talk and visual cues to prompt better coping.

Modeling:

- "I'm getting very frustrated, so I am going to take some deep breaths."
- "I'm nervous about the fire drill. Using a squeeze ball might calm down my muscles."

Prompting:

- "You seem upset. I wonder what tools you have learned in therapy that could help."
- "This might be a good time to use your calming-down kit."
- "Do you think bubbles or a squeeze ball would help you calm down more?"

Older children/teens may wish to develop a nonverbal cue or code word with parents that helps parents remind them to use techniques without embarrassing or "nagging" them.

(continued)

Reinforcing the Child:

- "I'm proud of you for trying your kit. Keep practicing and it will get easier."

Predicting and Problem Solving:

- "Let's pretend you are at the birthday party and you get upset because Carla is so busy with her other friends she doesn't seem to be interested in playing with you. What tools can you use to calm yourself down? Show me how you would do that."

Systematic desensitization is being used to help the child face feared situations in graduated steps. Systematic desensitization involves facing predetermined steps of a fear while using relaxation strategies to manage anxiety.

Modeling: You can model self-talk and other relaxation techniques to assist the child in using the techniques while facing the designated fear.

Prompting:

- "Remember, what will happen to your worries if you keep practicing?"

Reinforcing the Child:

- "Wow! You worked hard to stay calm while you practiced facing that fear."

Predicting and Problem Solving:

- "What if it is time to do an exposure and you start to worry you won't be able to do it? What can you do to solve the problem? What could you remember that could help?"

Social skills

Modeling:

- "I am a little nervous to start my new job, but I know if I remember to make good eye contact and smile, I will be able to start a conversation and make a new friend."

Prompting:

- "I see one of your classmates walking toward us. What have you been practicing that might help you start a conversation with him?"

Reinforcing the Child:

- "I really like how you are looking me in the eye when you talk to me."
- "I noticed you said hello and asked Aunt Mary how she was when she walked into the house. That was great."

Predicting and Problem Solving:

- "Your history project is a group project. If you don't know some kids in your group very well, what can you say to them?"
- "There will be a lot of students at the meeting after school today. What have you learned that can help you join in the conversation?"

Pleasant events scheduling

Modeling:

- "I was not looking forward to doing yard work today, but it was more fun than I thought it would be. I really enjoyed talking with you while we worked."

Prompting:

- "Would you like to choose to use the computer or a book during your free time?"
- "How much fun do you think you will have during free time?"

Reinforcing the Child:

- "I like how you tried [the activity] even though you guessed it would not be much fun. It looks like you are enjoying yourself now."

Predicting and Problem Solving:

- "What if you were planning to schedule going to the mall with a friend, but she couldn't go? How would you feel? How could you solve that problem? What if you complete the activity and you don't have much fun? What can you remember?"

Contingency management

Modeling:

- "I worked really hard to get my 'to-do list' done early, so I am going to reward myself by going to the movies this weekend."

Prompting:

- "Remember, if you follow the rules you will earn tokens that you can use for more computer time."

Reinforcing the Child:

- "Awesome job following directions the first time! Here are two chips."

Predicting and Problem Solving:

- "What if you really want to go to a friend's house after school today, but you realize you don't have enough chips to do so?"

CHAPTER 5

Self-Instructional and Cognitive Restructuring Methods

Self-instructional methods represent CBT's first-line intervention for coping with inaccurate and distressing thoughts. These methods involve training in self-talk techniques. Self-talk reflects "cognitive content or what people say to themselves when they are thinking" (Spiegler & Guevremont, 1998, p. 306). Self-talk procedures work to modify what children and adolescents say to themselves when experiencing a disturbing emotion or problematic circumstance. Cognitive restructuring teaches the child that if you change your thoughts, you can also change the way you feel (Deblinger et al., 2006). Thus, cognitive interventions deal with inner speech.

Self-talk and other cognitive restructuring interventions are used to build coping templates (Kendall & Suveg, 2006). The key in any cognitive intervention is not the extinction of negative cognitions and emotional distress, but rather its reduction and a shift toward more adaptive views. Padesky (1988) knowingly remarked that the goal of CBT is to "cast doubt where there was once certainty of belief."

Self-talk interventions enjoy a long tradition (Bailey, 2001; Kendall & Suveg, 2006). Anxiety disorders, depression, anger control problems, eating disorders, and even PDD have been treated with self-talk procedures. Research has shown that self-talk interventions emphasizing personal competence and coping worked well with children who were afraid of the dark (Kanfer, Karoly, & Newman, 1975). Kendall and his colleagues' seminal work on the Coping Cat program based on self-talk interventions is widely researched and its success is well documented (Flannery-Schroeder & Kendall, 2000; Kendall, Aschenbrand, & Hudson, 2003; Kendall et al., 1992, 1997). Moreover, the Coping Cat has spawned spin-offs such as the Coping Koala (Barrett et al., 1996) and the Cool Kids Program (Allen & Rapee, 2005; Rapee, Wignall, Hudson, & Schniering, 2000). The Coping Cat cognitive module employs the FEAR acronym (Feeling Frightened, Expecting Bad Things to Happen, Attitudes and Actions That Help, and Results and Rewards).

CBT for childhood OCD includes a significant cognitive restructuring module as a facilitative or primary strategy preceding the exposure-and-response prevention phase of treatment (March & Franklin, 2006; March & Mulle, 1998; Piacentini & Langley, 2004; Piacentini et al., 2006). These approaches make liberal use of sports metaphors (e.g., basketball, football) and cartooning to promote cognitive restructuring. Additionally, cognitive restructuring also serves to reinterpret the meaning of the obsessions and compulsions (D. A. Clark, 1999). More specifically, attributions of personal responsibility, overvaluing thoughts, thought–action fusion, overestimations of danger, intolerance for uncertainty, fears of loss of control, and perfectionism are targets for cognitive restructuring in OCD (D. A. Clark, 1999).

Flannery-Schroeder (2004) noted that children with generalized anxiety disorder (GAD) are effectively treated with cognitive restructuring techniques. Cognitive restructuring with GAD includes modifying anxiety-producing self-talk and building new strategies to cope with anxiety. The Coping Cat (Kendall et al., 1992, 1997; Mendlowitz et al., 1999) and Coping Koala (Barrett et al., 1996) CBT protocols mentioned above target GAD with cognitive restructuring procedures.

Wachtel and Strauss (1995) suggested self-instructional strategies for separation anxiety disorder. "I can do this on my own" and "My parents will be fine, and I am brave when I am alone" are examples of self-instructions offered by Wachtel and Strauss. Many treatment packages for social anxiety include cognitive restructuring techniques focusing on coping strategies and managing fears of negative evaluation (Albano, 1995, 2000; Beidel & Turner, 2006).

Cognitive restructuring interventions are used in the treatment of posttraumatic stress disorder (PTSD; Cohen, Deblinger, Mannarino, & Steer, 2004; Deblinger & Heflin, 1996). Deblinger et al. (2006) described the use of cognitive coping techniques for treating children who have experienced sexual abuse. They employ Socratic dialogues, tests of evidence, and the "best-friend role play."

Stark and his colleagues have applied self-talk interventions for childhood depression (Stark, 1990; Stark, Swearer, Kurowski, Sommer, & Bowen, 1996). Their self-talk module includes increasing positive self-statement, promoting productive problem solving, and replacing unrealistic thoughts with more realistic appraisals. The cognitive interventions include tests of evidence, self-instruction, self-control, reattribution, and decatastrophizing.

The Primary and Secondary Control Enhancement Training (PASCET) program for youth depression (Weisz, Southam-Gerow, Gordis, & Connor-Smoth, 2003; Weisz, Thurber, Sweeney, Proffitt, & LeGagnoux, 1997) is another well-established program making use of a self-talk module. They address "habits of thought," which characterize childhood depression. Cognitive restructuring is seen as a secondary control strategy. Young people are taught to alter negative cognitions, decatastrophize, develop multiple problem-solving options, and decrease rumination.

Clarke and colleagues' Coping with Depression for Adolescents (CWD-A) also includes a significant self-talk component (Clarke, DeBar, & Lewinsohn, 2003; Clarke, Lewinsohn, & Hops, 1990a, 1990b; Clarke, Rohde, Lewinsohn, Hops, & Seeley, 1999). Patients are taught to argue with negative thoughts in order to decrease exaggeration, overreactions, and unreasonable expectations. They learn pivotal questions to ask themselves when they are depressed.

Self-talk interventions are essential ingredients in Anger Control Training (Feindler & Ecton, 1986; Feindler, Ecton, Kingsley, & Dubey, 1986; Feindler & Guttman, 1994; Feindler, Marriott, & Iwata, 1984). The self-talk interventions focus on self-instruction, reattribution, and alternatives to hostile explanations. Lochman and his colleagues include an even heavier dose of cognitive interventions in their Anger Coping Program (Boxmeyer, Lochman, Powell, Yaros, & Wojnaroski, 2007; Larson & Lochman, 2002; Lochman, Barry, & Pardini, 2003; Lochman, Fitzgerald, & Whidby, 1999) and the Coping Power Program (Lochman & Wells, 2002a, 2002b). They focus on reattributing hostile biases, modifying distorted interpersonal perceptions, and decreasing hopelessness.

Attwood (2004) advocated cognitive restructuring to modify patients with Asperger syndrome's false assumptions about situations and other people. Moreover, self-talk interventions can help people decrease their overly literal interpretations. The characteristic cognitive rigidity of children with Asperger syndrome may also be loosened up with cognitive restructuring procedures. Self-talk interventions also help with managing anxiety, depression, and anger, which challenge these young patients. Attwood suggested comic strip conversations and storyboards to increase children's social interpretations. Myles (2003) also offered a variety of simple cognitive strategies for stress management for children with Asperger syndrome, such as the self-instruction "Walk Don't Talk" when provoked. Self-talk-based games and exercises include "Spot the Message," "Guess the Message," "Fix the Feeling," and "Emotional Toolbox." Anderson and Morris (2006) recommended heavy doses of visual material to accompany cognitive intervention.

Turk (2005) described the use of cognitive restructuring procedures for children with developmental disorders and disabilities. He stated that the main goal of treatment is to "coax and encourage the child and family to consider and test out alternative hypotheses in a practical fashion" (Turk, 2005, p. 246). Therapists focus on decreasing children's absolutistic all-or-none thinking, misattributions, and personalization. Cognitive strategies also promote affective education, managing special interests, and coping with anxiety in children with autism spectrum disorders (Sofronoff, Attwood, & Hinton, 2005). Sze and Wood (2007) used cognitive modules to treat an 11-year-old girl with high-functioning autism using the *Building Confidence Manual* (Wood & McCleod, 2007). Their approach emphasized role-playing and metaphors to facilitate cognitive restructuring.

Cognitive restructuring and self-talk interventions have recently been applied to eating disorders and obesity. Wilfrey, Passi, Cooperberg, and Stein (2006) described their cognitive approach to overweight children, which includes strategies to counter catastrophic, all-or-none thinking. Lock (Lock, 2002; Lock & Fitzpatrick, 2007; Lock, le Grange, Agras, & Dare, 2001) and his colleagues have developed innovative cognitive approaches to treating anorexia nervosa and bulimia nervosa. Lock and Fitzpatrick (2007) discussed the use of cognitive interventions to shift concerns about loss of control, feelings of guilt and shame, helplessness, and self-criticism. Stewart (2005) discussed her approach helping patients with eating disorders evaluate the evidence for their distorted thoughts regarding their shape, weight, and food.

QUALITIES OF EFFECTIVE SELF-TALK PROCEDURES

Spiegler and Guevremont (1998) noted that self-instruction involves six components: (1) preparation, (2) attentional refocusing, (3) guiding behavior, (4) providing encour-

TABLE 5.1. Cognitive Restructuring Techniques

Technique	Purpose	Age	Modality
Superhero Cape	Building self-efficacy, stress inoculation	5–10 years	Individual, family, group
Thought Crown	Visualizing the self-talk process	6–9 years	Individual, family, group
Toss Across	Cognitive restructuring, self-instruction	7–12 years	Individual, family, group
Coping Necklace	Cognitive restructuring	7–11 years	Individual, family, group
Handprint on Your Heart	Cognitive restructuring of beliefs associated with separation anxiety	7–11 years	Individual, family
For Now or Forever?	Cognitive restructuring for addressing pessimistic views	8–18 years	Individual, group
Caring or Control	Decreasing parent–child conflict through accurately discerning whether the parent's behavior is motivated by caring or control/coercion	8–18 years	Individual, family, group

agement, (5) evaluating performance, and (6) reducing distress. Self-instruction often combines self-talk with problem solving.

The goal of cognitive therapy is to develop productive and functional, albeit not always 100% positive, counterthoughts (Padesky, 1988). Friedberg et al. (2001) recommended avoiding overly positive, simplistic, and Pollyannaish self-talk. When implementing a self-instructional self-talk procedure, the alternative response should clearly address the stressor and include a problem-solving or coping response. The coping thought should approximate the actual language children and youth would use.

This chapter offers various innovative procedures based on conventional cognitive interventions. Cartoons, games, and engaging exercises make cognitive interventions come alive (Friedberg & Gorman, 2007; Stallard, 2005). The interventions that follow make use of crafts, artworks, song lyrics, and metaphors that help young patients more fully embrace the procedures. The procedures are summarized in Table 5.1

SUPERHERO CAPE

Ages: 5–10 years.

Purpose: Building self-efficacy, stress inoculation.

Materials Needed:

- Construction paper.
- Pens, crayons, sticker.
- Ribbons.
- Scissors.
- Aluminum foil.

- Glue stick.
- Hole punch.

Superhero Cape is a self-instructional intervention that is aimed at building children's self-efficacy and inoculating them against stressors. Identifying superhero characters as covert models is an established procedure (Kendall et al., 1992; Rubin, 2007). In fact, CBT with chronically ill children encourages young children to see themselves as superheroes and summon up their special powers to battle their pain, fear, and anxieties (Kendall et al., 1992; Rubin, 2007). Superheroes may include typical figures such as Batman, Spiderman, or Wonder Woman. One child with Asperger syndrome chose Dr. Who as a superhero character (Attwood, 2003, 2004). Other children may see celebrities and sports figures as their superhero. Allen and Rapee (2005) reported one anxious patient who chose Jennifer Lopez as a coping model. Thus, the range of models is limitless.

In our use of the Superhero Cape, we combine imagery, self-instruction, and craft making. The child is invited to create a superhero persona for him- or herself, complete with superpowers. The child can be asked to draw the character. This gives the therapist confidence that the child has a clear picture of the superhero. Once the superhero image is created, the child assigns the character superpowers. Any superpower that is not self-destructive, aggressive, or otherwise harmful to others is acceptable. Becoming invisible, being able to shrink or supersize themselves, tolerating frustration or other negative feelings, using self-control such as Stop and Think skills, communicating, and problem solving are also examples of special powers.

The fun part comes next. The therapist, the child, and sometimes caregivers/parents make the cape. The cape is for the child to wear so he or she can take on the superhero role. The cape is made of heavy-duty construction paper. The child draws empowering symbols or characters on the cape. Stickers and pictures may also be pasted on the cape. Aluminum foil may also be glued to one side of the paper as a shield. Two holes are punched in the top of the cape and a ribbon is placed through the holes so it can be tied. The child then tries it on for size!

The following example illustrates the use of the cape with Asher, a 7-year-old traumatized boy. Asher was repeatedly physically, emotionally, and sexually abused by his biological parents. These tragic circumstances left him feeling anxious and challenged by several persistent ruminations such as "I'm helpless," "I'm unprotected," and "I'm open to attack." He underestimated the coping skills he possessed that made him a genuine survivor.

The superhero procedure began with an introduction. Asher loved Spiderman, which made the explanation easier. The following dialogue shows you how.

THERAPIST: Asher, you are kind of like Spiderman.

ASHER: (*Smiles.*) Really? How?

THERAPIST: Well, you know that many bad things happened to Spidey. Just like you. And you know what? Spidey got special powers from all these things.

ASHER: (*Excitedly.*) Yeah, like his spidey senses and shooting webs.

THERAPIST: Exactly. So you are kind of a superhero too.

ASHER: I am? Can I have a superhero name?

THERAPIST: Sure. What name would you like?

ASHER: Cazooba.

THERAPIST: Now we need to name your superpowers and make a cape that shows off your powers and keeps you safe.

ASHER: OK!

After the introduction, Asher and his adoptive parents began listing his superpowers. Depending on the case, parents may be included or not. The family decided on strength, smartness, love, and speed. Each power was associated with a symbol that was drawn or pasted on the cape (strength = earth, smartness = lightning, love = heart, speed = fire). Then, the specific coping skills were listed under each symbol (smartness = being good at school, talking about feelings; love = being kind to others, hugging and kissing Mom and Dad, taking care of pet). After the skills were added, the construction paper was glued to a sheet of aluminum foil. The foil metaphorically represented an impermeable shield. Next, two holes were punched in the top that allowed a ribbon to be pulled through and tied. Asher then ran around the clinic with the cape flying unfurled behind him exclaiming, "I'm Cazooba. Made of fire, earth, heart, and speed!"

THOUGHT CROWN

Ages: 6–9 years.

Purpose: Visualizing the self-talk process.

Materials Needed:

- Construction paper or poster board.
- Scissors.
- Stapler.
- Pens, crayons.
- Tape, Velcro strips.
- Cut-out thought bubbles.

Thought Crown is a self-instructional procedure that helps children visualize automatic negative thoughts, as well as the self-talk process. The procedure begins with the creation of a poster-board crown. Next, the therapist should make several blank thought bubbles cut out of paper. The crown and thought bubbles are illustrated in Figure 5.1.

Once the crown is placed on the child's head, the therapist and child write down various automatic thoughts (ATs) on the thought bubbles. After the ATs are identified and recorded on the thought bubbles, they are placed on the crown by attaching them with tape or Velcro strips. When the thought bubble is placed on the crown, it gives the visual impression of the thought popping out of the child's head (see Figure 5.1).

The therapist then Socratically processes the experience with the child. The following dialogue demonstrates the procedure.

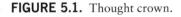

FIGURE 5.1. Thought crown.

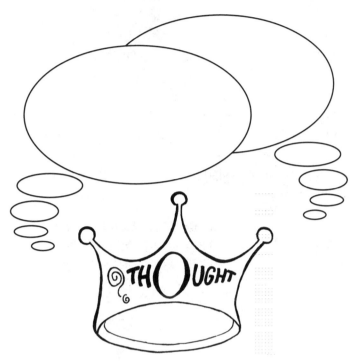

THERAPIST: Let's put your thought "I'm a loser" on your Thought Crown. (*Attaches it to crown.*) What feeling do you have?

ANDI: Sad.

THERAPIST: Make your face look like that. That sure makes sense. If "I'm a loser" popped into your head, you will feel sad. Should we see if we can come up with something to take its place?

ANDI: Sure.

The next step in the process represents the self-instruction or self-talk intervention. The child and the therapist work together to develop alternative coping thoughts to relieve the distress associated with the inaccurate thought. Once the alternative responses are constructed, they are recorded on thought bubbles. The therapist and child then proceed to concretize the thought replacement.

The following dialogue illustrates the process.

THERAPIST: OK, let's try this out. Let's take the "I'm a loser" out of your Thought Crown and put in this new thought, "Just because I didn't get to take the teacher's notes down to the office does not mean I am a loser." (*Therapist puts the new thought on the crown and takes the other thought off.*) Now how do you feel?

ANDI: Not so sad.

THERAPIST: Make a not-so-sad face. Now, let's put the old thought back. How do you feel now?

ANDI: Sad again.

THERAPIST: Now change your Thought Crown. How do you feel with the new thought in your head?

ANDI: Not so sad again.

THERAPIST: So what's the takeaway message?

ANDI: When I think I'm not such a loser if I am not the teacher's helper one day, I don't feel so sad.

THERAPIST: And how much in charge of your feeling does that make you?

ANDI: Really in charge.

The dialogue illustrates several points. First, Andi learned that when she changed things in the thought bubble, her feelings changed. Second, she discovered that she had greater control of her feelings. Consequently, her sense of efficacy increased.

TOSS ACROSS

Ages: 7–12 years.

Purpose: Cognitive restructuring.

Materials Needed:

- Bean bag/hacky sak.
- Slips of paper/index cards.
- Pen, paper.

Toss Across is a fun way to practice cognitive restructuring with young children. The technique involves nine negative automatic thoughts collected from children's thought records completed in the prior self-monitoring module (see Chapter 2). The nine automatic thoughts are written on index cards, laid on the floor, and arranged like a tic-tac-toe board. The child tosses a bean bag toward the cards. When it lands on a card, the child reads the automatic thought and must turn the thought around by constructing a coping statement. If the child crafts an appropriate response, it is written on the opposite side of the card. The coping side remains face up. The game continues until the child gets three in a row. The game can be played individually with the therapist and/ or in a group with peers.

Toss Across is handy because after the game, the child takes the coping cards home. Any cards that are left unresolved are assigned for homework. If peers or a therapist play, their responses also serve as models. The following dialogue gives you some hints for using Toss Across.

THERAPIST: Christian, toss the bean bag and see if you can land on a square. When you land on the square, see if you can turn the thought around and come up with a helpful new way to see things. If you can, you get to stay in the square. When you get three in a row in any direction, you win. Ready?

CHRISTIAN: I'm gonna win.

THERAPIST: That's a confident attitude.

This dialogue shows a brief but clear introduction to Toss Across. The therapist quickly moves to the game and reinforces the child's spontaneous positive self-talk.

THERAPIST: OK, Christian, throw your hacky. (*Christian throws.*) Look, you landed on "I must have things go my way or it is awful." How can you turn it around?

CHRISTIAN: That is a hard one. Can you do it?

THERAPIST: First, you try and I'll help if you need it.

CHRISTIAN: Umm, how about "Things don't have to go my way."

THERAPIST: Almost there. What else can you say to yourself to turn it around? What about the awful part?

CHRISTIAN: Well, it's not awful. I can stand it.

THERAPIST: What can you do?

CHRISTIAN: Just know that this too shall pass and wait it out.

The therapist walked Christian through the cognitive restructuring process. Despite his initial reluctance, Christian made a good stab at self-instruction. The therapist helped him flesh out his initial skeletal response and include a problem-solving component.

COPING NECKLACE

Ages: 7–11 years.

Purpose: Cognitive restructuring.

Materials Needed:

- Ribbons or plastic cord.
- Poster board or heavy-duty construction paper.
- Markers.
- Self-adhering play jewelry.

Coping cards are widely used in CBT. Typically, they are written reminders of constructive problem-solving strategies and helpful attributions. While coping cards are effective, children frequently forget, misplace, and/or lose them. The Coping Necklace is a way to make a coping card more memorable, fun, and easier to keep track of.

You will need ribbons or plastic cording, heavy-duty construction paper/poster board, self-adhering play jewelry, which can be purchased from a craft or educational supply store, and markers. On one side of the construction paper you write the problematic thought. On the other side, the coping thought is written. After the coping thought is written on the paper, the child begins to decorate it with the "jewels." A hole is punched on top of the paper and you place a ribbon or cord through the hole, completing the necklace.

The child is reminded that the productive strategy or coping response is the one with the jewelry. He or she is instructed to turn the negative thought around to view the jeweled coping thought whenever he or she is plagued by the distressing cognition. By having a necklace, the coping card can be displayed. Embellishing the coping card with jewels makes it more memorable. Finally, by wearing their coping "bling, bling," the children literally adopt and internalize the coping response.

HANDPRINT ON YOUR HEART

Ages: 7–11 years.

Purpose: Cognitive restructuring of beliefs associated with separation anxiety.

Materials Needed:

- Handprint on Your Heart Worksheet (Form 5.1).
- Markers or pens.

Handprint on Your Heart is a procedure for children and parents experiencing separation anxiety. It makes use of metaphors and concrete self-instructions. Moreover, the task is completed together, which connects parent–child warm emotions to the procedure. The necessary materials are quite simple; all you need is the Handprint on Your Heart Worksheet (Form 5.1) and some markers or pens.

Handprint on Your Heart is based on a song, "For Good," from the popular Broadway musical *Wicked* (Schwartz, 2003). The metaphor is apt because it concretizes a sense of emotional permanence (the handprint) for the young patient. Moreover, by mothers or fathers leaving their handprint, the procedure becomes a unique "stamp" of encouragement and self-instruction.

The procedure is quite simple. First, you present the metaphor of the "handprint on your heart." The following is a sample introduction.

> "Do you know what a handprint is? It's something that is totally special about a person. No two people have the same handprint. Your mom's handprint is totally her own. When someone places their handprint on your heart, you are touched and close to them always, even though you may be apart from them.
>
> "We are going to make Mom's handprint on your heart with this worksheet. It kind of means Mom is always near to you. On each finger on the handprint, we are going to put something that reminds you of Mom being close and how brave you can be on your own. How does this sound?"

Second, you invite the parent to trace his or her handprint. Next, the child, parent, and therapist develop some instructions to help foster separation (e.g., "Mom will be at home when I return from school. Dad can protect himself from the dangers. You can be brave without Mom or Dad being close."). Children then elect to keep the sheet in a special location at home, carry it with them to school, or both.

The following transcript illustrates the process with 8-year-old Kym and her mother.

THERAPIST: Look, Kym. Here's Mom's Handprint on the Heart.

KYM: That's cool.

THERAPIST: Now what I want you and Mom to try is to write something on each finger that will help you remember that Mom cares about you *and* you can be OK without her being always with you.

MOTHER: Kym, remember we always talk about your day when you come home.

KYM: I love that. We usually eat brownies and talk then.

THERAPIST: Which finger should we write that on?

(Kym and her mother pick a finger.)

THERAPIST: Now, what is something that helps you remember you are OK without Mom being with you?

KYM: I love school and do all my school work by myself.

MOTHER: You sure do, honey.

THERAPIST: How about making friends and playing during recess?

KYM: I have fun and do that myself too!

The process continued with the other three fingers. Kym and her mother learned to write down reminders and self-instructions for negotiating separations during the school day. The handprint represented a visual cue for coping that Kym carried in her backpack.

FOR NOW OR FOREVER?

Ages: 8–18 years.

Purpose: Distinguish between stressful events that endure and ones that are short lasting.

Materials Needed:

- Previously completed Thought Diary (see Chapter 2) or other paper.
- Pen or pencil.

For Now or Forever? is a simple cognitive restructuring intervention for young patients who see things as unchangeable and subsequently adopt a pessimistic stance. For Now or Forever? is based on the same premise as Permanent versus Temporary (Friedberg et al., 2001). Accordingly, it teaches children to distinguish problems that will always be present from problems that are more situational. Conceptually, For Now or Forever? works directly on the stable/unstable and global/specific attributional dimensions embedded in the attributional model of learned helplessness (Abramson, Seligman, & Teasdale, 1978). For Now or Forever? is inspired by the compelling song "For Now" (Lopez & Marx, 2003) from the Broadway musical *Avenue Q*. The simple song poignantly communicates that one inevitable thing in life is change. Since the procedure deals with the identified automatic thoughts, For Now or Forever? follows the completion of Thought Diaries described in Chapter 2.

The following introduction sets the stage for the technique.

> "Dylan, you have told me you feel trapped by many of your problems. You see them as lasting forever and never changing. I understand how helpless you see yourself to be. Sometimes it can be helpful to list the problems and decide whether these things will last just 'for now,' or will be there 'forever.'"

The procedure is completed in several stages. First, the therapist and the youngster list the troubling problems or issues on a piece of paper or in the child's Thought Diary. The therapist then creates two other columns alongside the list of the problems. One column is headed "For Now," the second "Forever." The patient is then asked to consider whether each problem is "for now" or "forever," and put a check by that problem in one of the columns. Some Socratic questioning may be necessary to help him or her discern the difference. When the patient is finished, the therapist asks which column has more checks. This is followed by synthesizing questions such as "What do you conclude from this?"; "What do you make of this?"; and/or "What do you take from this?" The conclusion is then written on a coping card.

The following dialogue illustrates the process with a 15-year-old depressed girl, Dylan, who sees herself as overwhelmed and incompetent.

THERAPIST: Dylan, let's list the things that you are struggling with.

DYLAN: You mean things that stress me out?

THERAPIST: Sure.

DYLAN: My grades, my mom's and dad's expectations, the shitty cliques at school, the bitchy girls, my soccer coach is pressuring me, homecoming and not having a date, eating too much junk food, my sister getting into my makeup. Is that enough?

THERAPIST: It's a start. Are these all the big things?

DYLAN: Well, getting into college, getting my driving permit, whether I'll ever not be depressed all my life.

THERAPIST: OK, let's take a look at these, OK? (*Writes down the items as Dylan states them.*)

DYLAN: Sure.

THERAPIST: Put an X on whether you see the problem as being something that just is bothersome for now in the present, or whether you see it as always being a struggle. (*Hands journal to Dylan.*) [See how Dylan completed the journal in Figure 5.2.]

THERAPIST: How many are problems for now, and how many are forever?

FIGURE 5.2. Dylan's For Now or Forever? journal.

Problem	For Now (something that bothers you just for now)	Forever (something that always will bother you)
Grades	X	
Parents' pressure		X
Cliques at school	X	
Bitchy girls	X	
Soccer coach pressure	X	
Homecoming	X	
Dating		X
Eating too much junk food	X	
Sister getting into makeup	X	
Getting into college	X	
Getting driver's permit	X	
Question about how long I will be depressed		X

DYLAN: There are nine in the "For now" and three in the "forever" column.

THERAPIST: What do you suppose that means?

DYLAN: I dunno. (*Pause.*) Maybe most of my problems are just for now ... but I still have the big three in the forever column.

THERAPIST: Let's talk about that. Your parents' expectations, worries about dating, and worries about being depressed.

DYLAN: I just want to be normal. My parents aren't going to change. I have to be perfect or else I'll disappoint them. Guys are always going to freak me out. I don't understand them.

THERAPIST: These are ongoing struggles for you. Are you learning ways to cope with them?

DYLAN: Some. It's just hard.

THERAPIST: So what can you say to yourself to summarize all this?

DYLAN: (*Pause.*) I dunno .... Most of my problems are for now. I guess that's not so abnormal.

THERAPIST: What about the others?

DYLAN: My parents are always going to pressure me. Dating sucks and is hard. I guess it's kinda natural for me to feel bad, but I'm working on it.

THERAPIST: When you say that out loud, how do you feel?

DYLAN: Less freaked.

THERAPIST: Then write that statement on a card.

This dialogue shows how the therapist systematically works through the For Now or Forever? procedure with Dylan. The therapist elicited a long list of problems in an unedited fashion. Then he asked Dylan a question to collect data: "How many are problems for now, and how many are forever?" Next, synthesizing questions ask the patient to interpret the data: "What do you suppose that means?"; "So what can you say to yourself to summarize all this?" The therapist then checked to see if there was an improvement in mood with the cognitive restructuring: "When you say that out loud, how do you feel?" Finally, Dylan wrote the statement on a coping card.

CARING OR CONTROL

Ages: 8–18 years.

Purpose: Decreasing parent–child conflict through accurately discerning whether the parent's behavior is motivated by caring or control/coercion.

Materials Needed:

- Previously completed Thought Diary or other paper.
- Pen or pencil.

Parents, teachers, and young people often become trapped in control battles. During these conflicts, both parties misinterpret each other's intentions. A teacher or parent may enforce limits, place demands, and/or ask nosy intrusive questions due to their concerns. Commonly, children are quick to misperceive the caring as control. Accordingly, they righteously fight the control. This leaves the caring parent befuddled, frustrated, and resentful of the children's rejection of their concern. This then leads to parental anger, an escalation of limits, and an expansion of parental involvement and authority. Not surprisingly, the conflict intensifies and the children's rebellion increases proportionately. Helping youngsters and their parents discriminate between control and caring deescalates conflict.

Similar to the For Now or Forever? technique, Caring or Control uses three columns on a separate sheet of paper or drawn in the child's Thought Diary. In the first column, children identify the parent/adult who may be viewed as either controlling or caring. Second, they rate (on a 10-point scale) the degree of control (column 2) and/or caring (column 3) they perceive in the adult's behavior. Finally, the therapist and child process the data collaboratively.

Annaleigh was a 15-year-old angry and depressed teenager who was resentful about her mother's behavior. Annaleigh saw her mother as totally coercive and domineering. On previously completed Thought Diaries, she recorded beliefs such as "My mom is a complete control freak," "She insists on me being her clone," and "She only cares for me if I am exactly who she wants me to be." Consequently, the therapist elected to do the Caring or Control procedure with Annaleigh to decrease her all-or-none thinking about her mother's behavior.

The therapist invited Annaleigh to list the behaviors that her mother did that annoyed her. Then the therapist explained, "We need to see how controlling and caring you see your mom to be. How should we rate this? On a 1–10 or a 1–100 scale?" Annaleigh chose a 1–10 scale. The therapist continued by saying, "Whenever your mom does something that makes you mad, list it, and then give it a control or caring score." Annaleigh then recorded her mother's behavior and the control and caring ratings as illustrated in Figure 5.3. The following dialogue demonstrates therapeutic processing with the Caring or Control Worksheet.

THERAPIST: Annaleigh, let's look at your Caring and Control Worksheet. How was it to complete?

ANNALEIGH: A little hard. I wasn't sure if I did it right.

THERAPIST: Let's talk it over. First on your list, you saw your mother's behavior at breakfast as more caring than controlling. Tell me about that.

ANNALEIGH: She just wants me to start the day right. She lets me eat pretty much what I want.

THERAPIST: OK. You also saw her questions about coming home, physics, and your sweatshirt as more caring than controlling.

ANNALEIGH: She worries a lot.

THERAPIST: You saw her comment about your skirt as a mix of caring and controlling.

ANNALEIGH: I'm 15! She wants me to dress like I'm 56. Things have changed in the world. She thinks boys are trying to get busy with me.

THERAPIST: The shower and IM things you saw as pretty controlling?

ANNALEIGH: She's a perfectionist and wants things just so. "Just so" means her way. It is my shower. Who cares how I clean? And she doesn't want me to be

FIGURE 5.3. Annaleigh's Caring or Control Worksheet.

Adult Behavior	Caring level (1–10)	Control level (1–10)
Mom told me to eat a roll for breakfast.	9	5
Mom asked when I would come home.	9	3
Mom asked about my physics test.	9	2
Mom told me to wear a sweatshirt to the football game.	9	2
Mom said my skirt was too short.	7	6
Mom corrected how I washed out the shower.	3	9
Dad told me to put the chips away.	2	9
Dad said to practice my speech.	7	3
Mom told me to get off the IM and do my homework.	4	8

involved with my friends. Sometimes I think she does not want me to have my own life apart from her.

THERAPIST: That's an interesting idea. Let's write that down. "My mom does not want me to have a life apart from her."

ANNALEIGH: That's her.

THERAPIST: For Dad, he was more controlling about the chips and more caring about the speech.

ANNALEIGH: He's a neat freak. I think he's psycho about crumbs. He does care about my grades, though.

THERAPIST: So what do you make of all this?

ANNALEIGH: I dunno. My mom is a control freak.

THERAPIST: Another interesting idea. Let's write that down too. Now how will we know if these ideas are on target?

ANNALEIGH: I dunno.

THERAPIST: If Mom was a control freak and did not want you to have your own life, how many of these would be more controlling than caring?

ANNALEIGH: I guess most would be control.

THERAPIST: Let's check it out. How many are mostly due to control?

ANNALEIGH: Two out of seven.

THERAPIST: So is it mostly about control and not wanting you to have a life of your own?

ANNALEIGH: I just thought so. Maybe she cares too much and needs to trust me more. I am older now and she just has to get that.

THERAPIST: What does that do to your anger?

ANNALEIGH: Makes it less.

THERAPIST: When you are less angry maybe you can teach Mom to trust you more and care for you like a 15-year-old.

The dialogue with Annaleigh demonstrates several important issues. First, the therapist facilitated the dialogue with descriptive comments as well as questions. Second, the therapist was patient and explored the data slowly with Annaleigh. Third, the therapist set up the cognitive restructuring with a specific synthesizing question: "If Mom was a control freak and did not want you to have your own life, how many of these would be more controlling than caring?"

FAIR OR WHAT I WANT?

Ages: 8–18 years.

Purpose: Decreasing children's frustration and anger due to confusing what is fair with getting/doing what they want.

Materials Needed:

- Paper.
- Pen or pencil.
- Ruler.

Angry, noncompliant, and oppositional children frequently adopt a view that the things that happen to them are unfair. They distort reasonable demands and see them as inequitable requirements. In short, they inaccurately equate fairness with things going their way. Like the preceding For Now or Forever? and Caring or Control, Fair or What I Want? uses a three-column format. The first column lists the situations or events that are upsetting. The second and third columns require the patient to consider whether the circumstances are unfair or just not what they want. After they complete the columns, the therapist and the patient process the data.

The following dialogue illustrates the process with Costas, an 11-year-old, who threw many tantrums and used high levels of emotionality to ensure his belief that "my needs must always be met even if it is at the expense of others."

COSTAS: (*Tearfully.*) Everything is so unfair! I hate my life.

THERAPIST: Costas, tell me what is so unfair.

COSTAS: My teacher gives me too much homework.

THERAPIST: I know homework can really stink.

COSTAS: I hate it. And on top of that, my mother makes me do chores at home. I need down time.

THERAPIST: So, that is unfair too?

COSTAS: Yeah, sometimes Edgar, Aron, and Anoop take my Yugi-Oh cards.

THERAPIST: You see that as unfair too?

COSTAS: That's right. Nothing seems to go my way.

THERAPIST: No wonder you are so teary and upset. You see fair as being the same as getting what you want.

COSTAS: Wait. What do you mean? I guess I do, sort of.

THERAPIST: Let me ask you, do you see most upsetting things as unfair or not what you want?

COSTAS: A little bit of both.

THERAPIST: That can be confusing. Let's see if we can help you see things clearer. Would that be OK with you?

COSTAS: OK.

THERAPIST: So, let's list the things that are upsetting you. You said the amount of homework your teacher gave was unfair?

COSTAS: Yes.

THERAPIST: Well, what makes it unfair?

COSTAS: I hate homework.

THERAPIST: I understand you don't like it, but how many other kids don't like it and still have to do it?

COSTAS: Everybody, I guess.

THERAPIST: So does that mean it is unfair, or just something you don't like?

COSTAS: I guess it is something I don't like.

THERAPIST: The next thing is Mom doesn't let you have enough down time because she makes you do chores.

COSTAS: Yeah, I need time for me.

THERAPIST: I see. Are you the only one who has to do chores in your family?

COSTAS: No, my sister Bridget does.

THERAPIST: How much homework does she get?

COSTAS: She's in 10th grade. She gets a lot.

THERAPIST: So are chores unfair or just not what you want?

COSTAS: Oh, crap, I see where you are going with this.

THERAPIST: Well, be patient. We still have a few items. What about Anoop, Aron, and Edgar?

COSTAS: They are bossy.

THERAPIST: They may be. Let's talk more. What's your arrangement with the cards?

COSTAS: We are supposed to trade, but they just take my cards.

THERAPIST: That sounds pretty unfair. What do you think?

COSTAS: It sucks. Totally unfair.

THERAPIST: So what do you make of this list?

COSTAS: Most of the time, I mix up what is unfair with what I want.

In the above dialogue, the therapist helped the child clarify the distinction between unfair and undesirable. The therapist elicited the child's beliefs in an empathic, nonjudgmental manner. Then Costas was gently questioned about his appraisals. Finally, "So what do you make of this list?," the synthesizing question, yielded the coping statement. Costas's completed worksheet can be seen in Figure 5.4.

FIGURE 5.4. Costas's Fair or What I Want Worksheet

Upsetting thing	Unfair	Just not what I want
Homework		X
Chores		X
Anoop and Edgar want turn	X	

ARE YOU READY FOR SOME CHANGES?

Ages: 8–18 years.

Purpose: Increasing children's motivation.

Materials Needed:

- Are You Ready for Some Changes? Questionnaire (Form 5.2).
- Pencil or pen.

Are You Ready for Some Changes? is a cognitive restructuring exercise aimed at motivating patients toward change. It is based on motivational interviewing (Miller & Rollnick, 1991), stages of change (DiClemente, 2003; Geller & Drab, 1999; Prochaska, 1979; Prochaska & DiClemente, 1992; Prochaska, DiClemente, & Norcross, 1992), and acceptance and commitment therapy (Schulte et al., 2002). The literature base indicates that patients differ in how distressing they see their problems, how well they see themselves able to make changes, and how much effort they direct toward these changes. In essence, patient resistance, avoidance, or "stuckness" in therapy is seen as ambivalence (Zinbarg, 2000). Are You Ready for Some Changes? tries to shift patients' ambivalence toward commitment. Many of the questions in Are You Ready for Some Changes? are based on the Readiness and Motivational Interview developed by Geller and Drab (1999) and the basic conditions of patient behavior noted by Schulte et al. (2002). A blank Are You Ready for Some Changes? Questionnaire is provided in Form 5.2.

The exercise begins with the youngsters' definitions of their presenting problems. The next seven questions address different perceptions of change elements. Each question is rated on a 7-point scale to discourage all-or-none responding. The first question ("It bothers me ... ") deals with level of subjective distress associated with the problem. More subjective distress is motivating (Schulte et al., 2002). The second question is conceptually similar to the first question and addresses a sense of helplessness and lack of control linked with the problems. The third question assesses the sense of abnormality or differentness caused by the problem ("I think _____ people my age have this type of problem."). Seeing oneself as outside the norm is motivating (Schulte et al., 2002). The next question deals with the patient's confidence in the treatment process and hopefulness about the outcome. Higher levels of confidence in treatment are more motivating (Schulte et al., 2002). The final three questions evaluate patients' subjective appraisal about their commitment to change and their perceived ability to make changes. Lack of commitment and low self-efficacy are demotivating (Bandura, 1977a, 1977b, 1986; Geller & Drab, 1999; Prochaska & DiClemente, 1992).

The pattern of youngsters' responses is revealing and provides a robust foundation for cognitive restructuring. For instance, if the problem is mildly distressing, the patient's effort is less likely. If the problem is distressing but the patient does not experience much helplessness or lack of control, this inconsistency should be Socratically processed: "Explain to me how _____ can really bother you, but you only feel a little helpless"; "How is it that you can be bothered a lot but you see yourself in control?" Confidence in the treatment process and perceived self-efficacy for change are particularly compelling areas for intervention. The problem may be very distressing and contribute to high hopelessness and a sense of being abnormal, but if the patient doubts treatment will help, he or she will get stuck in treatment. In this case, the therapist would focus on perceived confidence in treatment in order to increase motivation. Finally, patients may be in distress, helpless, seeing themselves as abnormal, confident in the therapist, yet remain ambivalent and unmotivated because they fundamentally doubt their ability to change. In this instance, increased patient self-efficacy for change is key.

The following dialogue illustrates how to increase self-efficacy for change with a 15-year-old patient with anorexia named Jasmine. She has not been progressing in treatment and has just filled out the Are You Ready for Some Changes? Questionnaire (Figure 5.5).

> THERAPIST: Thanks for filling this out, Jasmine. Let's take a look at what you circled. Not eating bothers you a lot; you feel out of control; you want to change your feelings, thoughts, and behaviors, but you don't think treatment will help and you think you are not able to change your feelings, thoughts, and behaviors. Is that pretty accurate?
>
> JASMINE: Yeah, you could put it that way.
>
> THERAPIST: Would you put it that way?
>
> JASMINE: Sure.
>
> THERAPIST: Well, this helps me understand how hard this is for you. This anorexia bothers you and makes you feel bad, so no wonder you don't really try the therapy.
>
> JASMINE: It won't help anyway.
>
> THERAPIST: I see. What makes you think treatment won't help you and you can't change your feelings, thoughts, and behaviors.
>
> JASMINE: I haven't changed them in the past and the other therapist and hospital didn't help.
>
> THERAPIST: What does that mean about you?
>
> JASMINE: I'm a lost cause.
>
> THERAPIST: So you don't want to put any energy into a lost cause?
>
> JASMINE: Exactly.
>
> THERAPIST: When you see things as hopeless, you sure don't want to try anything.
>
> JASMINE: Sure.
>
> THERAPIST: So what makes you a lost cause?
>
> JASMINE: This is going in circles. I can't eat!
>
> THERAPIST: It is exactly a circle. That's really the hard part. How possible is it that you don't know *how to change?*
>
> JASMINE: Possible, I guess.
>
> THERAPIST: OK. How much do you think you are able to keep progress going?

FIGURE 5.5. Jasmine's Are You Ready for Some Changes? Questionnaire.

My problem is _Not eating_   .

It bothers me (circle one number):

1	2	3	4	5	⑥	7
Not at all			Kind of			A lot

I feel out of control and helpless because of it.

1	2	3	4	5	⑥	7
Not at all			Kind of			A lot

I think people my age have this type of problem.

1	2	3	4	⑤	6	7
Not many			Some			Many

I am sure that my treatment will help.

1	②	3	4	5	6	7
Not at all			Kind of			Totally

I want to change my thoughts, feelings, and behaviors.

1	2	3	4	⑤	6	7
Do not			Kind of			Totally

I am trying to change my thoughts, feelings, and behaviors.

1	2	3	④	5	6	7
Not			Kind of			Really

I think I am able to change my thoughts, feelings, and behaviors.

1	②	3	4	5	6	7
Do not			Kind of			Really

JASMINE: I almost always slide back.

THERAPIST: So is it possible you lack confidence in your coping too?

JASMINE: I just don't think I am good at coping with things. I get freaked out a lot.

THERAPIST: So you don't know how to change and you can't keep it up?

JASMINE: That's me.

THERAPIST: How changeable are skills and confidence?

JASMINE: Changeable, I guess.

THERAPIST: So, if confidence and skills are changeable, how much of a lost cause are you?

JASMINE: I dunno. I never thought about it. ... Maybe not a lost cause. (*Smiles.*)

THERAPIST: You smiled just then.

JASMINE: I never thought about it that way.

THERAPIST: How willing are you to build some new skills and see if your confidence builds?

The dialogue illustrates how to use the worksheet with an avoidant young patient. First, the therapist used Jasmine's responses as data to clarify and empathize with her helplessness. Second, the therapist aligned with Jasmine against her lack of self-efficacy. Third, the therapist gently questioned Jasmine's belief that she was a lost cause by separating it from a lack of confidence and skills.

TRICK OR TRUTH

Ages: 8–15 years.

Purpose: Increasing children's identification of inaccurate thinking.

Materials Needed:

- Trick or Truth Diary (Form 5.3).
- A Dozen Dirty Tricks Your Mind Plays on You Handout (Form 3.1).

Based on A Dozen Dirty Tricks Your Mind Plays on You, Trick or Truth is a child-friendly version of naming distortions that also includes a restructuring component. The technique teaches children to examine automatic thoughts for distortions and it creates initial doubt regarding the absolute accuracy of their interpretations. The procedure interrupts the connection between automatic thoughts, distressing feelings, and problematic behavior.

Trick or Truth begins with the four columns (date, situation, feeling, thought) of the Thought Diaries presented in Chapter 2. A fifth column invites the child to identify the dirty trick, and column six asks the child to record whether the thought is trick or truth. If the thought is accurate, problem solving ensues. If the thought is a dirty trick, you begin to cast doubt on the thought's accuracy. The process ends either with a problem-solving strategy or a new coping thought written on a card.

The following dialogue demonstrates how Trick or Truth creates doubts. Anjani is a 9-year-old Asian Indian American child who feels lonely, is excruciatingly self-critical, and is isolated by peers who hurl racial slurs at her. Her Trick or Truth Diary is shown in Figure 5.6.

ANJANI: I filled out my Trick or Truth Diary. Wanna see?

THERAPIST: Of course. Let's see, when you were playing tag with the boys, they made you it because you are brown. You felt sad and thought you didn't fit in and that no one will ever see you as you really are. You said it was a trick.

ANJANI: One-eyed ogre.

THERAPIST: So if it is a trick, how much should you believe it?

ANJANI: Only a teeny tiny bit.

THERAPIST: When they were bullying you and teasing you, how much did you believe the one-eyed ogre.

ANJANI: A *lot*! I cried.

THERAPIST: Sure you did. At the time, it seemed true that no one will ever see the real you and you won't fit in, but when you thought it over, you didn't believe in the tricks.

ANJANI: Yep.

THERAPIST: Let's write that all on a card.

ANJANI: Should I write that I don't believe I won't fit in? It's just my one-eyed ogre.

THERAPIST: Absolutely.

The therapist then continued with the dialogue for the 12/7 and 12/11 entries. However, the 12/12 entry was accurate and required a problem-solving intervention.

ANJANI: We still have the last one to do.

THERAPIST: Let's look at this one. The kids were chasing you and calling you names. You felt sad, and thought they were mean, jealous, and scared.

ANJANI: But I think that is *true*.

THERAPIST: I think so too. You did a great job on this diary. Many kids are scared by someone who is different and they take out their scared feelings on them.

ANJANI: Like trying to make them feel scared?

THERAPIST: Exactly. So what can you do that doesn't make you feel hurt and bad?

ANJANI: Tell the recess aide and stay close to her. Play with girls I know are safer. Tell my mom too.

THERAPIST: Good ideas. Let's write them on a card.

FIGURE 5.6. Anjani's Trick or Truth Diary.

Date	Situation	Feeling	Thought	Dirty trick	Truth or trick	Problem solving
12/6	Boy teased me about being brown. I had to be it because I was brown.	Sad	I wish I wasn't brown. I don't fit in. No one will ever see the real me.	One-Eyed Ogre	Trick	
12/7	Left out during Christmas craft.	Sad	Tony said I couldn't help with the tree because I wasn't Christian and no one will like me then.	Disaster Forecaster	Trick	
12/11	Named best student of the month for getting all A's. The kids booed me.	Sad	There's something wrong with me.	Maxi-Me Thinking	Trick	
12/12	The kids chased me and called me names because I am brown and they say I talk funny.	Sad	Most of the kids are mean. I think they may be scared of me and a little jealous.		Truth	Tell the recess aide, stay close to her, play with girls who are safe. Tell mom.

144

IT'S ME, NOT OCD

Ages: 8–12 years.

Purpose: Separating children's personhood from OCD symptoms.

Materials Needed:

- Flat wooden sticks (e.g., tongue depressors, paint stirrers).
- Markers for drawing.
- Magazine pictures or clip art.
- Scissors.
- Glue stick.

Teaching children to talk back to OCD is a common restructuring technique used by many CBT-oriented clinicians (Chansky, 2000; March & Mulle, 1998; Piacentini & Langley, 2004). Moreover, March and Mulle (1998) recommend distancing the child from the OCD by objectifying the disorder through drawing or cartooning. It's Me, Not OCD is a cognitive restructuring technique that makes use of both the talk-back strategy and cartooning.

Like in March and Mulle's (1998) manual, the first step is to ask the child to represent the OCD visually. The child may draw a cartoon, select a picture from a magazine (e.g., ugly spider), or use clip art (e.g., a monster). Next, the child and you paste the picture on one side of a tongue depressor or paint stirrer; if you want to be fancy, craft stores offer wood cutouts of child figures.

On the reverse side, you paste a school picture of the child or a cartoon portrait of the child. Once the two sides are illustrated, write down some of the pivotal OCD thoughts on the OCD side. Then you help the patient conduct talk-back strategies on the "Me" side.

The following dialogue shows you how to use It's Me, Not OCD with a 9-year-old girl named Anise.

THERAPIST: Anise, I know you like to draw.

ANISE: I love to draw. I am great at art!

THERAPIST: OK. You see this? (*Holds up a wood cutout of human figure.*) I want you to draw a picture of what you think OCD looks like on this side.

ANISE: Remember we called OCD a real butt nugget insect. (*Draws it on one side.*)

THERAPIST: Great, now on the other side we need a picture of you. What can we do?

ANISE: Use my school picture! I just got them. (*Mother hands it to Anise.*)

THERAPIST: Paste it on the other side, the "you" side. Now you are on one side …

ANISE: Yeah, and the butt nugget is on the other side.

THERAPIST: Now on the smelly butt nugget side write down what OCD tells you.

ANISE: Like I have to say my prayers perfectly right from start to finish.

THERAPIST: Or what might happen?

ANISE: (*Softly.*) My family will get hurt.

THERAPIST: Write that down.

ANISE: (*While writing.*) Bad smelly butt nugget thought!

THERAPIST: Now on the "me" side with your school picture, write down something you can say to back off the butt nugget.

ANISE: I don't take orders from a smelly butt nugget insect like you.

THERAPIST: Great, now you can take this home and read it over. And for homework make some more of them with OCD on one side and you on the other side.

In the above transcript the therapist and patient aligned together against the OCD. The craft-like exercise engaged Anise's interests and competencies. She was able to identify the distressing OCD command and construct a self-talk strategy. The therapist gave her the homework assignment to continue to develop talk-back statements with the crafts.

CLEAN UP YOUR THINKING

Ages: 8–13 years.

Purpose: Cognitive restructuring.

Materials Needed:

- Clean Up Your Thinking Diary (Form 5.4).
- A Dozen Dirty Tricks Your Mind Plays on You Handout (Form 3.1).
- Pen or pencils.

Clean Up Your Thinking is a technique based on the Spot the Dirty Tricks procedure, and is also inspired by work with a precocious 8-year-old girl with severe performance anxiety. She progressed relatively quickly through the self-monitoring process and was quite able to identify the dirty tricks in her thinking. After reviewing the Spot the Dirty Trick Diary, Ricki spontaneously remarked, "I'll vacuum the dirty trick out of my head." Clean Up Your Thinking is a concrete way children can vacuum away their dirty tricks.

Clean Up Your Thinking includes the date, situation, feeling, thought, and dirty trick in columns 1–5. Column 6 includes the clean-up strategy or counterthought. Clean-up strategies are produced via Socratic dialogues with the patient. The diary allows you as the therapist to note what were productive questions, and then record them for the patient on the diary. The diary then aids generalization by helping the patient ask him- or herself questions to clean up his or her thinking. The following transcript illustrates its use with 13-year-old Paula, who struggles with self-criticism, fears of disapproval, sadness, and anger. Her Clean Up Your Thinking Diary is shown in Figure 5.7.

THERAPIST: Paula, let's look at your Clean Up Your Thinking Diary [See Figure 5.7].

PAULA: I did everything but the clean-up strategy. I just didn't know what to write.

THERAPIST: OK. Let's work together on it. On the first one you wrote, "I'm angry. I have to get rid of this feeling. I hate it. I should just hit her." What made you say it was a prisoner of feeling?

PAULA: It was like the anger took hold of me and I forgot to think through things and I hit her.

THERAPIST: OK, so clean it up. Who's stronger, you or the anger?

PAULA: Me. Feelings can't hurt people. Actions can. I can stand the feelings. I just don't like them.

THERAPIST: See, you can clean it up. Now, the second one. "I'm ugly. My nose is too big. I'm too short. My legs are too fat."

PAULA: Yeah, I'm not the prettiest, preppy girl. You know, the girls who are all that.

THERAPIST: So how come it is circus mirror thinking?

PAULA: Well, I'm not skanky or hideous.

THERAPIST: Well, isn't that what you are saying to yourself?

PAULA: Kind of. (*Sighs.*)

THERAPIST: How come?

PAULA: 'Cause Oscar is this boy I like and he ditched me.

THERAPIST: OK. So Oscar determines whether you are ugly and other ways you see yourself?

PAULA: (*Pause.*) I'm not giving that horny toad that much power. Just because Oscar didn't dance with me doesn't mean I am ugly. I feel sad and that is what is making me see my weaknesses.

THERAPIST: Now, the last one. "Mom should know I need her approval. She should pay more attention to me and what I want." What makes that a mules' rules?

PAULA: I have a lot of rules for her.

THERAPIST: How much does she know the rules?

PAULA: Not much. I keep the rules to myself.

THERAPIST: Silent rules.

PAULA: Yep.

THERAPIST: How can she know them?

PAULA: (*Laughs.*) Reading my mind, I guess.

THERAPIST: How good a mind reader is she?

PAULA: She sucks at it.

FIGURE 5.7. Paula's Clean Up Your Thinking Diary.

Date	Situation	Feeling	Thought	Dirty trick	Clean-up strategy	Fresh thought
11/7	Bree said I was a skank.	Angry	I hate being angry. I have to get rid of it. I should hit her. My anger has a hold on me.	Prisoner of Feeling	Who's stronger, you or your anger?	Feelings can't hurt others. Actions can. I can stand these feelings. I just don't like them.
11/8	Looked in mirror in gym class after Oscar ditched me.	Sad	I'm ugly. My nose is too big. My legs are too fat.	Circus Mirror	Just because Oscar ditched me doesn't mean I'm ugly.	This is just my depression talking. I'm not going to give that horny toad Oscar that much power.
11/9	Mom criticized my artwork.	Sad, mad	My mom should know that I need her approval. She should pay more attention to me.	Mules Rules	How do the rules work?	My rules are silent. They are not clear even to me. I can't make her do what I want.

148

THERAPIST: How do your mules' rules work for you?

PAULA: Not good. How could she know my rules? I never told her. They are not clear even to me. Maybe these rules I do have are no good. I can't make her do what I want.

In this dialogue, the therapist helped Paula construct a clean-up strategy with systematic questioning. The identification of each dirty trick produced the springboard for the questioning. The therapist also propelled the cognitive restructuring by peppering the questions with reflections so Paula would not see herself as being interrogated (e.g., "So Oscar determines whether you are ugly and other ways you see yourself?"; "Silent rules").

SWAT THE BUG

Ages: 8–13 years.

Purpose: Cognitive restructuring.

Materials Needed:

- Completed What's Buggin' You? Diary (Form 2.4).
- Swat the Bug form (Form 5.5).
- Pencil or pen.

Swat the Bug is a self-talk intervention that should follow the self-monitoring technique What's Buggin' You? (Chapter 2). The coping counterthoughts are presented as different "bug swatters" and act to silence the irritating bugs. This procedure is akin to March and colleagues' (March, 2007; March & Mulle, 1998) boss-back strategies. The talk-back strategies also distance the young patients from the judgmentalness associated with self-critical thinking, much like the clever cognitive defusion strategies (e.g., passengers on the bus, man in the hole) espoused by Hayes, Strosdahl, and Wilson (1999). Some of the coping thoughts may make use of the "just because" strategies pioneered by Elliott (1991), as illustrated in the dialogue below.

First, the cartoon swatters are presented (see Form 5.5). Then the child writes his or her own talk-back strategies on the blank swatters. The following dialogue illustrates the use of the Swat the Bug procedure.

THERAPIST: Remember when we wrote down your thoughts on the What's Buggin' You? sheet? Well, now we are going to learn how to stop the bugs from annoying you. Are you ready to do that?

EVAN: Sure.

THERAPIST: OK. The next tool I am going to show is called Swat the Bug. Take a look at the Swat the Bug sheet. See these bug swatters? There is a place to write something on them that will knock out the thought that bugs you. Some boys and girls think it is helpful to start the knock-out thoughts with the words "Just because." Let's try it with your thoughts. How does this sound?

EVAN: I want to knock out the thought!

THERAPIST: Let's start with the first thing you wrote on your What's Buggin' You? Diary. Your sister was annoying you when she kept drawing on your baseball magazine. You felt angry and thought: "She is trying to prove she is better than me and she is showing me who is the boss. I must hit her to show her who is boss or else she will know I am a punk." What else can we put on the swatter to knock out that thought and cool off your anger?

EVAN: She is a punk for drawing on my magazine!

THERAPIST: We could put that down, but would that cool off your anger?

EVAN: No, I would get madder.

THERAPIST: I think so too. How about we try the Just Because idea. I'll get you started and you finish. Just because I can hurt my sister does not mean I am her boss, I can show her I am in charge by _____. (Pause.)

EVAN: Pulling my magazine away and telling my mom. I am going to write *that* on my sheet.

This dialogue illustrates the graduated nature of many cognitive restructuring interventions. In the initial stages of the dialogue, the therapist asked open-ended questions, which did not elicit productive responses. When the therapist helped Evan craft a counterthought, the task became easier for him. This strategy is especially good for younger children and patients who are not skilled in depthful rational analysis.

TRASH TALK

Ages: 8–18 years.

Purpose: A talk-back technique.

Materials Needed:

- Trash Talk Worksheet (Form 5.6).
- Pen or pencils.

Trash Talk is a cognitive restructuring procedure based on the sports practice of the same name. When a player "talks trash" or "smack" to other competitors, he or she says irritating, untrue things to upset them and throw off their games. Negative automatic thoughts are smack talk or trash talk, which characterize distressing, internal dialogues. Essentially, Trash Talk is a talk-back technique. It is helpful with lame blame thinking and one-eyed ogre thinking. Therapists work with young patients to construct comeback statements to the trash talk.

To introduce the Trash Talk exercise, the therapist might say:

"Do you know what trash talk is? When someone talks trash, they say untrue things that are upsetting. It is important not to believe trash talk. Remember when we learned to catch the negative automatic thoughts that go through your mind when you are upset? Now it's our turn to talk back to the trash your sad, angry, and worried feelings send to you! How does this sound?"

The child and the therapist record the trash talk and come up with counterstatements. A sample Trash Talk Worksheet entry is shown in Figure 5.8 and a blank Trash Talk Worksheet is provided in Form 5.6. The following dialogue demonstrates the procedure.

THERAPIST: Remy, remember when we captured the things that run through your mind when you are upset?

REMY: Yeah, I still have them.

THERAPIST: Good. Today, we are going to work on them together using this Trash Talk Worksheet. How does this sound?

REMY: OK, I guess.

THERAPIST: Let's write down the trash talk that goes through your mind. What's one of the things you say to yourself that is trash?

REMY: I guess that I'm a loser and I'll never measure up to the other girls. No one will ever want to chill out and hang out with me.

THERAPIST: That is some strong trash talk your mind is sending you. Let's talk back to it.

REMY: I don't know what to do. You show me.

THERAPIST: It's hard, I know, to come up with new things because you've heard this trash for so long. But it usually works better if you take the lead in talking back.

REMY: I don't know what you want me to say.

THERAPIST: Whatever you think will help you quiet down the trash talk.

FIGURE 5.8. Remy's Trash Talk Worksheet.

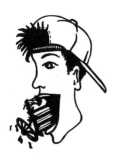

Trash I say to myself	My talk back
I'm a loser. I'll never measure up. No one will ever want to chill out and hang with me.	I'm more than my problems. When I feel bad, I forget my strengths and focus on what I lack. I can't tell for sure if people will think I'm not chill enough to be with.

REMY: "I'm not a loser."

THERAPIST: Will that quiet it down?

REMY: No.

THERAPIST: Maybe I can get you started. How about trying something like: "I'm more than my problems. When I feel bad, I forget my strengths and focus most on what I lack." Can you tell for sure no one will ever think you are cool enough to hang out with?

REMY: I kind of get it. Like we said before, this trash is the depression talking. I can't tell anything for sure.

THERAPIST: Now you're talking back to the trash! Does this type of talk-back seem to work?

The therapist began with a more nondirectional stance which tested whether Remy could construct a coping response on her own. When she got stuck, the therapist became more directive and modeled an initial response. Then the therapist asked the question "Can you tell for sure?," which cast doubt on the certainty of Remy's belief.

HOT SHOTS, COOL THOUGHTS

Ages: All ages.

Purpose: Cognitive restructuring for anger.

Materials Needed:

- Nerf basketball and hoop.
- Hot Shots, Cool Thoughts Worksheet (Form 5.7).
- Paper and pencil.

Hot Shots, Cool Thoughts is a basic cognitive restructuring task for angry children and adolescents. It also includes fun basketball action. It is a very simple procedure. All you need is a Nerf basketball, a hoop, the Hot Shots, Cool Thoughts Worksheet (Form 5.7), and paper and pencil.

The procedure begins with the child lined up to take a shot at the basketball hoop. Before he shoots, you ask him, "What goes through your mind when you feel really angry?" The angry cognition is recorded. Once he or she crafts his or her cool thought, it is recorded, and the child is permitted to take his or her cool shot. The following dialogue with a 9-year-old boy named Emilio illustrates the process (see Figure 5.9).

EMILIO: I am angry and proud of it.

THERAPIST: I see that! How willing are you to try something different?

EMILIO: I don't know. I'm pretty good with who I am.

THERAPIST: Emilio, I know you love to draw and do art. I thought you were creative.

FIGURE 5.9. Emilio's Hot Shots, Cool Thoughts Worksheet.

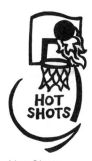

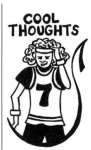

Hot Shots	Cool Thoughts
I will shut them up with my fists.	*I can draw them with their mouths stitched shut.*
I'll show them. Nobody is stronger than me. I am the fighting champ. I'll shove my foot up their ass.	*I want to put my foot up their ass to show them, but I lose power, strength, and control. Maybe I can stay in control by moving my seat and ignoring them.*

EMILIO: I am! My friends ask me to draw cartoons for them.

THERAPIST: So you are creative?

EMILIO: Sure.

THERAPIST: How about being creative with your anger?

EMILIO: How?

THERAPIST: With this game called Hot Shots, Cool Thoughts.

EMILIO: What is it?

THERAPIST: Here's what you do. You stand here on this line and take a shot at the basketball hoop and say one of your angry thoughts. That gets you one point. Then if you can turn the thought into a cool thought that doesn't get you fired up, you get two more points. You then take your shot. If you sink it, you get an extra point. The object is to get 20 points first.

EMILIO: OK. It is better than what we usually do.

THERAPIST: Good. Let's try one. Here's the ball. What goes through your mind when kids in your class make fun of you?

EMILIO: I'll shut them up with my fists.

THERAPIST: That's a hot thought for sure. One point for you. Now how do you get creative and cool off?

EMILIO: I can make them into a cartoon with their mouths stitched shut.

THERAPIST: So instead of hitting, you tell yourself to draw them.

EMILIO: Yeah.

THERAPIST: Good idea. Remember though, nothing violent in the drawing.

EMILIO: Yeah, you get an immediate out-of-school suspension for that.

THERAPIST: Two more points. Take your shot. (*Emilio misses.*) Good try. You've got three points already. Let's try another one. How about when you get angry on the bus?

EMILIO: They call me a faggot and poke pencils in my arm. They give me all sorts of shit.

THERAPIST: And what goes through your mind?

EMILIO: I'll show them. Nobody is stronger than me. I am the fighting champ.

THERAPIST: Anything else you can show them?

EMILIO: Like my foot up their ass?

THERAPIST: So do these hot thoughts work *on* you or *for* you?

EMILIO: I got bus suspension, so I guess *on* me.

THERAPIST: OK, one point for the hot thought. Then what else could you say to yourself for two more points?

EMILIO: I got nothing. You?

THERAPIST: How about I want to shove my foot up their ass to show them, but I lose control. Maybe I can stay in control by moving my seat and ignoring them.

EMILIO: Never thought about it that way.

THERAPIST: I guess you are doing something different. That is creative! Two points for you.

EMILIO: (*Shoots and then makes a basket.*) Cool. I've got seven points! When do you shoot?

In the work with Emilio, the therapist initially elicited Emilio's collaboration in the task. Then the therapist used Emilio's creativity as a tool to deal with his anger. When Emilio got stuck on a hot thought, the therapist modeled an appropriate self-instruction but then also reinforced Emilio's creativity.

EN FUEGO

Ages: 8–15 years.

Purpose: Cognitive restructuring with anger.

Materials Needed:

- En Fuego Diary (Form 5.8).
- Pencil or pen.

Angry children often seem like their minds and hearts are "on fire" ("en fuego" in Spanish). Cognitive restructuring aims to cool off hot-headed angry thoughts. En Fuego is an exercise where patients hose down their attributions, explanations, labels, and moral imperatives that fuel their angry fires. The patients work to exchange their "en fuego" thoughts with cool-headed interpretations.

In the first three columns of the En Fuego Diary, the child notes the date, the situation, and scales the intensity of the anger. Next, the child catches the thoughts that make him or her "en fuego," or on fire. Next, you and the child develop counterthoughts to put a chill on the en fuego thoughts. Like all of the cognitive restructuring tasks, it is best to use the child's wording. Last, the child rerates the intensity of the anger. We recommend that you coach the child to come up with a variety of coping statements. Having a supply of alternative thoughts gives the child more opportunity to cope. The children could carry a list of replacement thoughts to rely upon in "en fuego" moments in their life. They might use index cards or laminate a sheet of paper.

The following dialogue with 11-year-old Aubrey, who flies off the handle when her anger is ignited, steps you through the procedure (see Figure 5.10).

THERAPIST: Aubrey, do you know what *en fuego* means?

AUBREY: I heard it on that sports show my dad watches. I hate it when he watches because I want to watch *Hannah Montana*.

THERAPIST: Well, *en fuego* is Spanish for "on fire."

AUBREY: I don't take Spanish until next year.

THERAPIST: Well, I bet it seems like you are on fire when you get mad.

AUBREY: I really blow up.

THERAPIST: The other kids light you up.

AUBREY: I hate that.

FIGURE 5.10. Sample En Fuego Diary.

Date	Situation	How angry	En Fuego thought	Chill thought	New feeling
6/5	*Girls didn't play with me.*	*8*	*I hate them. I should throw a rock at them.*	*Rocks don't help me have friends. I can't count on rocks because they make things worse. I can't change them.*	*5*
6/6	*Girls didn't let me in group. I flipped the desk.*	*10*	*They hurt me so I should hurt them! I will get them back. I am helpless.*	*I can't change them by hurting them. If I go to the other group, I'm not so helpless and alone.*	

THERAPIST: For a take-charge girl like you, I am sure that sucks.

AUBREY: It does.

THERAPIST: Would you like to try this En Fuego Diary to see if it helps you not get lit up by the other kids?

AUBREY: OK.

THERAPIST: OK, let's write down some of the things that really make your anger catch fire. What happened today that made you mad?

AUBREY: Some girls did not play with me at recess. They were making a club I couldn't be in. I threw a rock at them. I hate them!

THERAPIST: Now comes the hard part. How do you cool that off?

AUBREY: I dunno.

THERAPIST: Did the rock make them want to play with you?

AUBREY: Duh … *no*!

THERAPIST: OK, what can you say about that?

AUBREY: Rocks don't help me make friends.

THERAPIST: Excellent start. What could you do to make friends or not get upset if they don't want to be friends.

AUBREY: Find someone else. Some girls are mean. I don't like it when they are that way.

THERAPIST: Can you change the other girls?

AUBREY: No, but *rocks can*!

THERAPIST: Now I see how you counted on the rocks. But did it work?

AUBREY: No.

THERAPIST: So rocks didn't help you. You couldn't count on the rocks and they even made things worse. Let's write that down. What does that do to your anger?

AUBREY: It goes down a little. I wish I could think like this on the playground.

THERAPIST: Me too. We'll work on that. It takes practice like what we are doing. Let's do another one. How about when you flipped the desk over in school?

AUBREY: You mean yesterday? That was a bad one. I melted down.

THERAPIST: Your en fuego flame melted you, didn't it?

AUBREY: Yeah, it did.

THERAPIST: So what happened and what went through your mind?

AUBREY: Kelsey, Michaela, Tori, and Elise all said they didn't want me to be in their group in language arts because my skirt and top didn't match. They said I dressed like a loser. They also said I didn't know how to use that stuff that goes under your arms. (*A little teary.*)

THERAPIST: You really felt hurt because they didn't let you in the group and made fun of you.

AUBREY: I wanted to hurt them.

THERAPIST: That's a hot en fuego thought! How can we cool it off?

AUBREY: (*Pause.*) I just hurt myself because I got sent to the principal.

THERAPIST: That's true. How much did you want to change their minds and make them let you in the group?

AUBREY: A lot.

THERAPIST: Could you change them?

AUBREY: No, I felt really bad.

THERAPIST: Did you feel alone and think you are helpless?

AUBREY: Yes.

THERAPIST: When girls like you feel alone and think they are helpless, they often count on being really tough and rough and flip desks. I get that, but here's the question—What did flipping the desk do to your helplessness and lonely feelings?

AUBREY: Made it worse, I guess.

THERAPIST: So what can you say to chill out when kids don't include you, you feel lonely, see yourself as helpless, and can't change them?

AUBREY: I can't change the girls. Maybe I should just be in a group with Bryn, Chelsea, and Abraham. They asked me and are my friends. Then I'm not so alone and helpless.

Several pivotal points are illustrated in this dialogue with Aubrey. First, the therapist engages Aubrey, but does not get sidetracked by some of her comments. The therapist is encouraging and uses Socratic questioning to help Aubrey shape her responses. As a result, the therapist and Aubrey work together to identify alternative thoughts through this cognitive restructuring technique.

MAD AT 'EM BALM

Ages: 8–15 years.

Purpose: Cognitive restructuring with anger; useful with inaccurate interpersonal perceptions.

Materials Needed:

- Anger Balms (Form 5.9).
- Mad at 'Em Balm Diary (Form 5.10).
- Pen or pencil.

Angry youngsters perceive themselves to be under attack by unfair rules and demands. Moreover, they see themselves as deliberately assaulted and injured by others. Their sense of justice and control are compromised. Moreover, angry and aggressive patients may see their self-esteem as threatened (A. T. Beck, 1976). Not surprisingly, feeling hurt and helpless may underlie their angry moods (Padesky, 1988). As a means to regain control and competence, angry youngsters externalize responsibility, blame others, and lash out aggressively.

Mad at 'Em Balm is a cognitive restructuring procedure focused on soothing the real or perceived hurts children experience. Moreover, by helping patients reframe their angry thoughts, they regain a lost sense of control. Mad at 'Em Balm is essentially a play on words older children and adolescents may find intriguing. It is recommended for older children who are predominately triggered by inaccurate interpersonal perceptions.

"Mad at 'Em Balm" sounds like "Mad Atom Bomb" until it is deconstructed and explained in therapy. While most youngsters know what an atom bomb is, few are likely to know the word *balm*. The explanation process primes the youngster for the procedure. The following dialogue illustrates the process with Talia, a very bright 11-year-old girl with an explosive temper and extremely low frustration tolerance.

THERAPIST: Talia, I want to explain something to you. Sometimes two words may sound alike but be spelled very differently and have very different meanings.

TALIA: I think we learned about this in language arts.

THERAPIST: Here is one that I hope you find interesting: *bomb* and *balm*. (*Writes on a white board.*) You know what a B-O-M-B is, but what is a B-A-L-M?

TALIA: Don't have a clue.

THERAPIST: B-A-L-M is something you put on a hurt or wound that makes it less painful.

TALIA: Kind of like Neosporin.

THERAPIST: Exactly. So there can be different meanings to the same word sound. Just like there are many ways to see a situation. You just have to be careful in understanding a situation.

In this introduction, the therapist primed Talia for the intervention by helping her see that the same-sounding word (e.g., *situation*) could have very different meanings. Talia learned that a "balm" is a soothing intervention that decreases pain. The therapist also reinforced the notion that Talia should be cautious in interpreting situations.

Once the priming is completed, the actual procedure is introduced using the Mad at 'Em Balm Diary (Form 5.10). Like En Fuego, the first four columns of the form record the date, situation, anger intensity, and angry attributions. The "balm" process involves teaching children to question the inaccurate interpersonal perceptions that shape aggressive behavior. These can include deliberate hostile attributions, a sense of unfairness, violation of moral rules and imperatives, all-or-none labeling of others, pressure to relieve the self from irritating emotions (e.g., embarrassment, anger, sadness), perceptions of helplessness, and a sense of victimization. The Anger Balms (Form 5.9) are questions that patients can apply to wounds associated with their aggressive behavior and impulsive emotional responding. The youngsters apply the balm in column five. The last column records the anger intensity accompanying these balm statements. Similar to En Fuego, patients should develop many balm statements to apply in multiple situations. The following transcript illustrates the cognitive restructuring component with Talia. Her Mad at 'Em Balm Diary can be seen in Figure 5.11.

FIGURE 5.11. Talia's Mad at 'Em Balm Diary.

Date	Situation	How angry	Thought that hurt	Balm statements that help	New feeling
3/7	Amber gave me the stink eye.	9	She's trying to make me look bad in front of Stacie.	I am only part sure that she is trying to make me look bad in front of Stacie.	6
3/8	Mom invaded my privacy.	10	She broke my rules for her. I must punish her by breaking her vase.	I want my mom to respect me but she will make mistakes. I would like to forgive her but I don't know how.	5
3/10	Teacher yelled at me.	8	This is unfair. She always picks on me and likes the Barbies more.	I could just pay attention to myself and my work. I don't have to compete with the Barbies. This is something I am in charge of.	3

THERAPIST: Talia, let's take a look at some of these questions that may be a balm for your anger. (*Shows Talia.*) These questions may help you come up with a balm to take care of the angry thought that hurts you and other people. Which one might fit with the first situation?

TALIA: The first thing that gave me trouble was when Amber gave me the stink eye and I thought she was trying to make me look bad in front of my new friend, Stacie.

THERAPIST: OK. What on the list can you ask yourself?

TALIA: How sure am I that my new guess is true?

THERAPIST: OK, how sure are you?

TALIA: Part.

THERAPIST: Let's write that down. What does that do to your anger?

TALIA: Makes it less.

THERAPIST: Let's try one of your other ones.

TALIA: My mother got on my phone and checked on my texts and she tries to listen when I talk to my friends when we hang out. I hate that. She invades my privacy, so I broke her vase to punish her.

THERAPIST: OK. Try a balm.

TALIA: There could be two. Am I expecting others to completely follow my rules? and How forgiving am I?

THERAPIST: So how do you answer your questions?

TALIA: I do expect my mom to obey my wishes, and I am not forgiving.

THERAPIST: I see. How can you soothe that pain?

TALIA: I guess I want my mother to respect me, but even she makes mistakes. She doesn't like me to make mistakes.

THERAPIST: Can you forgive her and not punish a mistake?

TALIA: I would like to.

THERAPIST: Let's write that down. What does that do to your anger?

TALIA: Helps me a little.

THERAPIST: Let's do one more.

TALIA: I flipped out when the teacher told me to stop talking and disturbing the class. She always picks on me and favors the popular girls. The Barbies.

THERAPIST: What balm can you use?

TALIA: What is my responsibility and how helpless am I?

THERAPIST: OK, so what do you think?

TALIA: I could just pay attention to my work and not compete with the Barbies all the time. This is something I am in charge of.

THERAPIST: What does that do to your anger and sense of control?

TALIA: It helps a lot. But I wish I could do this at the time.

THERAPIST: That's what we are going to do next. First, write down these new balm statements on these index cards and read them over three times per day. I want you to carry balm statements around with you and each time you feel yourself getting angry think of a question to soothe yourself. Last, do an entry in the Mad at 'Em Balm Diary every time you get angry.

The therapist's work with Talia illustrates how to use the balm questions to construct a coping response. Additionally, the therapist gave Talia a homework assignment so she could apply the acquired skills in naturally occurring situations.

TAMING THE IMPULSE MONSTER

Ages: 8–13 years.

Purpose: Cognitive restructuring for impulsivity and emotional reasoning.

Materials Needed:

• Taming the Impulse Monster Worksheet (Form 5.11).
• Pen or pencil.

Taming the Impulse Monster is a cognitive restructuring intervention for children directed by emotional reasoning (e.g., Prisoner of Feeling) and impulsive behavior. Impulsive behavior by nature refers to acting without forethought. Consequently, cognitive mediation is lacking. Taming the Impulse Monster is a way for impulsive children to build cognitive bridges that lead them forward to more productive and adaptive action.

Similar to the other tasks in the text, Taming the Impulse Monster is presented in several graduated steps. First, the impulse monster cartoon is presented and children's impulsive thoughts are recorded.

THERAPIST: Let's look at this cartoon, Lexi. When you feel like you have to speak out or touch somebody else's school supplies, it's like an impulse monster is telling you to do these things. It's a voice inside you that does not think about what happens next. How does this sound?

LEXI: A little confusing. Do I look like that inside my head?

THERAPIST: (Smiles.) No. We're just giving your inner voice a face to it. It might make it easier to catch your thought.

LEXI: Oh, OK.

THERAPIST: Now let's write down what goes on inside your head when you speak out of turn or take your classmate's gel pens. You see the gel pen on the desk and it looks really cool. What does your impulse monster say to you?

LEXI: Grab it. It looks really fun.

THERAPIST: Great. Let's write down what the impulse monster says here [see Figure 5.12].

FIGURE 5.12. Lexi's Taming the Impulse Monster Worsheet.

Situation *Sees Gel pens*

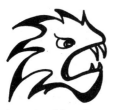	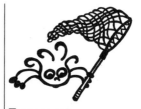
Impulse Monster says	Tamer says
Grab it. It looks fun.	*Look with your eyes and not with your hands.*

The therapist next introduces the trainer-or-tamer component. The trainer-or-tamer is the figure that represents the cognitive restructuring component.

THERAPIST: Let's look at this person. This is the tamer whose job it is to teach or train the impulse monster. How do you think she can train the impulse monster?

LEXI: (*Silent.*)

THERAPIST: What can she say to the impulse monster to help her not to take the gel pen?

LEXI: Maybe she could say, "Look with your eyes, not with your hands."

THERAPIST: That's a good start. Write that in the tamer column. You are starting to tame the impulse monster.

In the above dialogue the therapist patiently stepped Lexi through both the self-monitoring and self-instruction process. Lexi did not respond to the open-ended question, "How do you think she can train the impulse monster?" The therapist then self-corrected with a more concrete question, "What can she say to the impulse monster to help her not to take the gel pens?" Then the therapist reinforced her coping efforts.

RANK YOUR WORRIES

Ages: 8–18 years.

Purpose: Decreasing overestimation of magnitude and probability of anticipated dangers; decreasing catastrophizing.

Materials Needed:

- Rank Your Worries Worksheet (Form 5.12).
- Pen or pencil.

As stated in Chapter 2, anxious children tend to overestimate the probability and magnitude of danger and threats. Essentially, this tendency contributes to catastrophizing (e.g., Disaster Forecaster thinking). Rank Your Worries is a cognitive restructuring procedure that tests children's estimations of the danger's probability and magnitude. It makes use of scaling procedures and some simple Socratic questioning.

Rank Your Worries is completed in several phases. In phase 1, the worries and fears are listed. Phase 2 involves rating how bad or awful the event would be if it actually occurred. Phase 3 invites the child to rank the likelihood or probability of the danger. The scaling procedure in phases 2 and 3 sets up the restructuring process as well as simultaneously challenging the child's all-or-none reasoning (one-eyed ogre thinking). When children rank their estimations, they begin to see their worries on a continuum.

The restructuring process begins with an evaluation of the awfulness ratings. Then it moves to a review of the probability rankings. In the final synthesizing stage, the child compares the probability and magnitude rankings and builds a conclusion. The following dialogue illustrates the cognitive restructuring process with a 10-year-old girl named Idina, who struggles with generalized anxiety and separation anxiety.

THERAPIST: Idina, I see you finished the Rank Your Worries Worksheet [See Figure 5.13].

IDINA: (*Sighs.*) I did. I wrote down a lot of worries.

THERAPIST: How willing are you to take a fresh look at them?

IDINA: It'd be OK.

THERAPIST: Well, with all these worries going on inside your head, no wonder you feel so tired and your stomach hurts a lot. Let's see if we can make sense of this list. Let's take a look at how likely the worries are. How many of the worries are higher than 5 on the likely column?

IDINA: (*Counts.*) Five.

THERAPIST: How many are less than 5?

IDINA: 10.

THERAPIST: Which are more? The highly likely ones or the not very likely ones?

IDINA: (*Excitedly.*) Less likely by 2 to 1!

THERAPIST: So what do you take from this?

IDINA: Many of my worries are not very likely.

THERAPIST: Now write that on a card. Next, let's look at both the bad and likely column. Let's look at just the really awful worries, ones that are 7 or higher. How many are there?

IDINA: 10

THERAPIST: Now of these 10, how many are higher than 5 in the likely column?

IDINA: (*Surprisingly.*) None?

THERAPIST: It looks like that. Now, of the really less awful worries, how many are very likely?

IDINA: All of them!

FIGURE 5.13. Idina's Rank Your Worries Worksheet.

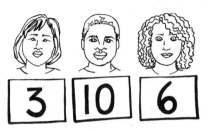

Worry	How bad/awful	How likely
Mom being bit by a snake	9	2
Dad having a heart attack	10	3
Mom and Dad being kidnapped	10	1
House catching fire	9	2
Car accident	8	3
Tornado	7	3
Tsunami	8	1
Getting an F	8	1
Throwing up	5	7
Friends being mean	5	7
Getting in trouble at school	8	3
Losing my favorite toy	5	8
Burglar breaking into the house	9	2
Mom yelling at me	4	9
Falling off my bike	5	9

THERAPIST: What do you make of that?

IDINA: All of my really *bad* worries are not very likely. The ones that are most likely are the not-so-bad ones.

THERAPIST: Let's put that on another card!

The therapist's work with Idina illustrates several key points. First, the therapist begins with an empathic response and then coaches Idina through the procedure with specific questions. The therapist stops midway through and at the end of the process to ask synthesizing questions (e.g., "What do you take from this?"; "What do you make of that?"). Finally, the therapist encourages Idina to record conclusions on cards.

CUT THE KNOT

Ages: 8–13 years.

Purpose: Breaking inaccurate contingencies involving self-worth.

Materials Needed:

- Construction paper.
- Scissors.
- Marker or pen.
- String or ties.

Cut the Knot is a self-instructional exercise that works to break inaccurate contingencies between patients' views of themselves and others and some unrealistic standard. The literature often speaks about this as a "contingent self-worth" (Kuiper, Olinger, & MacDonald, 1988). Moreover, most common cognitive errors or "dirty tricks" involve "magical thinking" (Einstein & Menzies, 2006) (e.g., Tragic Magic). In cognitive therapy, magical thinking posits a superstitious-like relationship between two elements based on chance correlations. Often, this process is all over OCD symptoms such as, "If I see a black spot on the sidewalk, I'll get cancer or if I move when the clock hands are on 7 or 3, I'll have bad luck my entire life."

In one form, Cut the Knot involves identifying various stems such as "If ..., then ...," "I am ...," and "People must ...." Often these stems and conditions are readily recognized through the case conceptualization processes detailed in Chapter 1. The second step involves determining the unreasonable conditions that must be met (e.g., "If I am perfect, I am always in control. Thus, perfection is determined by absolute control over everything."). Figure 5.14 provides some example stems and conditions. Once these stems and conditions are named, they are written on long strips of construction paper.

The next step involves punching a hole in the back of the stem and in front of the conditional statement. The stem and condition are then tied together and knotted with string, ribbon, or plastic cording. Once they are connected, the therapist initiates a Socratic dialogue aimed at breaking this spurious correlation. After the Socratic dialogue is completed, the therapist invites the child to cut the knot and replace the absolutistic demand with a more functional alternative.

The following sample dialogue with DeMarcus, a perfectionistic 11-year-old boy, illustrates the process.

THERAPIST: OK, DeMarcus, so we defined you "measuring up" as you being the best-behaved child in your family, as always winning the school spelling contests, being named to the Little League All-Star team every year, being the most popular boy in your class, and always getting all A's.

DEMARCUS: That's what I wrote.

THERAPIST: OK. Let's tie these things together. (*They tie these statements together.*) [See Figure 5.15.]

FIGURE 5.14. Sample stems and conditions for Cut the Knot.

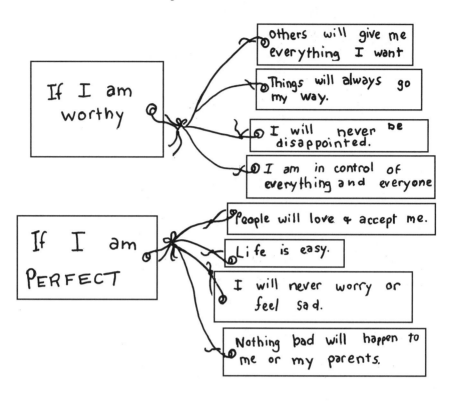

FIGURE 5.15. DeMarcus's Cut the Knot stem and conditions before cognitive restructuring.

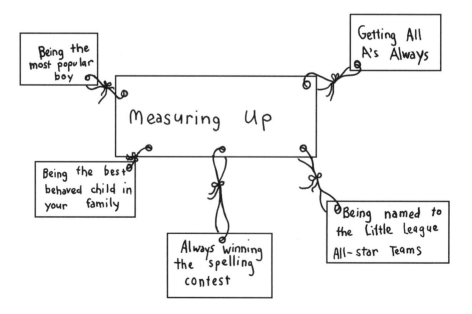

DeMarcus: Wow, this is heavy.

Therapist: Yeah, it's a lot of weight on you to carry these expectations. Would you like to cut some of the ties?

DeMarcus: Sure.

Therapist: Which one first?

DeMarcus: Always winning the spelling contests.

Therapist: OK, cut it. (*DeMarcus cuts it off.*) Now we have to replace it with something that won't weigh you down as much. What can you say to yourself about the spelling bee?

DeMarcus: Trying my best isn't the same as having to be the best all the time.

Therapist: Good, DeMarcus, write that on this paper. (*Therapist and DeMarcus punch holes in the paper and tie it to "measuring up."*)

The therapist used DeMarcus's sense that the construction was "heavy" to illustrate how unreasonable demands can "weigh him down." When these unrealistic demands were removed, they needed to be replaced rather than simply eliminated. Each of the conditions for "measuring up" (e.g., being the best-behaved child, always winning the spelling contests, being named to the Little League All-Star team, being the most popular boy in school, and always getting A's) was written on a separate piece of paper and then tied to a bigger strip of paper with "measuring up" written on it.

Through the Socratic dialogue, the therapist helped DeMarcus separate the burdensome conditions from the idea of measuring up. The process was concretized by cutting the string between measuring up and its dysfunctional conditions. The procedure concluded with the therapist and DeMarcus writing a more functional condition (e.g., "Trying my best isn't the same as having to be the best all the time.") to replace the burdensome one on a blank strip of paper and making a new connection to measuring up by tying it to the paper with "Measuring Up" written on it. The above dialogue and process with DeMarcus continued until all the absolutistic criteria were replaced (see Figure 5.16).

Another way to use Cut the Knot requires scissors, a pencil, and a sheet of paper. In step 1, the patient's goal is identified (e.g., What is it you want most of all? What do you most of all want to happen?). Then in a rectangle in the center of the page, the therapist writes the child's goals in terms of fundamental motivations, such as control, approval, success, perfection, and so on. Step 3 involves writing down, around the rectangle, the magical ways the patient is going about pursuing these goals (e.g., washing hands seven times, ordering Pokemon cards, avoiding conflict, choosing only particular pens; see Figure 5.17). In step 4, the therapist tries to create doubt regarding the child's hypothesized correlation between the goals and the way he or she goes about attaining them (e.g., "How much are these things truly tied to success? Do you think these things are the most powerful ways to get success? If there are more powerful determinants of success, are the things on the paper linked to it? What should we do?"). In the final step the therapist cuts around the rectangle, effectively separating the goal from its capricious determining factors. The therapist then "cements" the lesson of the procedure by handing the patient the goals contained in the rectangle (e.g., control). The process ends with

FIGURE 5.16. DeMarcus's Cut the Knot stem and cognitions after cognitive restructuring.

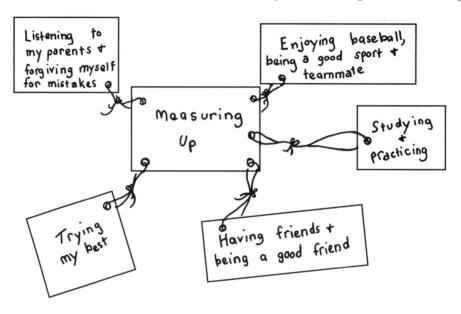

FIGURE 5.17. Cut the Knot for fundamental motivations.

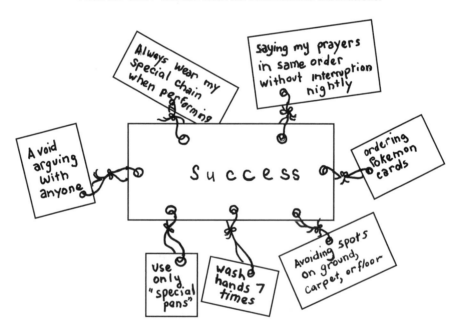

a Socratic dialogue (e.g., "So what do you have in your hand? So is it possible to hold on to control without having to _____? Does it seem like these behaviors and your goal are two separate things?").

We like this exercise because it does not blame the children for their symptoms. The procedure communicates that the child is well intentioned but misguided. The goal is a good one (e.g., success, control, approval), but the strategies designed to achieve it are flawed.

WANTING VERSUS WILLING

Ages: 8–18 years.

Purpose: Helping distinguish willingness from wanting; increasing willingness to confront discomfort and distress.

Materials Needed:

- Wanting versus Willing Worksheet (Form 5.13).
- Pencil or pen.

Most children and adolescents do not want to experience discomfort and distress. They often actively avoid emotional stimulation and negative affect in order to shield or protect themselves. Therefore, they may present in an emotionally absent and sanitized manner. They disengage from treatment tasks and work hard to keep their negative feelings at bay. They mistakenly believe they have to want to face their distress in order to confront it. However, they only have to be willing to approach distress. In our view, the task of the cognitive-behavioral therapist is to increase patients' willingness. The Wanting versus Willing exercise is a way to separate willingness from desire, and to increase willingness.

The notion that patients will confuse willingness with wanting is embraced by conventional cognitive-behavioral therapists as well as newer third-wave cognitive-behaviorally based approaches such as acceptance and commitment therapy (ACT; Hayes et al., 1999). We further believe willingness and wanting are situational and contextual. Thus, they may be scaled relatively and sequentially processed.

Wanting versus Willing begins with making a distinction between the two. The following dialogue with Dana, a 16-year-old female with depression, self-mutilation, emotional intolerance, and disruptive behavior, illustrates the initial stage. Her Wanting versus Willing Worksheet can be seen in Figure 5.18.

THERAPIST: Dana, it seems you are stuck. Kind of frozen in place and unable to move one way or another.

DANA: Nothing's changing. I hate this.

THERAPIST: So let's try to unfreeze you. What are you willing to work on?

DANA: I really hate talking and feeling bad.

THERAPIST: Are you willing to feel bad for a period of time before things change for the better?

FIGURE 5.18. Dana's Wanting versus Willing Worksheet.

Action	Wanting	Willing
Talk about negative feelings	2	5
Feel anxious, sad, angry	2	4
Stop cutting myself	5	6
Come in at curfew	2	5
Do homework	3	5
Stay in school without skipping	3	6

DANA: No, I don't want to.

THERAPIST: You sure are impatient. I understand you are in a hurry to feel better. But I didn't ask you if you wanted to feel bad. Few people want to feel bad, but are you willing to?

DANA: What's the fucking difference?

THERAPIST: Well, for me, wanting is liking or preferring to do something. How about you?

DANA: Sure.

THERAPIST: Willing is different. How do you see it as different?

DANA: I don't know.

THERAPIST: Willing seems to be about being open to new challenges, being agreeable to experiment. Maybe even a little adventurous.

DANA: Like risk taking?

THERAPIST: Sure.

In this dialogue, the therapist gently broached Dana's therapeutic paralysis. Since Dana is a highly emotionally reactive adolescent, the therapist proceeded slowly and liberally used empathy. He also used a frozen metaphor to illustrate Dana's inertia. Finally, he modeled a definition of wanting and willing and then encouraged Dana's collaboration. Wanting versus Willing continues with more specific processing, as illustrated below.

THERAPIST: Dana, let's list the things you feel stuck about.

DANA: Where should we start?

THERAPIST: That's up to you.

DANA: Like I said, I hate talking about negative feelings.

THERAPIST: How about actually having them?

DANA: That sucks too.

THERAPIST: What about the cutting on yourself?

DANA: Yeah, I'm stuck to that.

THERAPIST: We're developing a good-size list.

DANA: I keep breaking curfew and blowing off my homework.

THERAPIST: What else about school?

DANA: Skipping class is big.

THERAPIST: OK, now look at these columns. I titled them "Wanting" and "Willing." Let's rate them on a 1–10 scale. How does this sound?

DANA: OK, I guess.

THERAPIST: How much do you want to talk about negative feelings?

DANA: Umm, a 2.

THERAPIST: How willing?

DANA: Maybe a 5.

THERAPIST: How much do you want to feel anxious, sad, and angry?

DANA: A 1.

THERAPIST: How willing are you?

DANA: A 3.

THERAPIST: How much do you want to stop cutting?

DANA: A 5.

THERAPIST: And how willing?

DANA: 6.

THERAPIST: Coming in at curfew?

DANA: Wanting a 2, willing a 6.

THERAPIST: One more to do.

DANA: Not skipping. Hmm. Wanting is a 3 and willing is a 6. Now what?

THERAPIST: Let's compare the columns. Which column has the higher number?

DANA: The willing. So?

THERAPIST: What do you make of that?

DANA: I don't want to do those things.

THERAPIST: Do you think you have to want to do something to be willing to do it?

DANA: I don't know.

THERAPIST: Well, let's check out your ratings. If you believed that you have to want to do something to do it, would the numbers be the same or different?

DANA: The same, I guess.

THERAPIST: So let's look and check it out.

DANA: Hmm. They are all pretty much different.... I guess I don't have to want to do something to be willing to.

THERAPIST: Let's write that on a card.

During the work with Dana, the therapist maintained a collaborative stance. Then the therapist asked simple synthesizing questions to help Dana analyze complex information. ("Do you think you have to want to do something to be willing to do it?" "If you believed that you have to want to do something to be willing to do it, would the numbers be the same or different?")

DON'T AVOID, RATHER ENGAGE (DARE)

Ages: 8–18 years.

Purpose: Preparation for exposure and behavioral experiments.

Materials Needed:

- Paper.
- Pencil or pen.

Don't Avoid, Rather Engage (DARE) is a cognitive restructuring exercise that prepares young patients for exposure and behavioral experiments. Experiential avoidance characterizes many patients' approach to emotional challenges. Experiential avoidance includes maladaptive actions to escape from aversive private thoughts, feelings, and bodily reactions (Hayes, 1994; Hayes et al., 1999). Experiential avoidance exists on a continuum and becomes troublesome when excessive time and effort is spent escaping these thoughts, feelings, and physiological reactions (Kashdan, Barrios, Forsyth, & Steger, 2006). Kashdan and colleagues noted that this avoidance compromises goal attainment and distances oneself from others and their own experiences.

The more patients inhibit unwanted thoughts and feelings, the more they paradoxically intensify them (D. Clark, 2004; Gross, 2002). Then, because experiential avoidance worsens patients' disconnection to others as well as to their own experiences, there is also a loss of pleasure (Gross & John, 2003). Hayes and colleagues (1999) proposed that experiential avoidance intensifies and interferes with a person's ability to live and act in a way that is congruent with one's values. Thus, freedom is restricted and the person is less able to take productive action.

Experiential avoidance may be mediated by various beliefs (Leahy, 2007). Some patients may believe that if they allow themselves to feel certain emotions, they will lose control. Others may believe that negative emotions such as anger, shame, sadness, anxiety, and guilt are bad. Therefore, experiencing and expressing emotions may lead to self-punishment and/or punishment from others. Additionally, many patients hold a sort of emotional perfectionism, where negative emotions are seen as personal flaws. Simply, they neglect the reality that human distress is universal and inevitable (Hayes et al., 1999; Leahy, 2007).

DARE involves helping patients see the advantages of distressing emotions. You and the patient work to develop a number of coping self-statements about experiencing

FIGURE 5.19. Sample DARE statements.

- Everyone feels bad sometimes. It makes me more human.
- Coping with bad feelings makes me stronger than avoiding them.
- Distress is uncomfortable, not disastrous.
- Distress is time-limited; feelings change.
- It says more about me that I can handle feeling uncomfortable than if I always feel comfortable.
- Feeling uncomfortable means I am challenging myself.
- I can step into discomfort rather than walking away from it.
- Distress means I value something.

distress. Figure 5.19 contains a number of sample DARE statements. The patient next puts some DARE-prepared statements on cards and then constructs some original ones, which are also placed on coping cards. The following dialogue with 17-year-old Grace, a depressed and self-mutilating patient who engages in considerable emotional avoidance, shows how to use DARE.

THERAPIST: Grace, what makes talking about your thoughts and feelings so difficult?

GRACE: It's painful. I'd rather just not deal with it.

THERAPIST: And what's so bad about feeling bad?

GRACE: I just shouldn't. Bad feelings are a weakness. You shouldn't have any negative feelings. You should always be happy. Life should be like a Disney movie.

THERAPIST: A Disney movie? Which one?

GRACE: (*Smiles.*) I loved *Aladdin*. When I was a girl, Jasmine was my hero.

THERAPIST: Really? And in that story, everything was perfect for her?

GRACE: (*Pause.*) No. She was lonely and her father overprotected her.

THERAPIST: Kind of like you.

GRACE: I never thought about it, but yeah.

THERAPIST: So what do you think of this princess who was lonely?

GRACE: I thought she was cool.

THERAPIST: Cool?

GRACE: Yeah, she was so strong when she escaped from the palace.

THERAPIST: So her strength spoke to you.

GRACE: Yeah, she was kind of fearless and daring.

THERAPIST: Did her strength come from avoiding or from facing her bad feelings?

GRACE: She faced them.

THERAPIST: I really liked your word, *daring*. A tool I want to tell you about is called DARE. It stands for "Don't Avoid, Rather Engage." To DARE, you need to say certain things to yourself so you are willing to face what you run from. Here is a list of DARE statements. Let's see if together we are able to come up with some more.

The therapist first elicited the beliefs buttressing Grace's experiential avoidance ("It's painful. I'd rather not deal with it." "Bad feelings are a weakness."). The therapist then aligned with Grace's avoidance ("Life should be like a Disney movie.") and a coping model emerged (Jasmine). Further, Grace fortuitously used the word *daring*, which led nicely to the DARE technique.

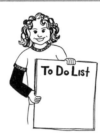

BOX 5.1 Summary Pad for Cognitive Restructuring/Self-Instruction

When to use:

- After the child/adolescent has been educated to the model (psychoeducation).
- After the child/adolescent has identified thoughts, feelings, and behaviors (self-monitoring).
- Before rational analysis.

For what purpose:

- Replacing inaccurate and unproductive self-talk with more accurate inner dialogue that guides productive behavior.

How to use it:

- Use simple engaging procedures that may include metaphors, stories, puppets, and toys.
- Make it fun.
- Make use of patients' own language.
- Be sure it addresses the patients' negative thoughts, problem situations, and distressing situations.
- Avoid absolutistic self-talk (e.g., "I'm a good person."; "Everything will be OK.").
- Include an action plan (e.g., "I am going to practice my thought skills.").

CONCLUSION

Many engaging and effective cognitive restructuring interventions are outlined in this chapter. It is up to you to choose the ones that will be most effective for the individual client. Keeping the case conceptualization in mind will guide you to the appropriate interventions. The case conceptualization will also provide you with important information for fitting the techniques to each patient, helping make each intervention come alive and be meaningful.

Matching techniques to clients' interests, skill level, and presenting problems is challenging. Keeping interventions fun, including the child's point of view and language, and frequently revisiting the case conceptualization is recommended. When you use the cognitive restructuring interventions to address the youths' "hot thoughts," the techniques will assist in modifying cognitions and developing a problem-solving plan, rather than simply replacing the negative thoughts with positive ones. Through this process patients create a change in their cognitive processes, behaviors, and emotional functioning.

Handprint on Your Heart

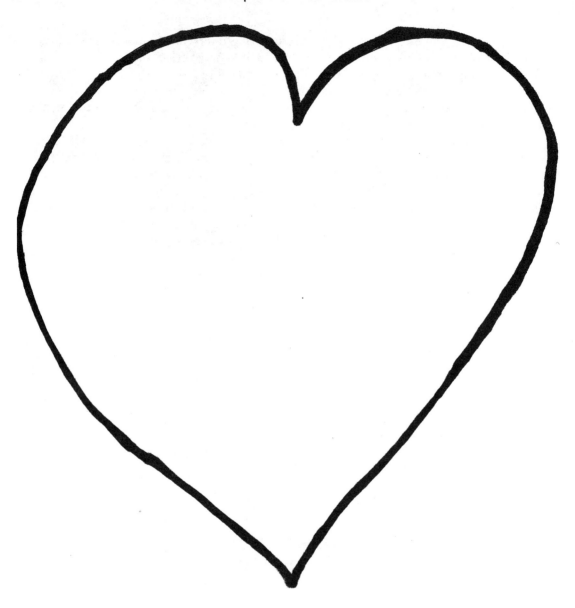

Are You Ready for Some Changes? Questionnaire

My problem is _____.

It bothers me (circle one number):

1	2	3	4	5	6	7
Not at all			Kind of			A lot

I feel out of control and helpless because of it.

1	2	3	4	5	6	7
Not at all			Kind of			A lot

I think people my age have this type of problem.

1	2	3	4	5	6	7
Not many			Some			Many

I am sure that my treatment will help.

1	2	3	4	5	6	7
Not at all			Kind of			Totally

I want to change my thoughts, feelings, and behaviors.

1	2	3	4	5	6	7
Do not			Kind of			Totally

I am trying to change my thoughts, feelings, and behaviors.

1	2	3	4	5	6	7
Not			Kind of			Really

I think I am able to change my thoughts, feelings, and behaviors.

1	2	3	4	5	6	7
Do not			Kind of			Really

Trick or Truth Diary

Date	Situation	Feeling	Thought	Dirty trick	Truth or trick	Problem solving

FORM 5.4

Clean Up Your Thinking Diary

Date	Situation	Feeling	Thought	Dirty trick	Clean-up strategy	Fresh thought

179

Swat the Bug

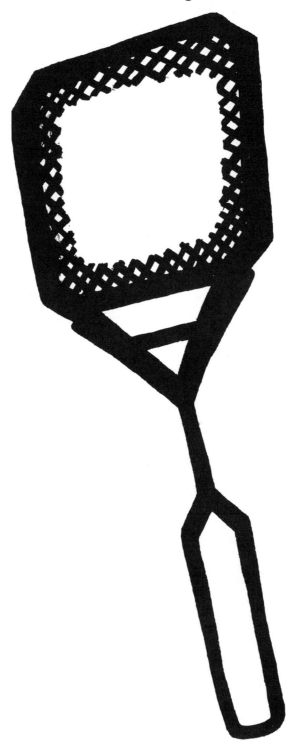

FORM 5.6

Trash Talk Worksheet

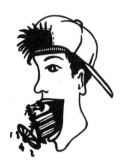

Trash I say to myself	My talk back

Hot Shots, Cool Thoughts Worksheet

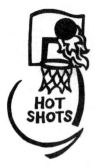

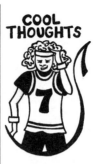

Hot Shots	Cool Thoughts

FORM 5.8

En Fuego Diary

Date	Situation	How angry	En Fuego thought	Chill thought	New feeling

Anger Balms

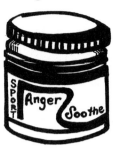

Am I confusing something done by accident with something done on purpose?

How sure am I that my guess about people's actions is true?

Am I confusing things being unfair with things just not going my way?

Do I think this is just happening to me or does this happen to everyone once in awhile?

Am I expecting others to completely follow all my rules?

Do other people know my rules?

How forgiving am I willing to be when people break my rules?

Am I seeing people in just one way? Can anyone be all one way all the time?

How accepting am I of my own bad feelings? Do I believe I must get rid of these feelings?

Am I getting rid of my own unwanted feelings by hurting other people?

How do I define power and control? Do I confuse self-control with controlling other people?

How helpless am I in the situation?

What is my responsibility for what happens to me?

FORM 5.10

Mad at 'Em Balm Diary

Date	Situation	How angry	Thought that hurt	Balm statements that help	New feeling

185

Taming the Impulse Monster Worksheet

Situation _____

Impulse Monster says	Tamer says

Rank Your Worries Worksheet

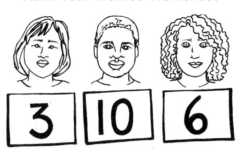

Worry	How bad/awful	How likely

FORM 5.13

Wanting versus Willing Worksheet

Action	Wanting	Willing

CHAPTER 6

Rational Analysis

R ational analysis procedures are the most sophisticated cognitive interventions. They are used to create doubt in children's firmly held beliefs. Bandura (1977b; 1986) stated that people's beliefs or personal rules are acquired logically and that rational processes are ways to validate the accuracy of conclusions. Moreover, Bandura cogently noted that logical errors may emerge from misleading appearances, insufficient evidence, overgeneralization, selection biases, and faulty inductive and deductive processes.

This chapter outlines various methods for evaluating the accuracy and usefulness of thoughts, assumptions, and beliefs, and for changing maladaptive and/or inaccurate patterns. Because rational analysis involves collecting and evaluating data, the process must remain collaborative rather than directive. Older children and adolescents with stronger verbal skills tend to benefit from rational analysis techniques. Metaphors make rational analysis more accessible for younger children. Basic skill acquisition in cognitive identification should occur prior to using rational analysis strategies to challenge and modify thoughts.

AN OVERVIEW OF RATIONAL ANALYSIS METHODS

There are different ways to conduct rational analysis (Beal, Kopec, & DiGiuseppe, 1996; J. S. Beck, 1995; Fennell, 1989). Tests of evidence, reattribution, advantages and disadvantages, problem solving, and decatastrophizing represent the major methods for rational analysis.

Tests of evidence encourage young patients to evaluate the factual basis of their beliefs, conclusions, and assumptions. It is a hypothesis-testing approach. Essentially, a test of evidence coaches children through the process of collecting the facts supporting and disconfirming their beliefs. Then they analyze the evidence and subsequently construct more accurate appraisals after a mindful weighing of the data.

Reattribution involves the search for alternative explanations. Reattribution teaches patients that there are always different ways of looking at the same realities.

The procedure requires children to examine their experiences from different angles. After reattribution, children learn to reframe their problematic interpretations from a new perspective.

Examining the advantages and disadvantages is cognitive cost–benefit analysis. When employing advantages and disadvantages techniques, children see what they gain and lose by holding on to a specific behavioral strategy, distressing emotion, or belief. After deliberating the pros and cons, children derive a reasoned conclusion.

Problem solving is yet another form of rational analysis. Generally, problem-solving efforts are directed toward making rigid thinking patterns more flexible. The search for alternative solutions and rewards for successful experimentation with productive strategies is a common approach. Generally, problem solving involves specifying the problem, brainstorming all possible options, evaluating the short- and long-term positive and negative consequences for each option, experimenting with an option, and self-rewarding for productive problem solving. Recently, Padesky (2007) crafted two creative Socratic questions that can be easily added to problem solving. The first is a simple query that states how well current problem-solving efforts do in resolving distress ("Does _____ make a positive difference in your life?"). The second question examines whether problem solving comes at a cost to self or others ("Is _____ a compassionate way to treat yourself? Other people in your life?").

Decatastrophizing focuses on logically evaluating the probability (How likely?) of a predicted catastrophe, predicting the magnitude of the disaster (How bad would it be?), and problem solving to either prevent it or cope with it once it occurs. The problem-solving component adds data for the rational analysis. If you can prevent or cope with the catastrophe, how bad could it be?

Rational analysis also makes use of the *universal definitions* process (Overholser, 1994). This process broadens children's narrow and limiting definitions of themselves and others. There are several steps in developing universal definitions. First, you elicit the specifics of the child's self-definition. Next, you rate the importance of each circumstance or characteristic. Then you work with the youngster to select a person who embodies the opposite of the child's self-definition. The child is asked to reflect on the similarities between these "opposites." Finally, you switch back to a personal perspective and broaden the child's self-definition. The steps in universal definitions are demonstrated in the Mirror, Mirror technique presented later in this chapter. It is particularly useful for self-blaming and other-blaming attributions that are punctuated by inaccurate labeling.

These primary means of rational analysis can be applied in multiple, creative ways for children and adolescents with various presenting problems and levels of functioning. As with other cognitive techniques addressed in this text, the selection of each rational analysis method should be grounded in the case conceptualization. Furthermore, the process of using the rational analysis technique is as important as the technique itself. Thus, the therapist is careful to use guided discovery and Socratic questioning while applying the rational analysis methods.

METAPHORS IN RATIONAL ANALYSIS

Metaphors and stories are good rational analysis strategies to help young people loosen up rigid thinking, feeling, and action patterns (Blenkiron, 2005; Friedberg & McClure,

2002; Friedberg & Wilt, in press; Grave & Blissett, 2004; Kuehlwein, 2000; Otto, 2000; Overholser, 1993; Stallard, 2005). Metaphors also render rational analysis accessible for young children and/or others who have limited logical reasoning abilities (Blenkiron, 2005; Stallard, 2005). Metaphors help children view their problems from an objective perspective. When children see therapy as more playful, their anxiety and avoidance lessen. Hopefully, they can forget they are "in therapy." Consequently, they feel more comfortable processing emotionally powerful material. In their review, McCurry and Hayes (1992) concluded that metaphors are apt tools for working with children. Metaphors and analogies may be medical, mechanical, strategical, or relational, or they may reference natural disasters. Linehan, Cochran, and Kehrer (2001) noted that metaphors facilitate understanding, alternative thinking, and cognitive reframing.

Cook et al. (2004) suggested that stories and metaphors promote cognitive restructuring, motivation, and vicarious learning (Kennedy-Moore & Watson, 1999; Samoilov & Goldfried, 2000). Simply, they should carry an emotional payload. Indeed, emotionally salient metaphors serve to shift processing from a purely intellectual level to an integrated cognitive–emotional–behavioral level. Evocative metaphors promote the transfer of cognitive-behavioral interventions from emotion and cognition to action.

Metaphors also lie at the core of ACT (Hayes et al., 1999; Heffner, Sperry, Eifert, & Detweiler, 2002; Murrell, Coyne, & Wilson, 2005). There are several aspects of metaphors that recommend them for clinical work with children. Hayes et al. (1999) remarked that metaphors are similar to simple stories and produce less psychological reactance. Metaphors are collaborative enterprises, and this collaboration minimizes power differentials. Hayes et al. (1999) continued by stating that metaphors are often associated with pictorial or visual images, which makes them especially useful for children. Finally, metaphors are memorable.

Friedberg and Wilt (in press) outlined the Magnificent Seven Guidelines for metaphor use with children. Not surprisingly, they state first that the metaphor must be embedded in a cognitive-behavioral case formulation. Second, metaphors and stories need to match children's developmental, environmental, and ethnocultural contexts. Third, good metaphors are concrete and foster experiential learning. Fourth, proficiency in traditional CBT procedures should accompany metaphorical communication. In CBT, concrete interventions are preferred over abstract ones. This rule directly guides the use of metaphors in CBT (Blenkiron, 2005). Fifth, meaning in metaphors needs to be unpacked and direct instruction should often accompany the metaphor. The intervention's impact is not left to chance. Sixth, a good metaphor speaks to children's emotional realities. Seventh, and last, but certainly not least, metaphors should increase fun and engagement in treatment.

Deliberate therapeutic processing via direct discussion of children's internal states (e.g., thoughts, feelings) is key. It is important that children translate the metaphor into productive action. Concrete and understandable metaphors bring CBT to life. Acting out metaphors allows children to try things out and see what happens. Curiosity and experimentation are highly valued in CBT. When metaphors and storytelling are accompanied by experiential activities, they enter the realm of immediate awareness and are more effective (Kuehlwein, 2000). Children may create a behavioral experiment or a written assignment based on the metaphor. Table 6.1 provides several examples of metaphors.

Jacquin, a 10-year-old boy with ODD, intense anger, and impulsive behavior, who lived in a violent neighborhood and suffered physical abuse, spontaneously offered a

TABLE 6.1. Metaphors and Their Potential Uses in Rational Analysis

Metaphor	Purpose	Ages
Spidey Sense	Self-protection, identify perceptions and predictions	10–18 years
Maze	Goal setting, problem-solving obstacles	10–18 years
Cat's Meow (Cotterell, 2005)	Teaches children the longer they resist an urge, the weaker it becomes	10–18 years
Half-Nelson Metaphor	Helps children and adolescents realize that the more they struggle against control, the tighter the control becomes	10–18 years
Bus Driver Metaphor	Helps children recognize they are in control of their behavior and they need to persist despite challenging circumstances, irritating thoughts, and distressing emotions	10–18 years

compelling metaphor in therapy. He loved Spiderman and the idea that someone could have special powers to cope with past, present, and future dangers. When discussing his interpersonal perceptions and strategies, Jacquin stated that he used his "Spidey sense" to evaluate circumstances. The therapist used Jacquin's Spidey sense to represent his interpersonal predictions. Together, the therapist and Jacquin designed a rational analysis procedure where he recorded the situation, his prediction (e.g., "Spidey sense says ... "), and what actually happened. The therapist and Jacquin evaluated how often his Spidey sense was correct. Since this child used his Spidey sense as a form of self-protection, it was important to replace one incorrect Spidey sense with another more adaptive Spidey sense or skill. Clearly, this metaphor can be generalized from Jacquin to other children who are Spiderman fans.

Twelve-year-old Amos spontaneously offered a metaphor for navigating difficult life circumstances. The patient was abused and abandoned by his biological parents, who left him homeless. He was placed in various foster homes and then adopted. He engaged in much testing behavior with his adoptive parents and pushed them to the point of reversing his adoption. During the course of a session, Amos spontaneously stated, "My life is like a maze. I think things will go well and then I walk blind into a blocked path."

Amos's metaphor profoundly communicated the puzzling and complex nature of his circumstances. The therapist and Amos made use of this theme and operationalized it. Amos drew a maze and labeled the blocked paths with the names of his various challenges (e.g., "I believe no one can be trusted"; "No one should tell me to do something I don't want to do."). Then Amos developed several strategies to cope with his blocked paths. His goal was placed at the center of the maze, and Amos listed the ways he could achieve success.

Cotterell (2005) offered a simple yet compelling metaphor illustrating reinforcing qualities associated with giving in to urges. The metaphor begins by asking the child to imagine a stray cat begging for milk at the back door.

> "Imagine a stray cat at your back door. She hasn't eaten in days and begins begging for milk and meowing. You try to ignore her but she gets louder and louder. MEOW, MEOW, **MEOW**! Finally, you give in and give her milk to quiet her down. What do you suppose happens then?"

Most children realize that the cat will stop meowing. The metaphor continues.

> "The cat does stop meowing for now. But you know what? She comes back again. She meows for more milk. *You are so annoyed that you try to ignore her. But the more you ignore her, the more she meows.* She gets louder and louder. MEOW, MEOW, MEOW. Until you finally give in and get her milk. So what have you taught her?"

Once the children recognize that they have taught the kitty that the louder she begs, the more likely she will be fed, you move onto the rational analysis. The following dialogue shows you how to process the Cat's Meow.

> THERAPIST: This is kind of the same with your anxiety. It keeps meowing at you to give in and you do. You never give it a chance to be quiet. So what can you say to yourself to quiet down your anxiety?
>
> AHMAD: Worry, you are annoying. You will go away if I just wait you out.
>
> THERAPIST: What convinces you of that?
>
> AHMAD: Well, the less I feed it, the less strong it gets. When I do wait it out, it does get less.
>
> THERAPIST: Does it ever get stronger the longer you wait?
>
> AHMAD: No, not really.
>
> THERAPIST: So, let's put this all together in a conclusion and write it down.
>
> AHMAD: It's like the cat. The more you feed it when it calls, the more it comes back. I need to not feed into my worries; they will get louder but won't stay loud for a long time. I just need to wait them out.

The therapist used a simple metaphor to help Ahmad learn that the longer you resist an urge, the weaker the urge becomes. Varying the loudness of the meow illustrated growing intensity, added humor, and made the point memorable. The Socratic questioning stepped Ahmad through the rational analysis process. Recording the conclusion concretized the process.

HALF-NELSON METAPHOR

Ages: 10–18 years.

Purpose: Helping children and adolescents realize that the more they struggle against control, the tighter the control becomes.

Materials Needed: None.

The *Half-Nelson* metaphor is inspired by a movie of the same name (Fleck, 2006). A half-nelson is a wrestling hold that makes escape difficult. The more one tries to break the hold, the tighter its grip becomes. Half-Nelson is an apt metaphor particularly for patients who are caught in control battles. The key is to relax and not fight the grip. Essentially, the metaphor conveys the message that the more you fight to escape, the more you are trapped. The metaphor is conceptually similar to the Chinese Finger Trap exercise presented in Chapter 7. The metaphor may be particularly apt for both rebellious youngsters and those burdened by unrelenting internal pressures. The following dialogue illustrates the Half-Nelson Metaphor in rational analysis with 15-year-old Eli, who repeatedly engages in self-protective but aggressive behaviors.

THERAPIST: Eli, you are really caught up in this fighting at school.

ELI: If people try me, they find out what's coming!

THERAPIST: What are you saying?

ELI: Look if people say bullshit things to me, I'll talk back. I walk through the halls and people call me rude names. They hit me in the back. I'm not going to take that!

THERAPIST: You feel attacked and then fight back. I get that. It's kind of like being trapped.

ELI: Exactly. They call me Spic and other things I don't want to hear. That is disrespectful to me and my family. I can't leave that.

THERAPIST: You are caught like in a wrestling hold.

ELI: Like what?

THERAPIST: Do you know what a half-nelson is?

ELI: No.

THERAPIST: It's a hold that an opponent puts you in and the more you struggle against it, the stronger the hold is. You can never get free of it then.

ELI: I just want to be free of these people bothering me. I want to get an education, but I can't without them fighting and disrespecting me.

THERAPIST: It's tough to be free of people who pick on you because of your skin color.

ELI: I could in my last school.

THERAPIST: That's what makes this hard. You are in a new school and this hasn't happened before. So, how do you get out of this hold?

ELI: The only way I know is to fight.

THERAPIST: And that makes it worse?

ELI: That's why I am here.

THERAPIST: So if you are in a hold where fighting against the hold makes it tighter, what is a way out?

ELI: I can't give in. That's weak! That's not the way I roll.

THERAPIST: I'm not saying surrender. To get out of the hold, what if you used their strategy against them?

ELI: Almost like in karate or something?

THERAPIST: Sure. Instead of fighting against their grip, use their grip against them.

ELI: Like their racist comments?

THERAPIST: Exactly. How could you use it against them and not get yourself caught in a trap?

ELI: Make it public. Like make them shout in the halls so the teachers hear their shit. Don't get into it with them after school where teachers can't see. Make them look bad in front of the teacher or principal.

THERAPIST: That would be kind of outsmarting them, wouldn't it?

ELI: Yeah, I am smarter than them. I can trick them into showing how stupid they are.

The dialogue with Eli uses the Half-Nelson Metaphor to communicate understanding and facilitate the rational analysis process. The therapist carefully conveyed understanding, introduced the metaphor, and crafted a Socratic dialogue. The use of the wording "caught up in this fighting" paved the way for the metaphor and spoke to Eli's dilemma. Through the Socratic process, the therapist helped Eli see that refraining from aggression doesn't have to mean surrender and weakness. The questioning facilitated Eli finding a way out of his predicament.

BUS DRIVER METAPHOR

Ages: 10–18 years.

Purpose: Helping children recognize they are in control of their behavior and they need to persist despite challenging circumstances, irritating thoughts, and distressing emotions.

Materials Needed:

- Bus Drawing (Form 6.1).
- Paper for map.
- Pencil, pen, or other markers.

The Bus Driver Metaphor is an ACT concept (Hayes et al., 1999; Heffner et al., 2002). Basically, the young patients imagine themselves as bus drivers who follow a self-defined route but must carry a load of unpleasant thoughts, feelings, and bodily reactions. The bus driver must follow the route and try to calm the passengers, deal with them, but not be hijacked. Heffner et al. neatly operationalized this metaphor by drawing a concrete, graphic map of an adolescent's goals, and having the patient keep a daily record of directions.

We augmented this metaphor to include more concrete cognitive strategies. The patient is presented with a bus drawing and then specifically adds passengers (problems). Then he or she draws a map filled with challenges and accompanying coping resources. We begin with the introduction:

"Have you ever been on a bus? I want you to imagine something with me. Pretend your brain is a bus. You are the bus driver and your problems are passengers on the bus. You have to pick up the passengers or stressors and you cannot let them off.

However, you have to keep control of the bus even when your passengers get unruly and bothersome. You also have to stay on your route and not let the passengers take control of the bus. Can you do that?"

The next stage concretizes the image and metaphor as the therapist says:

"Take a look at this bus drawing. In each window, I want you to write down the things that bug you or disturb you. Be as specific as you can."

After the passengers are loaded on the bus, a map (e.g., the bus route) is drawn. Caution signs, speed bumps, and pot holes representing challenges along the route are added. Finally, billboards representing self-instructions and emergency call boxes representing problem-solving and coping strategies are also included.

The following dialogue with 16-year-old Cheyenne, who presented with comorbid anorexia and major depressive disorder, illustrates the map-making process. (Cheyenne's Bus Drawing is shown in Figure 6.1.)

THERAPIST: Cheyenne, let's make a map for your bus.

CHEYENNE: I don't know how to start. What should the road look like?

THERAPIST: That's up to you. How do you see the road leading to your goals?

CHEYENNE: Kind of curvy and with a lot of bumps and pot holes.

THERAPIST: Yeah, life is pretty much a crooked road.

CHEYENNE: That could be a country song.

THERAPIST: So let's draw your crooked and bumpy road.

FIGURE 6.1. Cheyenne's bus drawing.

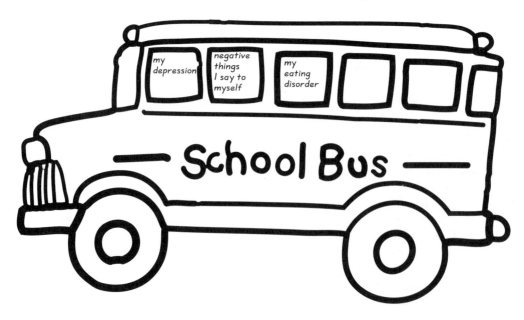

CHEYENNE: (*Draws.*) There ... Here it is ... I love to draw. [See Figure 6.2 for Cheyenne's map].

THERAPIST: I can see that! Now, have you ever seen the call or rescue boxes along the road?

CHEYENNE: Like on the turnpike?

THERAPIST: Exactly. Now I want you to make lots of call boxes that include problem-solving and support strategies for your bumps and curves.

CHEYENNE: I don't know what you mean.

THERAPIST: OK. Let's do the first one together. First, what is the first possible bump?

CHEYENNE: Maybe a breakup with my boyfriend.

THERAPIST: Good. What is going to happen to your passengers?

CHEYENNE: I know my depression and negative things about myself will act up.

FIGURE 6.2. Cheyenne's map.

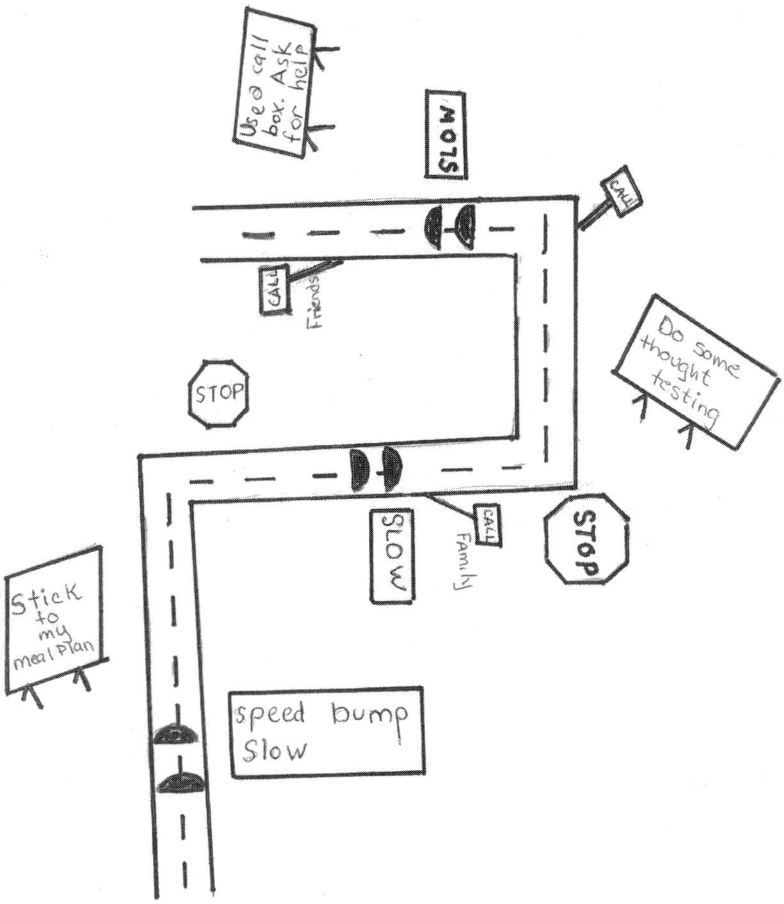

THERAPIST: What can you do then to keep your passengers in check and not take the bus off course?

CHEYENNE: Use my tools like the thought record and thought-testing skills. Maybe talk it out with my friends and some family members.

THERAPIST: Great. Draw the call box and write in the rescue factors. Now for the homework. I want you to add more things to the map. I want you to add bumps and rescue boxes. How many should we shoot for?

CHEYENNE: Maybe 10 or so.

THERAPIST: Sounds good.

Cheyenne then took the map home over the week and completed the homework for the next session. During that session, the therapist reviewed the homework with Cheyenne.

THERAPIST: Let's take a look at your map. You did a great job. Now, the next step is to add some billboards.

CHEYENNE: What are they for?

THERAPIST: They are self-instructions to encourage you and keep you going even when your passengers get unruly and distracting. Let's put some on your map.

CHEYENNE: OK. How about "Remember to use your call boxes"?

THERAPIST: Great. Now, what can you say to yourself when your eating disorder flares up?

CHEYENNE: Umm. Stick to my meal plan. I'm not defined by my weight. Weight changes, and don't freak if my jeans are too tight.

The therapist and Cheyenne worked on several more roadside billboards and then Cheyenne was assigned homework to come up with 10 more self-instructional billboards. In the above transcript, bumps, rescue boxes, and billboards are used as metaphors for problems, problem-solving strategies, and coping statements. The time spent drawing the map and augmenting it with the call boxes and billboards added to the fun of the session. Moreover, the pictorial icons were concrete reminders and cues for coping.

RATIONAL ANALYSIS GAMES

In our experience, young children tend to respond better to games that include rational analysis rather than direct paper-and-pencil methods for rational analysis. The games allow for concrete referents and direct experience with rational analysis. The following two games, Who's Got the Germ? and Control Dice, illustrate the procedure.

WHO'S GOT THE GERM?

Ages: 7–12 years.

Purpose: Test of evidence.

Materials Needed:

- Paper for game cards.
- Markers or crayons for drawing.

Who's Got the Germ? is a game that was individually constructed for several children who dreaded catching contaminants and getting sick. They excessively used hand sanitizers and panicked when other children in their class were sick. Naturally, school was frequently avoided since the other children were seen as "plague carriers." Not surprisingly, their peer relationships suffered since they saw interactive fun on the playground as profound threats to their health and well-being. The game begins with the therapist's introduction to "germ theory" as follows:

> "There are many types of germs. Some germs will make you sick, other germs make you strong and protect you from getting sick, and still others won't do a thing to you or for you."

After the introduction, the therapist and the child make the game cards after agreeing on what the three categories of germs should look like. The germs are drawn on strips of paper or index cards. The cards are then shuffled and dealt to the players (e.g., child, Mom, and therapist). Each player will inevitably get some good germs, harmful, sick-making germs, and harmless germs. The frequency of each type of card is recorded for each player. The cards essentially form the database for evaluating the belief that "all germs should be avoided." The following dialogue illustrates the process.

THERAPIST: Elle, let's count the types of germs you, Mom, and I got.

ELLE: OK, I have a lot.

THERAPIST: Great. Mom, how many do you have?

ELLE'S MOTHER: I have six germs that do nothing, three that get you sick, and five that help you.

ELLE: I have four germs that do nothing, four that get you sick, and six that help. What about you, Dr. Bob?

THERAPIST: I have four germs that do nothing, five that get you sick, and five that help. Elle, what do you make of that?

ELLE: You have the most bad germs!

THERAPIST: That's true, but what do we all have in common?

ELLE: We all have germs.

THERAPIST: So what does that mean?

ELLE: Well, you can't play the game without getting some germs.

THERAPIST: Do all the germs get you sick?

ELLE: No, just a few.

THERAPIST: So how can we put this together in one thought?

ELLE: You can't go around the world without germs and only a few of them get you sick.

THERAPIST: Great. Let's write that down on a card.

The dialogue with Elle illustrates the ebb and flow that characterize Socratic questioning with children. Elle and the therapist gathered data by counting the germs. Then the therapist erred by asking a synthesizing question that was too general too early in the process ("What do you make of that?"). The therapist corrected by following up with more specific and simple questions ("What do we all have in common?"; *Do all the germs get you sick?*). Finally, the therapist concluded the dialogue with a better-placed synthesizing Socratic question ("So how can we put this together in one thought?").

CONTROL DICE

Ages: 8–18 years.

Purpose: Test of evidence.

Materials Needed:

- Two cups.
- A die.
- Play chips or paper clips.

Control Dice is another rational analysis game that is especially useful for children who have overly valued notions of their own control. More specifically, these youngsters think, "I can control everything and everyone around me." The game requires two cups, a die, and playing chips or paper clips. The rules of the game are simple. The children always throw the die and guess. Children must accurately predict the number revealed on the die before it is thrown. If they are correct, they earn the number of chips shown on the die. However, if they are wrong, the chips go to the other player. Naturally, over many rolls, the children will guess incorrectly much more than they predict correctly. Like the germ game, the chips accrued form the basis for the rational analysis. The following transcript illustrates the procedure.

SHANNON: I am in control of everything.

THERAPIST: Wow! Is there anything you can't control?

SHANNON: Nothing important. I can get people to act in ways I want and make things happen the way I want.

THERAPIST: Can we try a game?

SHANNON: OK.

THERAPIST: Do you think you can predict what comes up on a roll of the die?

SHANNON: Sure. Once I get the hang of it.

THERAPIST: Here's how we play. You have to guess what number will come up on the die before you roll it. If you guess right, you get the number of chips shown on the die. If you are wrong, I get the chips. Do you understand?

SHANNON: Cool, I'll win.

Shannon and the therapist play for almost 20 rounds with Shannon guessing correctly only two rolls.

THERAPIST: Let's count up. I have 85 chips. How about you?

SHANNON: 12.

THERAPIST: You did horribly. I thought you were in control of everything.

SHANNON: This was unfair.

THERAPIST: And what is that like for you?

SHANNON: It sucks.

THERAPIST: When things are beyond your control, you see them as unfair?

SHANNON: Yep.

THERAPIST: What was it like for you to be in this situation?

SHANNON: I hate it.

THERAPIST: What went through your mind?

SHANNON: You are making the rules so I can't win. I hate it when I don't win.

THERAPIST: How close is that to what you think and feel when you fight with your parents?

SHANNON: Exactly.

THERAPIST: What's another way to look at situations that are truly impossible for you to completely control?

SHANNON: Avoid them.

THERAPIST: Most of the time that is impossible. How did you handle the dice game?

SHANNON: I just let it play out.

THERAPIST: What does that mean about always having to be in control?

SHANNON: I guess when I am not in control, I can let things play out like with my family. Maybe the next time things will turn in my favor.

THERAPIST: Maybe on the next roll?

SHANNON: Maybe.

THERAPIST: What would help you wait for the next roll?

SHANNON: Kind of trusting the next roll will be good for me.

THERAPIST: Sometimes you control things because you don't trust things will roll in your favor?

SHANNON: Yep.

THERAPIST: Let's add that to your coping thoughts. What do we have so far?

SHANNON: When I am not in control, I can let things play out. I have to trust that some things may turn into my favor and if they don't, trust that I can handle it.

The dialogue began with the therapist eliciting Shannon's overestimation of her control. Then they used the chip count as data to form conclusions. The data analysis portion elicited a strong emotional reaction ("This is unfair"; "It sucks"; "I hate it."). The therapist then bridged the game to her real-life context ("How close is that to what you think and feel when you fight with your parents?"). Similar to the example with Elle in the Who's Got the Germ? example, the first synthesizing question was placed too early in the Socratic questioning sequence ("What's another way to look at situations that are truly impossible for you to completely control?"). Shannon's belief that she cannot trust things to work out in her favor so she must overcontrol them was prompted by a very simple question ("What would help you wait for the next roll?"). Finally, Shannon and her therapist finalized this complex process by recording her conclusion on a card.

OTHER RATIONAL ANALYSIS TECHNIQUES

MASTER OF DISASTER

Ages: 8–13 years.

Purpose: Decatastrophizing, reattribution.

Materials Needed:

- Master of Disaster Worksheet (Form 6.2).
- Pen or pencil.

Master of Disaster is a cognitive restructuring procedure that targets catastrophic thinking (e.g., disaster forecaster thinking). Thus, it is a natural subsequent intervention for children who have previously completed thought records where they have identified disaster forecaster thinking. Master of Disaster guides the child through decatastrophizing and includes child-friendly Socratic questions based on the adult work by J. S. Beck (1995) and Fennell (1989). The procedure is also similar to Dreadful Iffy (Friedberg & McClure, 2002) and Making Lemonade (Friedberg et al., 1992).

The procedure starts with an introduction, during which the child learns about being a Master of Disaster. In step two, the catastrophic predictions are recorded. Then the questions on the Master of Disaster Worksheet (Form 6.2) help you and the child scaffold a Socratic dialogue that steps the child through the decatastrophizing process. First, the child assesses the probability of danger (e.g., "How sure am I the disaster will happen?"). Second, the child is asked about the historical precedence of the disaster (e.g., "When has it happened before?"). Third, if there is no historical precedence, you ask what is different this time that convinces the child it will happen. Fourth, you examine the youth's explanation for the disaster. The follow-up question creates doubt through reattribution (e.g., "What is another explanation for your sense it will happen now?").

The next three questions further address the historical precedence. The child's past capacity to deal with the disaster is queried (e.g., "If your disaster happened in the past, how did you handle it? What did you do?"). The questions lay the groundwork for highlighting the child's coping capacity. If the child's past coping efforts were unsuccessful, you move onto the next question (e.g., "If you did not handle it well before, what is different now?"). Since you and the child are in the rational analysis module, the child obviously has new skills developed through progress in the previous modules. The last question before the conclusion prompts a problem-solving strategy. *When a problem-solving strategy is in place, how disastrous could it be?* Finally, to complete the Master of Disaster conclusion, you help the child integrate all the information recorded and synthesize a conclusion. This can be a more difficult process. Accordingly, the following dialogue shows the process with Shoshanna, a 14-year-old patient with fears of humiliation and rejection. Shoshanna's worksheet can be seen in Figure 6.3.

THERAPIST: Shoshanna, let's look at your Master of Disaster Worksheet. You were worried about the girls at your lunch table.

SHOSHANNA: All they think about is getting with the guys they want and being rude to me.

THERAPIST: I see that. You had some trouble coming up with a conclusion.

SHOSHANNA: Yeah, it was confusing.

THERAPIST: So let's walk through it together. What is the reason you think the girls are mean and rude?

SHOSHANNA: I am ugly and people think I suck as a person.

THERAPIST: That hurts.

SHOSHANNA: No kidding.

THERAPIST: What might be another reason for their behavior?

SHOSHANNA: They are mean and are looking for someone to make feel bad.

THERAPIST: How much does that have to do with you?

SHOSHANNA: Not much.

THERAPIST: I see that you filled out what happened in the past but left what is different about you blank.

SHOSHANNA: I didn't know what to write.

THERAPIST: You stopped eating, cut yourself, and got depressed. That was before. But what about now?

SHOSHANNA: I am stronger now. I didn't think about that. It doesn't make sense for me to punish myself for their bullshit. Just because they treat me like crap doesn't mean I should do the same to myself.

THERAPIST: So you have a plan?

FIGURE 6.3. Shoshanna's Master of Disaster Worksheet.

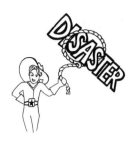

Disaster I can master: *The girls at my lunch table will continue to pick on me because my hair looks frizzy in my braids and I don't have a date to the dance.*

Master questions:

How sure are you that the disaster will happen? (Circle one.)

1	2	3	4	(5)
Not		Kind of		A lot

When has the disaster happened before? (Circle one.)

Never	Sometimes	(A lot)

If the disaster has not happened, what convinces you it will happen now? _____

_____

What was your explanation for the disaster happening before? *I am ugly and people think I suck as a person.*

What is another explanation for your sense it will happen now? *They are just mean and look for someone to pick on and make feel bad.*

If your disaster has happened in the past, how did you handle it?

(1)	2	3	4	5
Not well		Kind of		Really well

What did you do? *I really blew it. I got depressed, scratched on myself a little with an Exacto knife, and stopped eating for awhile.*

If you did not handle it well, what is different about you now? What could you do now that would be helpful? *I am stronger now. I really can't punish myself for other people's bullshit. Just because they treat people like crap doesn't mean I should treat myself like crap. Their opinions do not shape me. I'm not clay in their hands. I am just going to make myself who I am.*

If you have a plan for the disaster, how bad could it be? How in control are you? _____
Really in control.

Master of Disaster conclusion: *Although I let the girls control me before with their mean comments, I know not to let them do that again. What I do makes me who I am, not their opinions. I can handle their crap without cutting or stopping eating.*

SHOSHANNA: Yep.

THERAPIST: If you have a plan for a disaster, how in control are you?

SHOSHANNA: A lot.

THERAPIST: Let's put it together.

SHOSHANNA: I let the girls control me before. I'm in control now. I determine who I am. Their opinions don't shape me. I'm not clay in their hands.

THERAPIST: What about the cutting and not eating?

SHOSHANNA: I can handle their crap without that.

The therapist started the work with Shoshanna by eliciting the negative automatic thought and connecting it to her feelings. Then, the therapist asked for a reattribution ("What might be another reason for their behavior?"). Next, the therapist questioned Shoshanna's overly personalized conclusion ("How much does that have to do with you?"). The therapist also helped Shoshanna see that plans increase her perceptions of control. The dialogue concluded with a synthesizing conclusion ("Let's put it together.").

THOUGHT PROSPECTOR

Ages: 8–13 years.

Purpose: Evaluating overly critical self-definition.

Materials Needed:

- Thought Prospector Worksheet (Form 6.3).
- Pen or pencil.

Thought Prospector helps children discover neglected positive qualities and characteristics. They mine for positive and productive nuggets. Accordingly, Thought Prospector is especially useful for children who are depressed, have overly critical self-definitions, and hold low perceptions of their competence. Thought Prospector combines test of evidence and reattribution procedures.

Thought Prospector begins by eliciting the child's self-definition (e.g., "I'm a total loser."). The second step includes two Thought Prospector questions (e.g., "What is it that you do that a total loser would never do?" and "What is it that a total loser would do that you would never do?"). In step three, the synthesizing reattribution question is asked (e.g., "What's another way to look at yourself?"). The following dialogue with a self-critical and depressed 12-year-old named Jedadiah illustrates the process. His worksheet can be seen in Figure 6.4.

THERAPIST: Jed, do you know what a prospector is?

JED: Like in the Alaskan Gold Rush? We studied that.

THERAPIST: Exactly. A prospector keeps sorting through things.

JED: He shakes his pan around to get the gold out.

THERAPIST: Yeah, how come he does that?

JED: To see the gold.

THERAPIST: He has to separate out the real gold from the mud, stones, and fool's gold.

JED: Fool's gold isn't valuable. I have some of that!

THERAPIST: Well, I am going to teach you how to be a thought prospector and separate what is the fool's gold in your thinking from what is the real gold. How does that sound?

JED: Fun!

THERAPIST: Here's the Thought Prospector Worksheet. Now, you said you were a total reject. Let's see if that is real gold or fool's gold. Are you ready?

JED: OK.

THERAPIST: Now let's go prospecting. See this question?

JED: What does a "blank" do that you would never do? I don't get it.

THERAPIST: So we have to put in the thought we are prospecting. So you fill in "total reject."

JED: I get it.

THERAPIST: List some of the things a total reject does that you never do.

JED: Umm. Hurt people ... skip school ... disrespect the teacher ... cheat, lie, steal.

THERAPIST: Any others?

JED: Spread rumors about kids, fail in school, be greedy.

THERAPIST: Here's the second prospecting question. What do you do that a total reject never does?

JED: I'm on the honor roll. I play a lot of sports. I help kids who have trouble with their homework. I help others when I do church activities ... I help out my parents with chores on the farm. I'm invited to some parties, but not all of them. I invite some kids over to my house.

THERAPIST: Now we're prospecting! Last question. Look at the things you wrote down and ask, What is another way to look at yourself?

JED: I really don't have much in common with a total reject. Maybe when bad or sad things happen to me, I blow it up into too big a thing. Being a total reject may be just in my imagination. I may need to step back and sort through things.

THERAPIST: Look, you struck gold! Write this down.

The therapist initially explained the thought prospector metaphor. Once Jed understood the metaphor and the task, the therapist began the rational analysis. Jed's foundation for his belief that he was total reject was explored ("List some of the things a total reject does that you never do"; "What do you do that a total reject never does?").

FIGURE 6.4. Jed's Thought Prospector Worksheet.

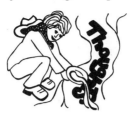

Thought you are prospecting: *I'm a total reject.*

What is it that you do that a *total reject* would never do?

Hurt people, skip school, disrespect my teachers, cheat, lie, gossip about kids, steal things, fail in school, be greedy.

What is it that a *total reject* does that you would never do?

Get on the honor roll, help kids in school, do church activities, help out my parents doing chores on the farm, be invited to some parties, have some kids come over to my house.

After prospecting, what's another way to look at yourself?

I really don't have much in common with a total reject. Maybe when bad or sad things happen to me, I blow it up into too big a thing. Being a total reject may be just in my imagination. I may need to step back and sort through things.

YOU STRUCK GOLD!

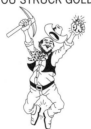

A subtle but important point in the dialogue is that the therapist varied the way he conducted the rational analysis. He used statements ("List some of the things …") as well as questions ("What do you do …?") so Jed would not feel interrogated. The therapist also repeatedly used the prospector metaphor throughout the dialogue to make the idea come alive ("Let's see if that is real gold or fool's gold"; "Now let's go prospecting"; "Now we're prospecting"; "You struck gold!"). Finally, the therapist concluded with a synthesizing question ("What is another way to look at yourself?").

COUNT DREADULA SAYS

Ages: 8–13 years.

Purpose: Rationally evaluating overly pessimistic attributions and predictions.

Materials Needed:

- Count Dreadula Questions sheet (Form 6.4).
- Count Dreadula Diary (Form 6.5).

Count Dreadula Says is for children plagued by overly pessimistic attributions and predictions. It is best suited to thoughts characterized by all-or-none thinking and catastrophizing. Many depressed children believe they will fail, nothing will work out for them, and nothing will change. Count Dreadula Says gives them questions to test their pessimistic thinking. It is a way for them to internalize the Socratic process. At the same time, the cartoon character of Count Dreadula helps children distance themselves from and objectify their distress. The character teaches children to rationally evaluate their beliefs in a graduated and sequential manner. Since these techniques are relatively more sophisticated than the cognitive restructuring procedures discussed in Chapter 5, they should be used after children have acquired and applied cognitive restructuring. Count Dreadula is similar to the Thought Digger exercise (Friedberg et al., 2001). Some of the Count Dreadula questions were inspired by the Thought Digger Diary as well as the work by Fennell (1989) and Resick and Calhoun (2001).

The procedure begins with introducing the Count Dreadula character as shown below. Then the child fills out the first four columns of the Count Dreadula Diary: date, situation, feeling, and automatic thought. The therapist presents the list of Count Dreadula Questions (Form 6.4). The child and therapist select a Count Dreadula question to ask and the question is written in the "Count Dreadula Asks" column next to the automatic thought. The child then responds to the question in the "Count Dreadula Says" column. In the final column, the child rerates the feeling. A blank Count Dreadula Diary is presented in Form 6.5.

The following transcript illustrates the above steps and makes use of the sample Count Dreadula Diary contained in Figure 6.5 with Armando, a 10-year-old depressed boy who sees himself and the world in harsh all-or-none terms.

THERAPIST: Armando, let me introduce a character that helps me teach boys and girls your age to test some of your thoughts. (*Takes out the Count Dreadula Questions sheet and Count Dreadula Diary.*) His name is Count Dreadula.

ARMANDO: Ooh, he's a vampire!

THERAPIST: Yeah, but he is a friendly one! He is called Count Dreadula because he helps you handle dreadful thoughts.

ARMANDO: Huh? I don't know what "dreadful" means.

THERAPIST: "Dreadful" means expecting the worst.

ARMANDO: OK.

THERAPIST: So, Count Dreadula helps you cope with thoughts that make you expect

FIGURE 6.5. Armando's Count Dreadula Diary.

Date	Situation	Feeling and rating	Automatic thought	Count Dreadula asks	Count Dreadula says	Rerate feeling
9/18	Taking a test	Worried (8)	If I make one mistake I'm doomed. People won't respect me.	Am I punishing myself? How forgiving am I being to myself?	Punishing myself for one mistake is too mean to myself. I can forgive myself for mistakes.	Worried (4)
9/21	Don't know	Worried (9)	It's horrible that I cannot tell the future. I can't stand the unexpected.	Am I letting my feelings trick me into thinking they are facts? Am I forgetting my strengths?	Yep. Feelings are not facts, they are just feelings. I am strong. I can stand it.	Worried (4)

209

the worst by asking yourself questions like these. (Shows the Count Dreadula Questions sheet [Form 6.4].)

ARMANDO: He kinda sucks out the bad things! (*Laughs.*)

THERAPIST: Yeah, exactly! The way he sucks out the bad things is by asking questions. Here are some. (*Shows Form 6.4.*) Let's pick out a few to use on your disaster forecaster thoughts like, "If I make one mistake, I'm doomed. People will not respect me anymore." What can Count Dreadula ask?

ARMANDO: Am I being too hard on myself? ... How forgiving of myself can I be?

THERAPIST: What's your answer to those questions?

ARMANDO: I guess I kind of am punishing myself and not forgiving myself for even one mistake.

THERAPIST: What's another one we can come up with?

ARMANDO: I worry that I can't tell the future. I can't stand when things happen I don't expect.

THERAPIST: What Count Dreadula questions can you ask for those thoughts?

ARMANDO: Hmm. Am I letting my feelings trick me into thinking they are facts? ... Am I forgetting about my strengths?

THERAPIST: And your answer is?

ARMANDO: Count Dreadula says yes. I am tricking myself. I can stand it. I am forgetting how I can handle unexpected stuff.

The therapist's work with Armando illustrates the way a child can be coached in thought testing. Armando is guided through the rational analysis procedure. He is prompted by the therapist to select and respond to salient questions ("What can Count Dreadula ask?"; "What's your answer to those questions?")

WHETHER REPORT

Ages: 8–18 years.

Purpose: Testing evidence; follows from Your Brainstorm.

Materials Needed:

- Whether Report Worksheet (Form 6.6).
- Previously completed Your Brainstorm Diary (Form 2.5).
- Pencil or pen.

Whether Report is a test of evidence procedure that conceptually follows directly from the self-monitoring technique Your Brainstorm. It is similar to techniques such as Finding Proof (Friedberg et al., 1992) and Private I (Friedberg & McClure, 2002). Finding Proof is a therapist-friendly worksheet that guides clinicians through the test of evidence procedure with adolescents using the five steps below. Private I is a child-friendly worksheet that encourages children to be detectives sorting through clues to find evidence that supports or disconfirms their beliefs. Like a traditional test of evidence, Whether Report includes five basic steps (Padesky, 1988):

- Step 1. Elicit data supporting the belief.
- Step 2. Elicit any data disconfirming the belief ("What makes you doubt this is totally true?").
- Step 3. Ask if there are other possible explanations for the data supporting the inaccurate belief. As an alert cognitive therapist, you probably realize that Steps 2 and 3 are designed to elicit doubt. Essentially, only one piece of data is needed in Step 2 to cast doubt and one alternative explanation in Step 3 dilutes the data in column one.
- Step 4. Invite the youngster to consider the data obtained in Steps 1 through 3 and make a synthesizing conclusion.
- Step 5. The child rerates the feeling.

The following dialogue illustrates the procedure with 13-year-old Claudia, who fears rejection and is very perfectionistic (see Figure 6.6 for Claudia's Whether Report Worksheet).

CLAUDIA: When the other girls are sitting together and laughing during school work, I feel very, very sad.

THERAPIST: How sad on a scale of 1–10?

CLAUDIA: 8.

THERAPIST: What runs through your head?

CLAUDIA: I have to be perfect, cheery, and full of answers for everyone to like me. I can't have one single thing wrong with me or I won't fit in.

THERAPIST: Claudia, remember when we used the Brainstorm Diary?

CLAUDIA: Yeah, I still have some of them.

THERAPIST: I have another diary just for brainstorms like you just had. How would you like to do one with me?

CLAUDIA: OK.

THERAPIST: This diary is called a Whether Report. It is based on the brainstorm idea, but it is about whether the storm is really true or not.

CLAUDIA: Oh, I get it. It's a homonym. You know, *whether* and *weather*.

THERAPIST: You know your language arts! Now, to tell we have to fill out these columns. One is titled "What convinces you this is totally true" and the other is "What makes you doubt this is totally true." Let's do the one about the thought being totally true first. What convinces you it is true?

CLAUDIA: Well, the girls talk a lot to each other.

THERAPIST: What else?

CLAUDIA: Sometimes they don't save a chair for me at lunch.

FIGURE 6.6. Claudia's Whether Report Worksheet.

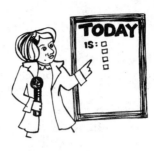

What is happening when you have a brainstorm? *We are all in class. The other girls are sitting together and laughing during the work.*

What feeling do you have? *Sad*

How strong? (Rate 1–10) *8*

What is running through your head during the brainstorm? *I have to be perfect, cheery, and full of answers for everyone to like me. I can't have one single thing wrong with me or I won't fit in.*

What convinces you this is totally true?	What makes you doubt this is totally true?
The girls talk a lot to each other.	*I play with the girls at recess.*
Sometimes there isn't a chair for me at lunch.	*When I cry, the other girls help me.*
When I make a mistake in class, they smile at me.	*I forgot the rules of a game at a party and they still included me.*

Make a conclusion on your Whether Report. *I may not be included all the time, but I am included many times. Being perfect does not seem to make me more included and maybe they accept me more when I am not so perfect. Being perfect is pressure I am putting on myself.*

What is your new feeling? *Sad (3)*

THERAPIST: Anything else?

CLAUDIA: Hmm. Sometimes when I make a mistake in class they smile at me.

THERAPIST: Any more?

CLAUDIA: No, that's it.

THERAPIST: Let's move on to the next column. What makes you doubt you have to be perfect and cheery all the time to be accepted?

CLAUDIA: Well, I do play at recess with the girls sometimes.

THERAPIST: What else?

CLAUDIA: That's it.

THERAPIST: Wow, a short list. What things do the girls do when things don't go well for you?

CLAUDIA: They help me when I cry.

THERAPIST: Let's write that down. When have they included you and you made a mistake?

CLAUDIA: Hmm. One time at a party I forgot the rules and they still wanted me on their team.

THERAPIST: Can you think of anything else?

CLAUDIA: No. These questions are hard. I'm getting tired.

THERAPIST: I understand. This is hard work. Hang in there for a little bit longer with me. You said something very curious before—that the girls smiled at you when you made a mistake in class. Do they say anything mean to you?

CLAUDIA: Not usually. Sometimes they pat me on the back.

THERAPIST: What might be another explanation for their smiles?

CLAUDIA: I never thought about that!

THERAPIST: Please take the chance to think about it now. (*Smiles.*)

CLAUDIA: (*Laughs.*) They might want to make me feel better.

THERAPIST: Claudia, I am going to ask you to do one last hard thing. How can you put all these new things together?

CLAUDIA: That's hard.

THERAPIST: Let me help you get started. Are you left out most of the time?

CLAUDIA: No. I am not always included, but most of the time I am.

THERAPIST: Is being perfect the most important thing that causes you to be included?

CLAUDIA: No ... I may be included more when I am not trying to be perfect. It's kind of a pressure I am putting on myself.

THERAPIST: How are you feeling now?

CLAUDIA: Less sad. Maybe a 3.

The transcript shows how difficult the rational analysis procedure is for many children. The dialogue begins with identification of feelings. Then the test of evidence is started. First, the evidence supporting the negative thought is elicited. It was important for the therapist to collect *all* of the evidence for the negative belief. Care should be directed *not* to preempt this part of the process. Be patient and get all the data the patient is using to reinforce the belief. Like most depressed patients, Claudia had trouble coming up with evidence that casts doubt on her belief. The therapist spent time helping her obtain this data.

Rational analysis is often a perplexing and sometimes emotionally exhausting experience for young people. It is hard work! Nonetheless, gentle persistence is indicated (e.g., "Hang in there for a little bit longer with me"; "I am going to ask you to do one last hard thing."). After all the evidence has been sorted, the therapist asked a concluding synthesizing question (e.g., "How can you put all these new things together?"). However, Claudia initially could not respond to the question. The therapist then stepped her through the process and cued her with a simpler question (e.g., "Is being perfect the most important thing that causes you to be included?").

MIRROR, MIRROR

Ages: 10–18 years.

Purpose: Structured analysis of negative self-definition.

Materials Needed:

- Mirror, Mirror Worksheet (Form 6.7).
- Pen or pencil.

Children form idiosyncratic self-definitions where they apply unforgiving rules and harsh standards only to themselves. Mirror, Mirror is a rational analysis procedure based on universal definitions and inspired by metaphors used by several young female patients on an inpatient psychiatric unit. Mirror, Mirror integrates the Socratic process inherent in universal definitions (Overholser, 1994), the double-standard technique (Burns, 1980), and Padesky's (2007) resilience model. Mirror, Mirror provides a structured way to navigate the seven steps in developing universal definitions (Overholser, 1994) as follows:

- Step 1. Elicit the adolescent's absolute self-definitions.
- Step 2. Record the elements upon which the absolute definition is built.
- Step 3. Measure the Weight of each component.
- Step 4 involves the mirror component. The adolescent is invited to nominate someone who he or she believes is at the other contrasting end of the continuum. Then the factors that figure into the adolescent's comparisons are listed.
- Step 5. The adolescent reflects on the degree to which he or she has the same characteristics as those listed in Step 4. The mirror is now established!
- Step 6. The adolescent is asked to reflect on what degree he or she has the same

characteristics as his or her counterparts (e.g., "Would someone who is totally worthless have any similarity to someone who is completely worthy?").

- Step 7 involves inspecting the mirror's reflection for the presence of the most significant element in the negative self-definition completed back in Step 3. Then, based on all the data, the therapist and patient construct a more accurate self-image.

The following dialogue demonstrates the procedure. Giselle is a 17-year-old patient with depression who unfavorably compares herself to others (see Figure 6.7 for Giselle's Mirror, Mirror Worksheet).

THERAPIST: How do you see yourself?

GISELLE: Pretty much as a scum of the earth who is unlovable.

THERAPIST: Those are some strong and painful words to describe yourself. On a scale of 1–10, how much of an unlovable scum are you?

GISELLE: Totally a 10.

THERAPIST: What is it that makes you see yourself as so unlovable?

GISELLE: I don't know. I'm ugly, fat … an emotional basket case. Kind of a psycho.

THERAPIST: Let's unpack this a little. What do you mean by ugly, fat, and a psycho?

GISELLE: Well, I'm not skinny like those cheerleaders in my school. My nose is too big for my face and I have emotional problems. I mean, I do see a shrink.

THERAPIST: OK. What else defines you as an unlovable scum?

GISELLE: I play sports, but I'm not a star. I'm OK at school work, but not like a brain.

THERAPIST: And if you were a star athlete and a brain?

FIGURE 6.7. Giselle's Mirror, Mirror Worksheet.

View of myself	Who is my standard?	How I see him/her	How do I compare?
Scum of the earth who is unlovable.	Amber	Pretty Athlete Good grades/smart Chill person (Perfect 8)	Pretty (7) Athlete (3) Good grades (8) Chill (3) (Perfect 7)

GISELLE: I don't know. I'd be in the paper or something. Brains have a perfect GPA. I know I am hard on myself, but it's just the way I feel and the way it is.

THERAPIST: This is what I wrote. You are not as skinny as the cheerleaders. Your nose is too big and you think you have flaws in your appearance. You see a shrink and have emotional problems. You are not the star of the team and you have a less than perfect GPA. Am I getting at your self-definition?

GISELLE: Quit reminding me of this shit. Aren't you supposed to build me up?

THERAPIST: I understand that this is painful. I am trying to hold up a reflection of you, like in a mirror. This tool I am going to teach you is called Mirror, Mirror. Here, take a look. I wrote down how you see yourself [see Figure 6.7]. Now which one of these things is the strongest part of your definition?

GISELLE: The part where I have things wrong with my appearance. Sometimes I look at myself and see hair out of place or a zit and I get so disgusted with myself that I get the urge to cut or burn myself.

THERAPIST: I see. Let me ask you, who do you know that you see as completely lovable?

GISELLE: Hmm … I guess my friend Amber. She's got it together.

THERAPIST: Now, let's look at the other side of the mirror. What makes Amber so lovable?

GISELLE: She's really pretty. She's smart and athletic. She gets good grades. She's a chill person.

THERAPIST: What does that mean?

GISELLE: (*Laughs.*) She's got it together. She does not get freaked out much.

THERAPIST: So this is the other side of the mirror. Take a look—does this seem like what you said?

GISELLE: Yeah. Amber is cool. Everybody loves her.

THERAPIST: OK. Now I want you to rate yourself on these qualities of Amber— the other side of the mirror. So how pretty do you think you are on a scale of 1–10?

GISELLE: I'm OK. I guess I'm a 7.

THERAPIST: How athletic?

GISELLE: I play three sports.

THERAPIST: So what number?

GISELLE: A 7, I guess.

THERAPIST: How smart?

GISELLE: I make the honor roll, but I don't get all A's. So maybe an 8.

THERAPIST: How chill?

GISELLE: I'm not chill. I'm hyper.

THERAPIST: So how much?

GISELLE: A 3 at most.

THERAPIST: Giselle, look at this mirror of unlovability. What does it say to you?

GISELLE: I feel like I should say "Mirror, mirror on the wall." (*Smiles.*) I don't know, what should it say?

THERAPIST: I'm not sure what it should say. But let me ask you, would someone who is a totally unlovable scum have any of these characteristics?

GISELLE: Probably not.

THERAPIST: So, let's do the math. How many of these things do you have more than a 5 on?

GISELLE: Three out of five.

THERAPIST: So if Amber is totally lovable and you have three out of five of her characteristics, how is it possible that you are totally unlovable?

GISELLE: I don't get it. I'm confused.

THERAPIST: Me too. Maybe that is a good sign. Would someone who is totally unlovable have over half of what it takes to make someone lovable?

GISELLE: I guess not.

THERAPIST: So write this all down. How do you feel now and what is your urge to cut?

GISELLE: A little better, I guess. I'm still not perfect, though.

THERAPIST: Wait, that's not on the mirror list.

GISELLE: That's what I meant by all that stuff.

THERAPIST: OK, so we'll add that. How perfect are you?

GISELLE: I'm OK, but not perfect. Maybe a 7.

THERAPIST: Fair is fair in Mirror, Mirror. Let's hold the perfect mirror up to Amber.

GISELLE: Well, nobody's perfect.

THERAPIST: I see. So, what number?

GISELLE: Maybe an 8.

THERAPIST: Let me get this. So a totally lovable person is 8 on the perfect scale and you, who are totally unlovable, are a 7. How does that add up?

GISELLE: I never thought about it that way.

THERAPIST: That's what we shrinks do. We try to change around the way you think. So what can you conclude?

GISELLE: Well, I am probably not a totally unlovable scum, no matter what my faults are. Nobody's perfect, not even Amber, and everybody loves her.... Maybe it's not so bad to be me.

This dialogue illustrates several points. In its first phase, the negative belief is elicited and scaled. Then the specific components of the belief are unpacked. Because this is a demanding procedure, the therapist took care to summarize the first phase ("This is what I wrote."). Giselle's belief is emotionally "hot" and her vulnerability is revealed in the early part of the transcript ("Quit reminding me of this shit."). The therapist was also careful to repeatedly communicate understanding.

In the second phase, Giselle's mirror opposite is identified (Amber) and Amber's complete lovability is operationalized. Once this task is accomplished, the therapist asked Giselle to rate herself on Amber's characteristics. Giselle initially had difficulty with the synthesizing question ("What does it say to you?"). This question may have been a bit too abstract and Giselle withdrew ("I don't know, what should it say?"). The therapist took the opportunity to simplify the process (e.g., "Would someone who is a totally unlovable scum have any of these characteristics?"; "So, let's do the math. How many of these things do you have more than a 5 on?"; "Would someone who is totally unlovable have over half of what it takes to make someone lovable?"). The therapist also reinforces Giselle's cognitive dissonance ("I'm confused.") by replying, "Maybe that is a good sign."

Giselle then added the perfection criterion when the process was nearly over. Fortunately, the therapist welcomed the addendum rather than excluding it. The therapist rightly stayed on target with the procedure rather than being thrown off ("Fair is fair in Mirror, Mirror. Let's hold the perfect mirror up to Amber."). The dialogue concludes with a simple and direct synthesizing question ("How does that add up?").

3-D THINKING

Ages: 8–18 years.

Purpose: Testing and modifying catastrophizing and emotional reasoning.

Materials Needed:

- 3-D Thinking Worksheet (Form 6.8).
- Pen or pencil.

3-D Thinking is a technique based on a patient-generated metaphor (Friedberg & Wilt, in press). It is useful for anxious children who engage in disaster forecaster (catastrophizing) and prisoner of feeling (emotional reasoning) thinking. Essentially, the procedure is designed to test and modify beliefs such as "Difficulty/discomfort is disastrous." Many of the children who engage in experiential avoidance or extreme anxiety sensitivity believe that any sign of discomfort signals catastrophes. Because their self-efficacy is so low, they see struggles or difficulty as signaling failure and vulnerability.

3-D Thinking is based on the notion that discomfort does not equal disaster. The technique helps children compare difficulty/discomfort and the level of disaster. On the 3-D Thinking Worksheet (Form 6.8), children record information in the first four columns as follows:

- Step 1. Children record the difficulty or discomfort they encountered.
- Step 2. They rate the level of discomfort (1–10, 1–100, etc.).
- Step 3. They write down the ways they cope with the difficulty or discomfort.
- Step 4. They rate the level of disaster associated with the difficulty.
- Step 5. During the Socratic processing, the therapist asks the child to compare

columns 1 and 2 (the difficulty and his or her rating of it) with column 4 (how much of a disaster). If there is a direct relationship between difficulty and disaster, there should be a high correlation between the columns. Inevitably there is a less-than-perfect correlation, and so a new conclusion is developed.

The following dialogue shows the procedure with Seamus, a 13-year-old boy with GAD.

THERAPIST: Seamus, let's try something with your areas of discomfort. How adventurous are you willing to be?

SEAMUS: In the middle.

THERAPIST: OK, let's list all the things you see as difficult and uncomfortable.

SEAMUS: Having a substitute teacher. Getting a throat swab when I have a sore throat. Having a blood test. Getting my seat moved in class.

THERAPIST: That's a good start. You have talked about some others.

SEAMUS: I hate it when my clothes get water on them or when a tag on my clothes gets itchy. Sometimes it gets too hot in class or in the car. I worry I will pass out and swallow my tongue. I also hate when we switch gym activities. I never know what to expect. I also don't like it when the homework gets switched.

THERAPIST: Great, now let's rate how uncomfortable these things are on a scale of 1–10 [see Figure 6.8].

SEAMUS: (Rates each one.)

THERAPIST: Even though each of these things happens, you handle them.

SEAMUS: I do!

THERAPIST: What did you do when you had a substitute teacher?

SEAMUS: I got nervous, but I checked my planner.

THERAPIST: So on a scale of 1–10, how much of a disaster was it?

SEAMUS: 4.

THERAPIST: How about the throat?

SEAMUS: I held my mother's hand, took a deep breath, told myself it only will last a few seconds.

THERAPIST: So how much of a disaster?

SEAMUS: Another 4.

THERAPIST: How did you handle the blood test?

SEAMUS: Kind of the same. I looked at the poster with a kitty on it and thought how it looked like my kitten.

THERAPIST: You distracted yourself.

SEAMUS: I distracted myself from disaster. It was a 3.

THERAPIST: How about the next ones?

SEAMUS: I talked to the other kids at the table. That wasn't too bad. Maybe a 3.

FIGURE 6.8. Seamus's 3-D Thinking Worksheet.

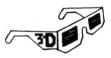

Difficulty/discomfort	How much discomfort?	How did you handle it?	How much of a disaster?
Substitute teacher	7	Got nervous Looked at planner	4
Get strep throat swab	8	Took deep breaths Held Mom's hand	4
Blood test	9	Looked away Focused on picture of kitty	3
Seat moved	9	Talked with new kids	3
Shirt being wet	8	Watched cartoons	2
Tag itchy	6	Played with cards and toys	2
Feet too hot	7	Thought my feet would run out of sweat Focused on spelling	5
Homework being changed	8	Wrote myself a note	2
Gym activities changed	7	Patient even though I freaked out a little	2

THERAPIST: And spilling water on your shirt?

SEAMUS: I thought it would dry soon and I kept watching the cartoons. That was a 2. Kind of the same thing with the tag. I just kept playing with my Pokemon cards and my toy figures. That was a 2.

THERAPIST: How about when you wore your heavy wool socks?

SEAMUS: Yeah, my feet got hot. I worried that I couldn't concentrate on the spelling test because I was thinking about my feet sweating. But I thought about my feet running out of sweat and stopping sweating. I put my mind on track so I could do spelling. This was maybe a 5.

THERAPIST: What about the gym activities and the homework bin?

SEAMUS: I got nervous that I would not find the bin in time. I wrote a note to myself and I found it. That was a 2. The gym activities changed and I worried I wouldn't do well and be picked for a team. I just was patient and things worked out even though I freaked out a little. I just let my freak pass. So maybe a 2.

THERAPIST: That is great work. Now, let's look at your sense or guess that if you have discomfort it is a disaster. If discomfort equals disaster, what would you see when you compare the discomfort and disaster columns? (*Points to the columns.*)

SEAMUS: The numbers would be the same.

THERAPIST: And what do you see?

SEAMUS: The disaster numbers are much lower.

THERAPIST: So what do you make of that?

SEAMUS: I guess just because I feel uncomfortable, it doesn't mean it is a disaster.

The therapist began the dialogue with the idea that the work was going to be an adventure and invited Seamus to list all his areas of discomfort. The discomfort was scaled and coping strategies were recorded. The level of disaster was rated. Then the therapist asked a very specific synthesizing question ("If discomfort equals disaster, what would you see when you compare the discomfort and disaster columns?").

FAKE MATH

Ages: 8–18 years.

Purpose: Reattribution to break inaccurate mental contingencies.

Materials Needed:

- Pen or pencil.
- Paper.

Children and adolescents often package their cognitions as mental equations (e.g., perfection = competence, never showing anger = approval, happiness = control and certainty). Fake Math is a reattribution procedure that includes an arithmetic metaphor and is founded on a central question, "What's the equation?" (Sokol, 2005). Once the equation is elicited, you use reattribution to modify the improper equation or contingency. The following dialogue begins with identifying the equation and proceeds with rational analysis. Meredith is an anxious and perfectionistic 14-year-old.

THERAPIST: Meredith, you spent tons of time trying to be perfect always and with everyone. What does it get you?

MEREDITH: A lot of stress, I guess.

THERAPIST: It sure does. But many young people like you create an equation in their minds about things.

MEREDITH: An equation? Like in math where something equals something else?

THERAPIST: Exactly. So in your mind what does perfection equal?

MEREDITH: Control and safety, I think.

THERAPIST: That makes sense, doesn't it? You would pursue perfection if it absolutely guaranteed or equaled control. I'm going to write this out like an equation. [See Figure 6.9.] What we have to figure out is whether this equation is accurate or not.

MEREDITH: How do we do that?

THERAPIST: Just like in math. We have to test the equation. For example, your equation says perfection absolutely determines your safety and control.

MEREDITH: It makes me feel in charge and nobody judges me then.

THERAPIST: OK. Let's test that equation. When have you done something perfectly and felt completely in control of your thoughts, feelings, and behaviors as well as everything and everyone around?

MEREDITH: Well, when you put it that way … never.

THERAPIST: Is that how you would put it?

MEREDITH: Yeah.

THERAPIST: OK, when have you been perfect, yet never feared disapproval or felt safe from others judging you?

MEREDITH: Never.

THERAPIST: How is the test going?

MEREDITH: Not too good for the equation. (*Smiles.*)

THERAPIST: Let's keep testing. When have you been imperfect, yet felt in charge and safe from judgment?

MEREDITH: When I made mistakes on my art project, I felt OK about that and my friends really rallied behind me. It was nice. They said it was cool to see me not be perfect.

THERAPIST: OK. Now what does that do to the equation?

MEREDITH: It changes it a lot.

THERAPIST: So, let's take all the information from the tests and rewrite the equation. What is a good rewrite?

MEREDITH: I'm going to try to do a good one. Not a perfect one. (*Smiles.*)

THERAPIST: Right!

MEREDITH: OK. Sometimes perfection makes me feel more in control and safe but it is kind of like a mirage in the desert. It seems like it is there, but not really. Most of the time trying to be perfect makes me more worried about others' judgments of me and I actually feel out of control. Perfection isn't what it's supposed to be. It's just a mirage.

FIGURE 6.9. Meredith's Fake Math equation.

$$PERFECTION = \begin{matrix} SAFETY \\ CONTROL \\ NO \; JUDGING \; BY \; OTHERS \end{matrix}$$

The therapist introduced the equation metaphor early in the dialogue ("But many young people like you create an equation in their minds about things."). The therapist elicited Meredith's equation ("So in your mind what does perfection equal?"). Once the equation was revealed, the testing process started ("When have you done something perfectly and felt completely in control of your thoughts, feelings, and behaviors?"; "When have you been perfect, yet never feared disapproval or felt safe from others judging you?"; "When have you been imperfect, yet felt in charge and safe from judgment?"). Finally, the therapist concluded with a synthesizing question ("Now what does that do to the equation?").

PLAYING CENTERFIELD

Ages: 8–18 years.

Purpose: Decreasing all-or-none thinking.

Materials Needed:

- Playing Centerfield Worksheet (Form 6.9).
- Pen or pencil.

Playing Centerfield is a way to teach the rational analysis continuum technique to younger children. Like the Newton's Cradle procedure used for adolescents (see p. 226), Playing Centerfield helps patients decrease their all-or-none thinking (one-eyed ogre thinking) so they see things in relative rather than absolute terms. It makes use of a baseball metaphor where the extremes are in right and left field. The middle ground is found in centerfield. The procedure begins with an explanation of the metaphor. Then Socratic questioning guides the patient in defining the extremes as well as the middle ground. The following dialogue is with Isaac, an 11-year-old boy troubled by depressive moods, guilt, and self-recriminations about real and perceived wrongs (see Figure 6.10 for Isaac's Playing Centerfield Worksheet).

ISAAC: I just have buckets of wrongs about me. I belong in the trash with all the garbage. I am a burden to my family. Maybe they should just throw me out. I'm horrible.

THERAPIST: I see how sad you feel. Do you remember what we called these types of thoughts?

ISAAC: It's my one-eyed ogre thinking popping up.

THERAPIST: It sure is, Isaac. You're a baseball player, right?

ISAAC: Yeah, third base.

THERAPIST: I want to show you something that may help you with your one-eyed ogre thinking. (*Takes out Playing Centerfield Worksheet [Form 6.9].*) Do you see this?

ISAAC: It's a baseball outfield. How is that going to help?

THERAPIST: I am going to teach you to play centerfield with your thinking.

FIGURE 6.10. Isaac's Playing Centerfield Worksheet.

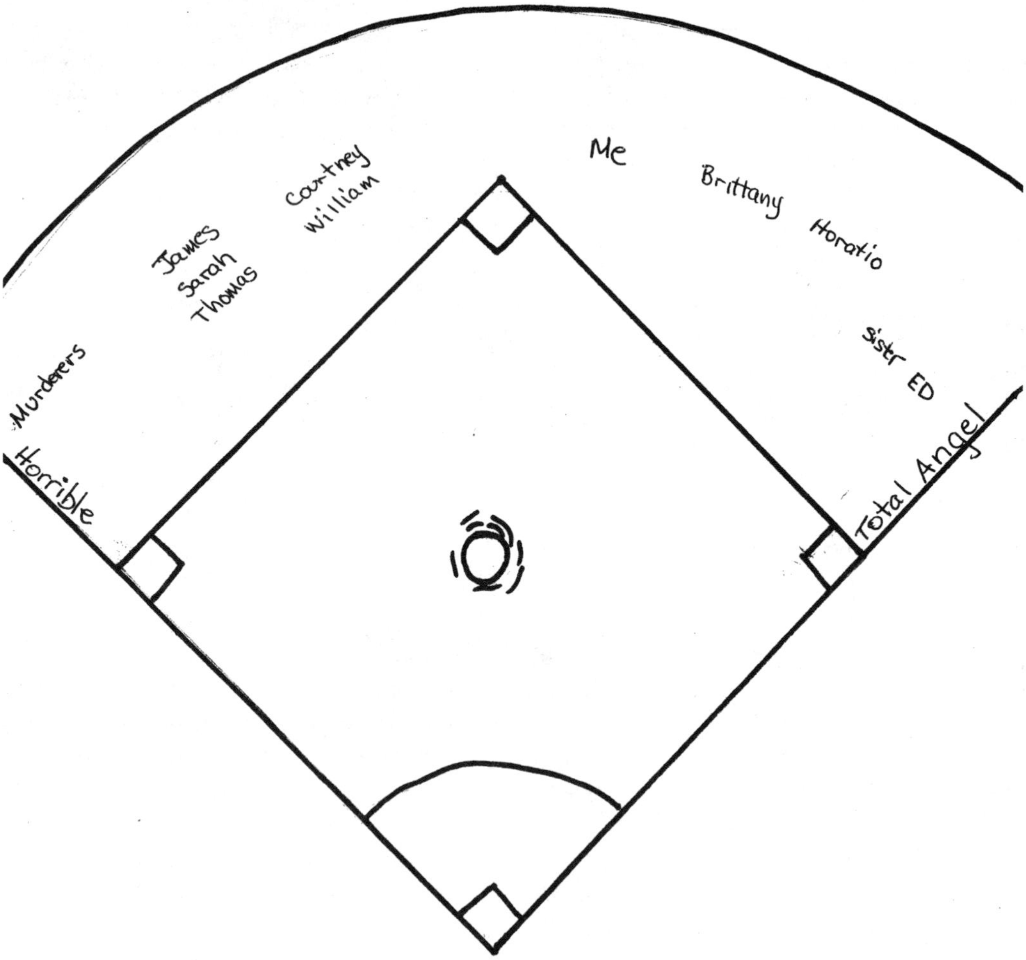

ISAAC: How do you do that?

THERAPIST: You said that you were horrible because of your big bucket of wrongs. Let's put this on the left field line and then what's on the opposite side of the field?

ISAAC: Right field!

THERAPIST: True, but what is the opposite of being horrible?

ISAAC: Being a total angel and never doing anything wrong.

THERAPIST: Let's write that down in right field. Now I want to put the players on the field.

ISAAC: What do you mean?

THERAPIST: Let's start in right field. Who do you know who is completely 100% an angel and never does anything wrong?

ISAAC: Maybe my cousin Ed.

THERAPIST: He never gets in trouble? There's nothing in his bucket of wrongs?

ISAAC: He makes a mess of some things. He does stay up late sometimes.

THERAPIST: So if he was a complete angel, he'd be exactly on the right field foul line. He does have some wrongs, so you position him.

ISAAC: Maybe here.

THERAPIST: Who else?

ISAAC: Maybe my younger sister.

THERAPIST: Where does she go?

ISAAC: She isn't as bad as me, but she does get on my parents' nerves. Maybe here.

THERAPIST: Who else?

ISAAC: My best friend, Horatio. He is a good student, but he acts up a lot.

THERAPIST: Where in the field is he?

ISAAC: Here.

THERAPIST: Who is the best, most popular, and most well-behaved student in your class?

ISAAC: Brittany—she thinks she is great.

THERAPIST: Where does she go?

ISAAC: Well, here ... because she also is mean sometimes to the kids who need extra help.

THERAPIST: Now who do you know who is horrible?

ISAAC: The people I see on the news who murder people.

THERAPIST: Where do they go?

ISAAC: Right on the left field line.

THERAPIST: How about people who you know who you see as horrible?

ISAAC: I don't like to judge people. I don't like to call others horrible.

THERAPIST: You just use that word for yourself.

ISAAC: (*Laughs.*) That's right.

THERAPIST: How about the bullies in your school?

ISAAC: James, Sarah, and Thomas. They're here.

THERAPIST: How about kids you see as disrespectful?

ISAAC: Courtney and William. They're here.

THERAPIST: Now looking at all these people, where on the field do you fit?

ISAAC: Maybe here.

THERAPIST: That's kind of in centerfield. What do you make of how far you are from the horrible side of the field.

ISAAC: I'm not that close. I have some wrongs and I'm not an angel, but I'm not that bad.

THERAPIST: What about that idea that you are horrible because you have many wrongs and your parents should throw you out with the trash?

ISAAC: That's coming from way out in left field. Maybe it's in foul territory. It's a foul thought!

In the above dialogue, the therapist worked with Isaac to define each end of his all-or-none thinking along the right and left field lines. Then Isaac positioned people along the continuum in the outfield based on how angelic or bad they were. After many people were placed on the field, Isaac positioned himself. The therapist then concluded with a synthesizing question ("What about the idea that you are horrible because you have many wrongs and your parents should throw you out with the trash?").

NEWTON'S CRADLE

Ages: 10–18 years.

Purpose: Decreasing all-or-none thinking.

Materials Needed:

• Newton's Cradle desk toy.

Newton's Cradle is a popular desk toy based on the laws of physics. The toy consists of five steel balls arranged in a horizontal line and vertically suspended from a frame. When a ball on one end is pulled and strikes the ball sitting next to it, the ball on the far end of the cradle moves but the balls in the middle remain at rest and motionless. The toy is a concrete demonstration of Newton's Third Law of Physics, which states that for every action there is an opposite and equal reaction.

Indeed, this is the physical science equivalent of all-or-nothing thinking. Extremes are placed at the opposite ends of the spectrum and patients bounce between these two poles, neglecting the middle ground. This all-or-none thinking (one-eyed ogre) results in emotional lability and impulsivity. Newton's Cradle is a concrete way to help youngsters appreciate the middle ground. The following dialogue shows you how to use Newton's Cradle with 14-year-old Morgan who is prone to dramatic outbursts.

THERAPIST: Morgan, we've been working with these all-or-none ways you see things and I want to show you something that may help with these beliefs. (*Pulls out Newton's Cradle.*)

MORGAN: I like this toy. I've seen it before.

THERAPIST: You know how it works?

MORGAN: Sure. You pull one ball out and the one on the end goes out too.

THERAPIST: And nothing happens to the ones in the middle?

MORGAN: Right.

THERAPIST: That's what happens in all-or-none thinking. Each end bounces off each other. That's how come you have such strong opposite feelings. What is the problem with that?

MORGAN: I just keep bouncing back and forth.

THERAPIST: You have to find the middle ground.

MORGAN: So I don't have so many mood swings?

THERAPIST: Pretty much. Each side is a trigger for the other side, so it keeps going on and on. How can you make each end less extreme and move to the middle with your thinking?

MORGAN: I don't know. It's how I am wired, I guess.

THERAPIST: First, let's define each end in a more balanced way. Let's use the example of the way you see your feelings. Do you remember what was on your Thought Diary?

MORGAN: Yes. I have it written down right here. One time I wrote that emotions are my private business and I should keep total control of them and keep them to myself. I also had the thought that emotions are uncontrollable. I should just explode and get rid of them. Put them on someone else so they have to deal with them.

THERAPIST: What's a less-than-total way to see emotions as completely uncontrollable private business that always has to be kept to yourself?

MORGAN: Sometimes I can keep emotions to myself.

THERAPIST: What do you mean when you say "total control"?

MORGAN: You don't show anyone how you feel.

THERAPIST: What would it be like for you to show some, but not all, that you are feeling?

MORGAN: I would cry or scream but not withdraw or go off on anyone.

THERAPIST: Is that complete control?

MORGAN: I guess not. At least I would loosen up some.

THERAPIST: We're getting closer to middle ground. What about your sense that the emotions are totally uncontrollable and you have to get rid of them and put them on someone else?

MORGAN: They get too strong for me.

THERAPIST: If they are too strong, does that mean they are totally uncontrollable?

MORGAN: I guess not.

THERAPIST: If you put them on someone else, does it decrease their strength?

MORGAN: It seems so at the time, but not much really.

THERAPIST: What's another way to look at it then?

MORGAN: It seems like they aren't uncontrollable, but they are just stronger than I like.

THERAPIST: What about putting them on another person?

MORGAN: It doesn't help.

THERAPIST: Just because you don't like them, do you think you should get rid of them?

MORGAN: No. I can hang onto them if I want.

THERAPIST: Where would you have more control? Hanging onto to them or putting them on someone else?

MORGAN: Hmm … Good question. I never thought about it that way. If I hang onto them, I'm in control.

Like many of the procedures discussed in this text, the therapist began by carefully introducing the metaphor. The metaphor was referenced throughout the dialogue (e.g., "We're getting closer to middle ground."). The therapist tested many of Morgan's absolutes with very specific Socratic questions ("If they are too strong, does that mean they are totally uncontrollable?"; "If you put them on someone else, does that decrease their strength?"; "Just because you don't like them, do you think you should get rid of them?").

CONCLUSION

In this chapter we have outlined a variety of rational analysis methods that clinicians can apply in fun, memorable, and effective ways (see Table 6.2). As we stated throughout, choose techniques based on the conceptualization of the case. Particular metaphors should be selected based on the patient's interests and/or life experiences. The timing of the rational analysis strategy must be thought out and based on identified thoughts, beliefs, and assumptions, as well as matched to patients' skill level. Socratic questioning is a key component of the rational analysis procedures, and thus the therapist must know and use varying types of questions so as not to put off the youth. Adding empathy and attending carefully to the youth's verbal and nonverbal responses will alert the therapist to any modifications that need to be made in the questions or process. Overall, these rational analysis techniques can be fun, active, and meaningful components of CBT.

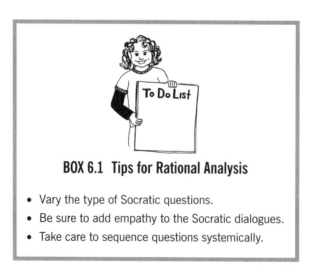

BOX 6.1 Tips for Rational Analysis

- Vary the type of Socratic questions.
- Be sure to add empathy to the Socratic dialogues.
- Take care to sequence questions systemically.

TABLE 6.2. Rational Analysis Techniques

Technique	Purpose	Ages	Modality
Who's Got the Germ?	Test of evidence	7–12 years	Individual, family
Control Dice	Test of evidence	8–18 years	Individual
Master of Disaster	Decatastrophizing; reattribution	8–13 years	Individual, group
Thought Prospector	Evaluate overly critical self-definition	8–13 years	Individual, family, group
Count Dreadula Says	Rationally evaluate overly pessimistic attributions and predictions	8–13 years	Individual, family, group
Whether Report	Testing evidence; follows from Your Brainstorm	8–18 years	Individual, group
Mirror, Mirror	Structured analysis of negative self-definition	10–18 years	Individual, group
3-D Thinking	Tests and modifies catastrophizing and emotional reasoning	8–18 years	Individual, family, group
Fake Math	Reattribution to break inaccurate mental contingencies	8–18 years	Individual, family, group
Playing Centerfield	Decrease all-or-none thinking	8–18 years	Individual, group
Newton's Cradle	Decrease all-or-none thinking	10–18 years	Individual, group

Bus Drawing

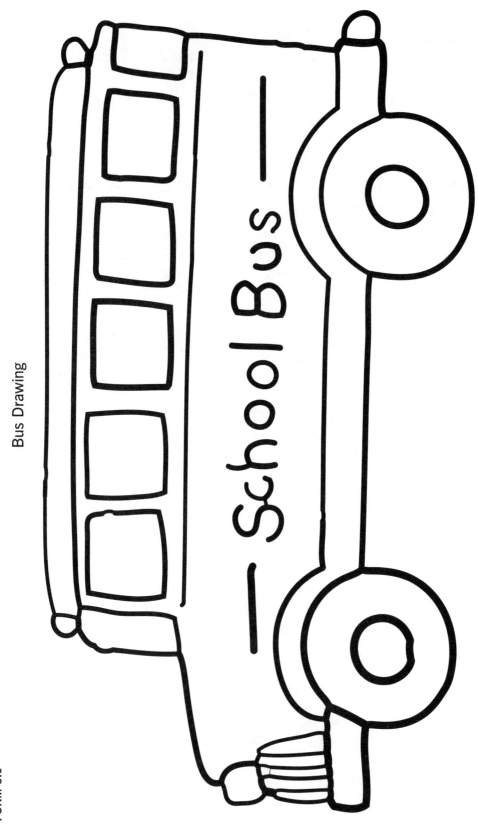

Master of Disaster Worksheet

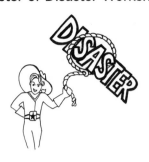

Disaster I can master: _____

_____

_____

Master questions:

How sure are you that the disaster will happen? (Circle one.)

1	2	3	4	5
Not		Kind of		A lot

When has the disaster happened before? (Circle one.)

Never   Sometimes   A lot

If the disaster has not happened, what convinces you it will happen now? _____

_____

_____

What was your explanation for the disaster happening before? _____

_____

What is another explanation for your sense it will happen now? _____

_____

If your disaster has happened in the past, how did you handle it?

1	2	3	4	5
Not well		Kind of		Really well

(continued)

What did you do? _____

_____

_____

_____

If you did not handle it well, what is different about you now? What could you do now that would be helpful? _____

_____

_____

_____

If you have a plan for the disaster, how bad could it be? How in control are you? _____

_____

_____

_____

Master of Disaster conclusion: _____

_____

_____

_____

Thought Prospector Worksheet

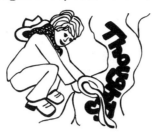

Thought you are prospecting: _____

What is it that you do that a _____ would never do? _____

_____

_____

_____

What is it that a _____ does that you would never do? _____

_____

_____

_____

After prospecting, what's another way to look at yourself? _____

_____

_____

_____

_____

YOU STRUCK GOLD!

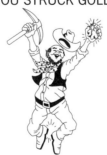

Count Dreadula Questions

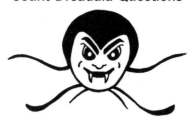

Am I punishing others for my mistakes?

Am I punishing myself for others' mistakes?

Am I confusing accidental with on purpose?

Am I confusing fair with what I want?

Am I confusing for now with forever?

Am I confusing possible with likely?

Am I being too hard on myself?

Am I forgetting about my strengths?

Am I being too hard on other people?

Am I letting feelings trick me into thinking they are facts?

How forgiving of myself can I be?

How forgiving of others can I be?

Are things all or none for me?

What could be worse?

Count Dreadula Diary

Date	Situation	Feeling and rating	Automatic thought	Count Dreadula asks	Count Dreadula says	Rerate feeling

Whether Report Worksheet

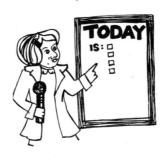

What is happening when you have a brainstorm? _____

_____

What feeling do you have? _____

_____

How strong? (Rate 1–10) _____

What is running through your head during the brainstorm? _____

_____

_____

What convinces you this is totally true?	What makes you doubt this is totally true?
_____	_____
_____	_____
_____	_____
_____	_____
_____	_____
_____	_____
_____	_____

Make a conclusion on your Whether Report. _____

_____

_____

_____

What is your new feeling? _____

_____

Mirror, Mirror Worksheet

View of myself	Who is my standard?	How I see him/her	How do I compare?

3-D Thinking Worksheet

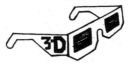

Difficulty/discomfort	How much discomfort?	How did you handle it?	How much of a disaster?

FORM 6.9

Playing Centerfield Worksheet

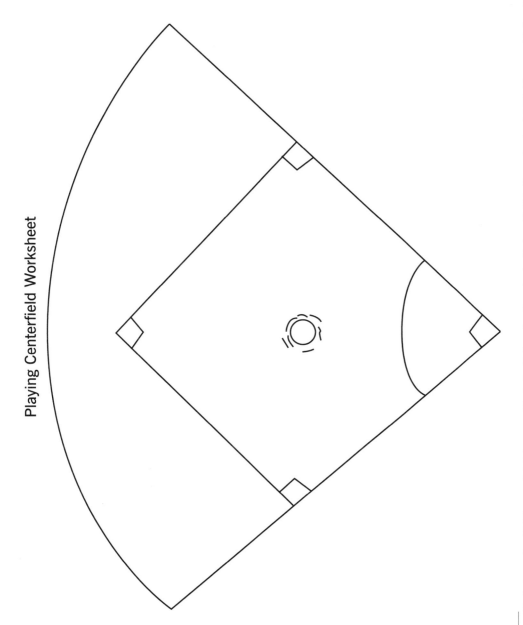

CHAPTER 7

Performance, Attainment, and Exposure

Popular culture recognizes the importance of demonstrating competence through performance or behavioral attainment. Phrases such as "Walking the walk instead of talking the talk," "Let your playing do the talking," and "Make it happen" reflect the value of doing. The Nike slogan, "Just do it," as well as *Star Trek*'s Captain Picard's command to his lieutenant, "Make it so," are based on the notion of engaging in difficult tasks despite the emotional obstacles. Finally, the axiom that when you fall off your horse, you have to get right back on speaks to the value of persistence in the face of discomfort or fear.

This last module brings the book full circle in many ways. In Chapter 1, we wrote about the crucial role emotional arousal and experiential learning play throughout CBT. Experiential learning helps the "head and heart reach consensus" (Padesky, 2004, p. 434). Behavioral experiments and experiential learning explicitly evoke emotional arousal so that new explanations, interpretations, and action plans can be learned (Barlow, 1988; Moses & Barlow, 2006). This chapter describes the rationale and procedures for constructing, implementing, and evaluating behavioral experiments that facilitate children's and adolescents' active experiential learning.

Behavioral experiments are powerful interventions due to their focus on experiential learning, emotional arousal, encoding experience, reflective learning, and the practicing of new plans (Bennett-Levy et al., 2004). Behavioral experimentation aims to change emotional states, promote flexible problem solving, make hidden beliefs more visible, and decrease the believability of negative assumptions (Rouf, Fennell, Westbrook, Cooper, & Bennett-Levy, 2004). Often, our young patients are convinced that their negative thoughts are absolutely true. Rather than seeing this as resistance or avoidance, Padesky (2004) sees it as a healthy skepticism for alternative views. She (p. 433) wrote, "Patients bring the healthy skepticism to experiments that true experimental science requires."

Patients require powerful disconfirming experiences to free themselves from strangling cognitive distortions, behavioral disturbances, and distressing emotions (Bandura, 1977a, 1977b). Padesky (2004, p. 434) concluded, "The first thoughts that occur to people in times of misfortune are most likely to rise from the experiential mind. Thus, to help ensure lasting change it is important that the experiential mind is convinced of new beliefs."

Powerful behavioral experiments often include some form of exposure. Barlow (1988) referred to exposure as a form of affective therapy. In exposure, the key element is developing new action tendencies. Instead of avoiding or freezing when confronting stressors, young patients learn to cope and endure. Barlow commented that exposure helps children develop adaptive senses of power and control. Through repeated emotionally arousing experiences and experiments, the patients learn to free themselves from the "holds old habits and beliefs place upon them" (Samoilov & Goldfried, 2000, p. 380). Exposure is a powerful way to ease patient avoidance and reservations (Padesky, 2004). Emotion is a focus for exposure tasks and the aim is to reduce emotional avoidance (Barlow, Allen, & Choate, 2004; Suveg, Southam-Gerow, Goodman, & Kendall, 2007). For example, anxious children withdraw from emotionally provocative situations, whereas children high in self-efficacy persist in distressing situations and consequently build adaptive coping skills (Suveg & Zeman, 2004).

Many young patients engage in experiential avoidance. "Experiential avoidance" refers to the unwillingness to have unpleasant private experiences. Exposure is the antidote to this avoidance. Greenberg (2006) astutely summarized the basic premise of exposure-based treatment. He (p. 90) wrote: "There is a strong human tendency to avoid painful emotions. To overcome emotional avoidance, clients must first be helped to approach by attending to their emotional experience and by changing the cognitions governing their avoidance."

Exposure teaches children to change their expectations about negative emotional arousal (Leahy, 2007). Leahy (p. 355) rightly asserted that this learning requires cognitive reappraisals and creates propositional ideas such as "When I have that feeling of anxiety, it doesn't overwhelm and destroy me" or "I am in a safe place even though I imagined what was terrible."

Experiential learning depends on the notion that transfer of learning from one situation to another is best achieved when the emotional contexts in the two situations are similar (Safran & Muran, 2001). Thus, if a coping state is acquired and practiced only in a calm state, it may not transfer to distressing circumstances. Clinical experience teaches us that anxious children are much more willing to "talk" about their fears than to actually face them. Additionally, our experience suggests that almost every angry child can acquire a variety of anger management strategies, but far fewer are able to apply these skills when they are actually pissing me off! Therefore, it is crucial to design experiments where children can practice their newly acquired skills in the appropriate emotional context.

Exposure, behavioral experiments, and experiential learning emphasize making changes rather than talking about change. Hayes et al. (1999) remarked that experiential exercises avoid the flaws inherent in purely verbal interventions. Experiential exercises create the genuine mastery required for enduring behavioral change. They augment and transcend rational analysis, cognitive restructuring, and other forms of verbal interventions. Hayes et al. wrote that experiential learning prompts the essential question, "What does your experience tell you?"

Behavioral experiments are reality-testing and discovery opportunities. They allow young people to evaluate and disconfirm their expectations. Accordingly, their predictions should be elicited ahead of time and then evaluated after the experiment. Therefore, Wells (1997) reminds us to help patients make specific predictions before any experiment is attempted. Vague expectations should be avoided ("I'll feel uncomfortable.") and more testable predictions are crafted ("People will smirk at me.").

Behavioral experiments then need to be cognitively processed (Rouf et al., 2004; Zinbarg, 2000). Emotion should not just be experienced, it should be understood (Boal, 2002). Boal rightly asserted (p. 37), "We cannot talk about emotion without reason or conversely, about reason without emotion; the former is chaos, the latter pure abstraction." Rouf et al. (2004) suggested a four-point sequence where behavioral experiments are planned, experienced, analyzed, and synthesized. In other words, experiments are designed, they are emotionally experienced, data are collected, and then conclusions are drawn. Rouf et al. (p. 31) cautioned, "Experience can be wasted, however, if patients do not take time to consider what they have observed."

The strategies in this chapter will provide clinicians with action-based interventions to propel the experiential learning phases of treatment. Ideas for designing and implementing the experiments with children and adolescents, as well as strategies for evaluating the outcomes of the experiments, are provided. These strategies will help bridge the gap between knowing and doing. Since anxious children have a tendency to withdraw from emotionally provocative situations, clinicians need to be comfortable guiding them through this process. The behavioral experiments presented in this chapter will help cast doubt on patients' maladaptive beliefs and expectations, thus opening the door for more effective cognitive restructuring and more lasting changes. Table 7.1 lists a number of examples of traditional exposures and experiments.

BASICS OF EXPOSURE

There are several important points to remember about conducting exposures and experiments (Craske & Barlow, 2001; Persons, 1989; Richard, Lauterbach, & Gloster, 2007). First, psychoeducation must occur before the exposure is begun. Patients and their families should have a clear understanding of the anxiety cycle, why exposures are used, and how the exposures will be collaboratively designed and completed. This education will decrease anxiety about the exposures, as well as give patients a sense of control. Specific ways of educating patients and families are outlined below, as are guidelines to help ensure that exposures are well thought out and tailored to fit the specific needs, interests, and skill set of the patient.

Educating Patients and Families about Exposure

Patients and families need to be prepared for exposure. Many of the psychoeducational materials presented in Chapter 3 can form the basis for the rationale. Collaboration is an important prerequisite. Remember, exposure is something you do *with* the patient rather than *to* the patient. Educating the patient about the rationale and process of

TABLE 7.1. Examples of Traditional Exposure Techniques and Experiments

Technique	Use
Play a board game where the therapist changes the rules (Kendall et al., 2005)	GAD, perfectionism, control, rigidity
Purposefully make a mistake (Kendall et al., 2005)	GAD
Blow up and burst balloons (Kendall et al., 2005)	GAD
Read in front of others in a funny voice (Kendall et al., 2005)	Social anxiety, fear of negative evaluation
Watch or read the news (Kendall et al., 2005)	GAD
Write something with nonpreferred hand (Kendall et al., 2005)	Perfectionism
Ask for directions (Kendall et al., 2005)	Social anxiety, fear of negative evaluation, perfectionism
Call a classmate on the telephone and ask for help on an assignment (Kendall et al., 2005)	Social anxiety
Try to remember 10 cards while being teased by peers (Lochman et al., 2003)	Anger management
Build a domino tower with nondominant hand while being teased by peers (Lochman et al., 2003)	Anger management
Practice losing things (Sze & Wood, 2007)	Hoarding

exposure without jargon may prevent young patients from feeling victimized (Lauterbach & Reiland, 2007). Exposure is best pursued with you, the patient, and the family forming a willing coalition.

Exposure is a scary experience for children and adolescents. After all, you are inviting them to face their threatening and dangerous situations. Since few patients *want* to do the exposure, the key to success is getting them to be *willing* to confront their distress (Hayes et al., 1999; Huppert & Baker-Morissette, 2003). As described in Chapter 5, the Wanting versus Willing exercise is a cognitive restructuring procedure that readies the patient for exposure. Additionally, your therapeutic alliance with children built upon the work completed in the previous modules provides the secure base upon which therapeutic adventures are pursued.

Hembree, Rauch, and Foa (2003) identified crucial components that should be included in a rationale for exposure. First, that avoidance is worse than encountering the anxiety is an important point. Second, that anxiety may initially increase, but that over time with repeated exposure the distress will decrease, should be communicated. Third, persistence and patience are learned skills. Finally, the outcome of positive exposure is a sturdier sense of competence and control.

Like many other procedures in this book, exposure is augmented by metaphors and analogies (Hembree et al., 2003; Huppert & Baker-Morissette, 2003). For example, Hembree et al. (2003, p. 24) offered a wound metaphor for trauma and explained, "The trauma may be viewed as a wound that has scabbed over but is not healed and remains sensitive to the touch. Prolonged exposure is the process of opening up and cleaning that wound and cleaning it thoroughly so while it may leave a scar, it will not hurt when something touches it." They also recommended a cave metaphor:

> Avoidance can be described as a cave where the patient retreated to heal from the trauma. While this safe cave has allowed [him or] her to function on some level, it also has significantly restricted the client's life. Exposure involves longer and more extensive journeys outside of the cave and that feels risky and dangerous. However, in order to completely heal from the trauma, the client must learn to live with the risks outside of the cave. (Hembree et al., 2003, p. 27)

Huppert and Baker-Morissette (2003) suggested two additional metaphors to educate patients about exposure, "learning a new language" and a roller coaster. Patients are learning a new language (approach) to replace an old language (avoidance). Continued practice fosters greater fluency. The roller coaster metaphor communicates the peaks and valleys of anxiety as well as the sense of control. Moreover, the roller coaster metaphor allows the therapist to explain that excitement/thrill and fear are essentially similar physiological reactions. Interpretations determine whether this state is seen as excitement or anxiety.

Hembree and Cahill (2007) offer some suggestions for strengthening the therapeutic relationship. First, you should reinforce the fact that you are aligned with the patients against their distress. Naming the Enemy and It's OCD, Not Me lay the groundwork for this notion. Second, collaboration and partnership are essential. Children get to set the pace and intensity of the exposure. Inviting the child to take the lead in designing and implementing adventures is a specific example of collaboration (Ginsburg & Kingery, 2007). We suggest that you avoid prescribing and/or assigning challenges to children but rather enlist the child and perhaps the family as coengineers. Children should guide the process and the therapist should takes cues from their young collaborators. This fosters a sense of control and builds the belief that children are "in charge" of their distress. Mineka and Thomas (1999) argued that exposure helps restore emotional order and control in peoples' lives. In fact, exposure's positive effects seem due to the increased perceived control. The increase in perceived control acts as a "safety signal" that cuts across situations. Kendall and Suveg (2006, p. 272) emphasized, "In vivo exposures that result from a collaborative effort between the therapist and child are often among the most memorable and meaningful to the child."

Collaboration may also include appropriate self-disclosure (Gosch et al., 2006). For instance, if the exposure creates some distress in you, it may be helpful to share this with a patient.

I (R. D. F.) was working with a 16-year-old female patient who feared contamination. She compulsively washed her hands, doggedly avoiding contact with any coins. After progressing through levels up the hierarchy, we reached the item regarding picking up change from the bathroom floor. We set up the experiment in the vacant clinic bathroom and designed it so we dropped change on the bathroom floor, picked it up, held it for a period of time, placed the change in a pocket/purse, and then washed hands once. This experiment created an increased sense of anxiety, discomfort, and even some dread in me. I shared this with the patient by saying:

"Radha, I have to tell you something. For better or worse, you have a therapist who is not so crazy about doing this experiment. However, I am going to do this with you anyway. Together, we are going to try to face down the discomfort. How does this sound to you?"

Modeling also is a form of collaboration (Hembree & Cahill, 2007; Kendall & Suveg, 2006). Encountering fearful situations with children bolsters their confidence. When therapists act as coping models, they demonstrate that they practice what they preach to patients. Moreover, when therapists accompany the children during their adventures, they are a genuine team who fights the fears side by side. Finally, children are comforted by the notion that they are not alone in their fearful context.

Dull experiments seem like work for youngsters. Thus, boredom as well as anxiety may combine to strengthen anxiety. Stimulating children's curiosity and adventurousness is key in encouraging emotional risk taking. Kendall and Suveg (2006) agree that creative and fun exposures are especially meaningful. They described several fun experiments—for example, a socially anxious child who feared public speaking pretended to give a speech after winning an award, and an overly inhibited child strutted through the library singing her favorite song aloud accompanied by a parent or therapist. Therefore, we generally refer to exposures and experiments as "adventures."

The Exposure Procedure

Effective exposure is comprehensive (Persons, 1989; Richard et al., 2007). Exposures need to address all the salient aspects of the avoided situations: cognitive, behavioral, emotional, physiological, and interpersonal. The therapist needs to construct experiments that resemble the actual experiences patients encounter. Fidaleo, Friedberg, Dennis, and Southworth (1996) noted that if the therapist creates an experiment with a worm to help a snake-phobic, it is unlikely to be effective because the worm and the snake do not share the same threatening properties. Clinicians must attend to variables such as who is present in the situation, the time of day, the patients' physiological state (e.g., sweaty, clammy/cold skin temperature, respiration rate), as well as various sensory experiences (e.g., room temperature, smell, sound).

Repeated or prolonged exposure sessions are generally indicated (Barlow & Cerny, 1988; Craske & Barlow, 2001; Persons, 1989; Richard et al., 2007). One-shot trials are less likely to be effective. Repeated exposure allows habituation and cognitive restructuring to take hold. While exposures are typically begun in session, patients and their families are invited to continue practicing their new skills during additional experiments in their real-world contexts.

Exposure is very present-focused and makes use of here-and-now experience (Richard et al., 2007). Exposure requires emotional engagement. However, as stated earlier in the chapter, many patients avoid this emotional contact. Hembree et al. (2003) recommended several strategies to promote emotional engagement. For instance, when conducting imaginal exposure, Hembree and colleagues recommended that patients keep their eyes closed, talk in the present tense, and include all sensory (visual, smell, and tactile) and response variables (cognitive, physiological, emotional, interpersonal). In this way, Hembree et al. concluded that patients experience all the aspects of distress, but remain firmly entrenched in the present context. Questions asked during the exposure should be brief and nonintrusive so as not to distract the patient. Useful questions recommended by Hembree, as well as questions from our own work for augmenting engagement, include:

"Describe what you see."
"What do you smell?"
"What emotions are you feeling?"
"What is running through your head?"
"Who is there with you?"
"What is happening inside your body?"
"What is the temperature in the room?"

To be effective, the exposure should not stop until the anxiety/distress decreases. Beidel and Turner (2006) recommend a 50% decline in responsiveness as a rough benchmark. The point of exposure is to gain confidence in coping with discomfort. Premature ending of the exposure strengthens avoidance and the sense that anxiety is dangerous.

Exposure may be compromised if the patient is overengaged with the emotional material (Hembree et al., 2003). In overengagement, the patient becomes overwhelmed and loses perspective. An overengaged patient loses contact with the present context during imaginal exposure, and traumatized patients may dissociate (Hembree et al., 2003). Children who become overengaged are asked to keep their eyes open (Hembree et al., 2003). The therapist may also ground the patient in the present through various techniques. First, the therapist may ask the patient to focus on his or her voice. Additionally, the therapist may direct the patient's attention to immediate physical sensations such as feeling the solid armrest on the chair or the firmness of the floor beneath his or her feet. Hembree et al. also recommended the cautious use of touch as a grounding technique. Physical touch should be discussed prior to the beginning of the procedure. Additionally, you should always ask permission (e.g., "May I touch your hand?").

Wells (1997) suggested the helpful PETS template to guide clinicians through the experiment-and-exposure procedures. First, clinicians prepare (P) the child and family through psychoeducation, rationale for the procedure, and self-monitoring (SUDS scaling, eliciting expectations/predictions). Then, the exposure (E) occurs and in the cognitive-processing phases the youth tests (T) or evaluates his or her predictions. Finally, the patient and therapist summarize (S) the experience and form conclusions to further enhance cognitive processing.

Rewarding Children's Efforts

Doing exposures and experiments is hard work for children and adolescents. They are emotionally provocative and challenging procedures. Therefore, efforts toward exposure should be reinforced (Gosch et al., 2006). Rewards may include praise, extra privileges, and small prizes. Videotapes (Kendall et al., 1992) and photographs (Kearney & Albano, 2000) depicting the child completing tasks are also rewarding. Ticket to Glide is a fun exercise designed to reward experimentation.

TICKET TO GLIDE

Ticket to Glide is a fun way for children to record and be reinforced for approaching their distress. It follows nicely from Up Up and Away (Chapter 4). Ticket to Glide combines self-monitoring, contingency, and craftmaking in one activity. The first step is recording the hierarchically arranged steps toward coping with their distress. Early steps are placed on the bottom of the ticket, with more difficult encounters placed on the top of the ticket. When each step is completed, the ticket is punched with a hole punch. When all the holes are punched, the goal is achieved. The ticket metaphor is helpful on several levels. First, most children do not like therapy in general and typically are avoidant of exposure. Ticket to Glide provides a concrete record of progress and represents their "ticket" out of therapy. Second, the ticket provides children and their families with a map to guide treatment direction. Third, punching tickets is a familiar experience for most children. Finally, the ticket can be decorated with drawings, stickers, and ribbons.

TYPES OF EXPOSURE AND EXPERIENTIAL LEARNING

Graduated Exposure

Graduated exposures make use of the hierarchies described in Chapter 2, which facilitate a stepwise approach to coping. Graduated exposures help children learn that situations are not threatening and that they possess adequate coping skills (Allen & Rapee, 2005). In gradual exposure, children learn that they tackle relatively easy situations first and then progress to increasingly emotionally challenging situations when their skill level permits. Kendall and Suveg (2006, p. 265) concluded that "gradual exposures help the child build experience upon experience and develop a sense of mastery over time." Graduated exposure is often referred to as a form of graduated practice. In most cases, we recommend a graduated approach to exposure training, whether imaginal, *in vivo*, or virtual reality, where the child systematically marches toward increasingly greater emotional challenges.

Imaginal Exposure

In imaginal exposure, young people recall events in imagination, and reexperience their distressing thoughts and feelings. Indeed, A. T. Beck et al. (1985) emphasized that imagery enhances patients' experience of anxiety. When conducting imaginal exposures, it is important to make the imagery as "real" as possible. Make sure descriptions occur in the present tense (e.g., "I am seeing" rather than "I saw" or "I will see") and include multiple sensory experiences (Richard et al., 2007; Padesky, 1988). Saigh, Yule, and Inamdar (1996) recommend a direct assessment of children's imagery skills. If the imagery is not "real" enough, the exposure will not produce the emotional arousal necessary for the exposure to be effective. Imaginal exposure may also be facilitated by the use of dolls, puppets, and other toys or props (Deblinger et al., 2006). Further, photographs, videos, audiotapes, and articles of clothing may also prompt imaginal exposure (Faust, 2000; Saigh, 1987). A vivid scene is characterized by a specific description of its situational context, emotions, cognitions, physiological responses, behaviors, sensory experiences, and interpersonal circumstances (Hembree & Cahill, 2007). Imaginal exposures are well suited to children with abstract fears, such as those with generalized anxiety (Kendall et al., 2005). Imaginal exposure may also be practiced as a step toward *in vivo* exposure.

In Vivo *Exposure*

In vivo exposure is confrontation of the situation "live and in person" (Kendall et al., 2005, p. 141). Generally, *in vivo* exposure follows coping skills training and imaginal exposure (Kendall & Suveg, 2006). *In vivo* exposure tests youths' acquired skills in the natural environment (Craske & Barlow, 2001). Real-life situations are scaled and hierarchically arranged. The child gradually progresses from mildly challenging situations to more intensely challenging situations. Various *in vivo* tasks can be constructed in the office. For instance, Kendall and Suveg (2006) gave taking tests, reading poems, and introducing oneself to office staff as examples. Most of the adventures in this chapter are *in vivo* exercises.

Virtual Reality Exposure

Virtual reality exposure is an alternative to imaginal and *in vivo* exposure (Forsyth, Barrios, & Acheson, 2007; Lauterbach & Reiland, 2007). Virtual exposure allows behavioral experimentation with stimuli and circumstances that may be otherwise inaccessible or uncontrollable (Koch, Gloster, & Waller, 2007). Patients are fitted with a head-mounted device that provides a visual image to each eye. The equipment eliminates visual contact with the real world and so narrows the patients' focus of attention. Sensors detect patients' movements so that they perceive they are moving in the virtual environment. The technique provides therapists with opportunities to monitor patients' reactions as well as to give feedback and support via headphones.

Hirai, Vernon, and Cochran (2007) identified several advantages of virtual reality. First, it reduces the likelihood of negative unanticipated events. Second, the properties of fearful circumstances can be individually tailored. Most children are infatuated with video games and so virtual reality may be very attractive to young patients. Bouchard, Côté, and Richard (2007) commented that virtual reality exposure enjoys the advantage of better protection of confidentiality, reduced costs, and focusing attention on avoidance behavior.

Flooding

Flooding is repeated or prolonged nongraduated exposure to the feared stimulus. Flooding does not include hierarchies and patients are exposed to intense aversive stimuli all at once. Patients remain in contact with the fearful stimulus until their anxiety decreases. Flooding is generally more distressing than graduated exposure (D'Eramo & Francis, 2004). The difference between flooding and graduated practice is akin to the difference between diving into the deep cold end of the pool on a hot summer day and gradually wading into the deep end with slow steps from the shallow end as your body temperature adjusts to the changing conditions (Shapiro et al., 2005).

Survey Experiments

Survey experiments can be applied to a number of clinical problems (Rouf et al., 2004). Survey experiments are simple to carry out. In our experience, many children find them fun. They are a way of "testing the evidence" for a belief in an active, experiential manner. To conduct a survey experiment about a specific belief, the children first make predictions about the survey results. Second, they write the survey questions. Frequently, we help them craft nonleading questions. Next, they collect opinion data from "real people" such as staff people in the clinic and/or others in the child's life (e.g., friends, family). We start the survey in the clinic to ensure that the child is "objectively" collecting data, and we give the child a "clipboard and pad" so the survey seems official. Once the survey data is collected, the children compare their observed results with their expectations and predictions. Following this comparison, a conclusion is formed.

Traditional Board and Sports Games

Traditional board and sports games are excellent forms of behavioral experiments. Games simulate the urgent win-or-lose dramas that emotionally punctuate children's lives. They are particularly apt for anxious, perfectionistic children who believe any failure or performance deficit is catastrophic, as well as for externalizing aggressive children who see losing as a threat to their competence and their sense that the world must work according to their unyielding rules.

Children's board games that require practice, patience, and frustration tolerance such as Bull's-Eye Ball (described later in this chapter) can be used in sessions. Games that involve "setbacks," such as Candy Land, Chutes and Ladders, and Hi-Ho-Cherry-O, are also useful tools to address frustration tolerance while conducting behavioral experiments regarding win/lose situations.

Improvisational Theater Games

Role playing traditionally assumes a central position in CBT. However, role playing frequently lacks spontaneity and emotional intensity. Improvisational theater games combine the cognitive-behavioral rehearsal procedures of conventional role playing with the immediacy of gestalt and experiential techniques such as the empty chair. Such theater games and creative dramatics are fun and potentially powerful ways to increase creativity and behavioral flexibility.

Behavioral rehearsal requires action, and dramatics bring action into an immediate emotional context (Landy, 2008). Improvisational theater occurs in real time and in urgent circumstances. Theatrical scholars (Boal, 2002) argue that this urgency propels genuine action, which is what we try to accomplish in exposure and experiential tasks. Authentic action gives patients a true sense of self-efficacy.

Improvisation also promotes a variety of skills including cooperation, listening, speaking, problem solving, tolerating imperfection, embracing spontaneity, creativity, and flexibility (Bedore, 2004). Bedore (p. 8) rightly contends that improvisation teaches children to change their routines and wrote, "Since our daily lives are unscripted, we are really doing improv all the time." Rooyackers (1998) noted that drama games help children get along better with others, develop better attention and concentration, practice self-control, and learn self-expressiveness. Improvisational theater games can be applied to social skills deficits, emotional tolerance, impulsivity, overcontrol, and fears of imperfection. Thus, they are suitable as an experiential exercise for children and adolescents with externalizing disorders such as ODD, ADHD, and PDD, as well as with patients with anxiety, depression, and eating disorders. Books by Bedore (2004), Rooyackers (1998), and Boal (2002) are stocked with fun exercises. The two games Counting on You and One Word Story, described later in this chapter, are just two examples of the way theater games can promote teamwork and cooperation (Bedore, 2004).

Family Crafts

Family crafts are favorite behavioral experiments. In essence, family members make something together. The details can be highly flexible. The therapist may assign the craft or provide craft options and have a family member choose. Family interaction patterns reveal themselves through the exercise, providing the therapist with opportunities for effective cognitive-behavioral intervention.

There are several important considerations in setting up and carrying out the experiment. First, decide who gives the directions. If one parent tends to take charge, invite the parent who stands back more to read the directions and assume responsibility for the task. The reactions of all the family members to changes in roles are cues for intervention. Pay particular attention to the thoughts, feelings, and behaviors produced at salient moments such as giving instructions, spilling of materials, and noncompliance. Further, take care to process the members' thoughts, feelings, and behaviors associated with taking the more dominant and submissive roles. Friedberg (2006, p. 163) identified several questions such as:

> Are the parents overly intrusive and protective?
> Do they fear the child will make a mess?
> Does the family work as a team to complete the task or are they competitive or sabotaging?
> How do they include the child in the task?

A case example will illustrate the process. Toni is a 10-year-old girl whose mother is highly coercive and controlling. Toni and her mother become entangled in intense power struggles where Toni sees herself as caught in a helpless situation where she can never please her mother. Therefore, she either becomes depressed and gives up or gets angry and acts out. Toni's mother does not recognize her role in this dysfunctional interaction. Talking about the problematic patterns yielded little progress. Therefore, we decided to try an experiment where mother and daughter made a craft together.

In the experiment, Toni was the leader and director. She decided what and how to make the craft. Her mother was instructed to follow Toni's lead. Not surprisingly, this was exceedingly difficult for Toni's mother. She became quite anxious and was given a thought record to complete. On the thought record, her mother listed a number of distressing hypotheses such as, "What is she making? Does she know how to do this? What if she messes up? What if she spills the beads and glue? She'll make a mess. I should help her or she'll never finish." The therapist invited Toni's mother to treat her own anticipatory-like hypotheses. Toni's mother continued to observe and intervene only if directed by Toni. Toni completed the task rather expertly. After the experiment, the therapist asked Toni to derive a conclusion (e.g., "What do you make of this?"). Toni replied, "I can do things well on my own if my mother lets me."

Toni's mother's hypotheses were also tested. Since her negative predictions failed to reach fruition, Toni's mother needed to reach a more accurate conclusion. The therapist helped Toni's mother synthesize the data from the experiment ("What does this say about all your worries?"). Toni's mother concluded, "If I trust her and let go of my worries, she will do fine."

This example shows how the family craft makes the hidden interaction pattern more transparent. Toni and her mother learned through the experience that Toni's competence was not determined by her mother's protection or control. The task was nonthreatening and ended with a small tangible reward for Toni, which may also serve as a visual reminder of the experiment and outcome.

Writing

Writing and journaling can also be forms of exposure. Cognitive processing therapy (Resick & Calhoun, 2001) makes extensive use of narratives. Patients write about the trauma or fear in detail. The therapist and patient then systematically process the exposure. The child develops a script of the event and describes it in a first-person, present-tense manner. Drawings may augment the process (Perrin, Smith, & Yule, 2000; Smith, Perrin, & Yule, 1999). Saigh et al. (1996) recommended asking traumatized children to draw their depictions of stressful circumstances and then verbally recount them. Deblinger et al. (2006) suggested using poems and songs in children's writing. Moreover, they noted that a book or other narrative form creates a permanent record that can be repeatedly reviewed.

THERAPEUTIC ADVENTURES: EXPOSURES AND EXPERIMENTS FOR DIFFERENT CLINICAL PROBLEMS

Traditional exposure methods may be applied to a variety of disorders ranging from mood and anxiety disorders to eating disorders, aggressive behavior, inattention, and PDD. In this section, we explain the ways in which exposure and experiential learning are applied to children's problems such as anger, control issues, depression, eating disorders, OCD, perfectionism, PDD, simple phobias, separation anxiety, and social anxiety. Table 7.2 summarizes the experiments and exposure techniques recommended in this chapter.

Anger/Aggressive Behavior

Therapeutic adventures are well suited to anger management problems. As most clinicians recognize, many children can readily acquire anger management skills. However, few youngsters apply these skills when they are actually mad. The key is to help them practice what is taught in real-world circumstances. Fortunately, there are several well-established experiments with angry and aggressive children in the literature (Feindler & Guttman, 1994; Lochman et al., 2003).

TABLE 7.2. Experiments and Exposure Techniques Described in This Chapter

Technique	Purpose	Ages	Modality
Circle of Criticism	Anger management skills, graduated practice	8–18 years	Group
Barb Technique	Anger management skills, graduated practice	8–18 years	Individual, family, group
Bull's-Eye Ball	Tolerating frustration and loss of control	8–18 years	Individual, family, group
Pop-Up Monkeys	Tolerating frustration and loss of control	5–18 years	Individual, family, group
Chinese Finger Trap	Learning to accept loss of control	5–18 years	Individual, family, group
One-Word Story	Teaching cooperation, reciprocity, and that no one is always in total control	8–18 years	Family, group
Family Meals	Testing inaccurate beliefs, practicing new family interaction patterns	5–18 years	Family
Picture Perfect	Decreasing all-or-none thinking about beauty, worth, and/or attractiveness	8–18 years	Individual, group
Germ Scavenger Hunt	OCD treatment	6–15 years	Individual, family, group
Musical Contaminants	Multiple-player game for OCD treatment	6–10 years	Family, group
Sharing the Persian Flaw	Modifying beliefs that mistakes are terrible and completely visible to others	5–18 years	Individual, family, group
Palm Print Your Mistakes	Decreasing conviction that mistakes are bad and must be avoided	6–15 years	Individual, family, group
Counting on You (Bedore, 2004)	Teaching listening, patience, and perspective taking, and noticing subtle cues associated with turn taking	6–18 years	Family, group
Battleship (Bergman, 2005)	Experiential game for selective mutism	6–12 years	Individual, family, group
Hansel and Gretel Technique (Shapiro et al., 2005)	Treatment of separation anxiety	5–10 years	Family
Let's Go Shopping	Graded exposure for social anxiety	5–10 years	Individual
Reading Allowed	Graded exposure for social anxiety	7–18 years	Individual, family, group
Museum Piece	Decreasing performance and evaluation anxiety	12–18 years	Individual

Feindler and colleagues (Feindler & Ecton, 1986; Feindler & Guttman, 1994) designed the Circle of Criticism and the Barb Technique to facilitate practice with anger management skills. Both of these procedures help patients respond to provocations in a calm, productive manner.

CIRCLE OF CRITICISM

Ages: 8–18 years.

Purpose: Anger management skills, graduated practice.

Materials Needed:

• Paper, pencil, bowl (optional).

In the Circle of Criticism, youngsters sit in a circle and are invited to serve up a criticism to the person on their right. The recipient then responds to the criticism with an anger management strategy (e.g., ignoring, agreeing, fogging, humor, assertive comment, calming self-talk). Feedback on the practice strategy is given by other patients and the therapist. Like all experiments, the task may be delivered in a graduated manner. In the early stages, the criticisms could be mild and supplied by the therapist. The criticisms could be placed in a hat or a bowl. As the patients progress, the supplied criticisms get harsher. In the final trials, the criticisms are spontaneously supplied by the youngsters themselves.

BARB TECHNIQUE

Ages: 8–18 years.

Purpose: Anger management skills, graduated practice.

Materials Needed: None.

The Barb Technique is a somewhat more intense behavioral experiment. Barbs are comments, questions, commands, and/or directives that typically provoke anger and aggression in the patient. The children's challenge is to respond to the provocation calmly using common anger management techniques. In the first phase of practice, a barb is explained and warnings are given ("I'm going to barb you"). Next, the barb is delivered ("You are so lazy. You'll never amount to anything."). The patient then applies an anger management strategy and is given positive and corrective feedback. Like in the Circle of Criticism, the barbs can be scaled in intensity. Repeated practice would then involve increasing the harshness.

Lochman et al. (2003) describe two other creative experiments for anger management. In one exercise, children are required to remember 10 cards in 5 seconds while being taunted. The second exercise involves children building a domino tower while being teased. Like Circle of Criticism and the Barb Technique, these experiments provide children with opportunities to apply anger management techniques in the context of emotional arousal.

Control Issues
BULL'S-EYE BALL

Ages: 8–18 years.

Purpose: Tolerating frustration and loss of control.

Materials Needed:

• Bull's-Eye Ball game.

Bull's-Eye Ball is a table game for children that is modeled after the skeeball arcade game. The object is to bounce small ball bearings into different numbered holes. The task requires eye–hand coordination, concentration, patience, frustration tolerance, and practice. The tiny balls are somewhat hard to control and they frequently spray all over. It is not uncommon for children to become quite frustrated at their initial attempts to earn points. These moments provide excellent opportunities for coaching patients through their distress and discomfort.

POP-UP MONKEYS

Ages: 5–18 years.

Purpose: Tolerating frustration and loss of control.

Materials Needed:

• Three pop-up toys with different timing mechanisms.

Pop-Up Monkeys is a behavioral experiment designed to help children accept the distress of being in a situation that is impossible for them to control. Moreover, Pop-Up Monkeys builds children's frustration tolerance. Accepting lack of absolute control and managing frustration are difficult tasks, but Pop-Up Monkeys is a fun, nonthreatening game. Young patients are frequently engaged by it. To play Pop-Up Monkeys, you need pop-up toys. We use monkeys, but pop-up toys come in many varieties. You can buy the toys at a store or online. Game play involves several set-up rules. First, the child walks from a chair to a table approximately 10–12 feet apart from each other, carrying the pop-up in his or her hand. At the table, he or she pushes the pop-up down. The child must get back to a chair walking slowly and not running before the pop-up pops. If the toy pops, he or she must return to the starting point. If by chance he or she makes it back to the chair before the monkey jumps, he or she can grab a second monkey and repeat the process, except that two monkeys are now pushed down at the table. If either of them pops on the way back to the chair, the child must start over with the first monkey. The therapist stops the game at emotionally salient points, such as when the child demonstrates frustration, anxiety, and/or any other emotional reaction. Socratic processing is applied at these moments (e.g., "What is it like for you to play this game?"; "What is running through your head?"; "How frustrated are you?"; "How in control do you see yourself?"; "How are you dealing with your frustration?"; "What are you doing to handle your lack of control?"). Next, alternative ways to deal with the frustration are practiced. Once the therapist senses that the child is constructing a new way to deal with frustration and lack of control, the game ends.

Of course, it is important for you to preload the task by selecting three monkeys that have different timing mechanisms so it is virtually impossible for the child to successfully control the task and so win the game. Similar to most of the procedures in this chapter, Pop-Up Monkeys is done in several phases. First, the task is explained and introduced. Second, Pop-Up Monkeys is initiated. Third, the experience is processed and the patient forms a conclusion or interpretation.

The following dialogue with Jackson, a 10-year-old who tightly held the rule "I must be in perfect control of everything and everyone," is a good example. Moreover, he connected his incompetence to his ability to control. The dialogue shows you how to process the experiment.

JACKSON: I hate this game! These monkeys are evil!

THERAPIST: This is really hard.

JACKSON: I want to break these evil things. (*Tries to break the toys.*)

THERAPIST: You may not break them. (*Jackson hands toy to therapist.*) What is running through your mind?

JACKSON: These darn things have a mind of their own. I can't make it work out.

THERAPIST: This is a good thing, Jack. This is a way to practice letting things be out of control and not have it eat at you.

JACKSON: It's one thing to talk about it. But doing it is a whole different story.

THERAPIST: That's why we are doing this. What things have you practiced with some of our exercises?

JACKSON: Well, I remember in Fake Math [Chapter 6] we came up with the thought that being in control does not mean you are a good person. I can still be seen as smart and stuff and let go of control.

THERAPIST: I'll write that on the card. So you say that to yourself while we continue to play Pop-Up Monkeys. What else can you tell yourself?

JACKSON: These monkeys won't get the best of me.

THERAPIST: That's two. See if you can come up with one more. Although you don't like the monkeys being in control, how able are you to deal with it?

JACKSON: Oh, I get it! Just because I don't like not being in control doesn't mean I can't deal with it.

The game successfully aggravated Jackson. Although he became agitated, the therapist set firm limits (e.g., "You may not break the toy."). The therapist reinforced the importance of practicing cognitive reappraisals and new action tendencies in the context of negative affective arousal ("That's why we are doing this!"). Following the above dialogue, Jackson played the game several more times while using coping statements.

CHINESE FINGER TRAP

Ages: 5–18 years.

Purpose: Learning to accept loss of control.

Materials Needed:

- Chinese finger trap.

The Chinese Finger Trap, like Pop-Up Monkeys, is an experiential exercise to help children and adolescents learn to let go of uncontrollable events (Hayes et al., 1999; Heffner et al., 2002). A Chinese finger trap is a toy made of woven straw and shaped like a tube with openings at both ends. When children put their index fingers in and try to pull out, the trap tightens. The way to escape is to give into the trap and push the fingers inward. Children learn that surrender is sometimes a winning strategy.

Surrender is often a tricky concept for rigid children who overly value control and dominance. They view surrender and/or submission in all-or-nothing terms. Further, they may mistakenly believe that surrender absolutely means defeat and so inaccurately tie their self-worth or perceived competence to their ability to control. Therefore, teaching them to see the advantages of surrender is crucial. Shifting their firmly rooted beliefs is a key task of the processing phase of the experiment.

The following is a dialogue with Alyx, a 14-year-old embattled adolescent girl who stubbornly refuses to submit to generally reasonable parental demands. The finger trap metaphor is initially introduced to Alyx.

THERAPIST: Alyx, do you know what a Chinese finger trap is?

ALYX: No, I don't think so.

THERAPIST: OK, this is it. (*Shows the trap to Alyx.*) You put your left and right index finger in the trap and try to get out. (*Demonstrates.*) See, you have to give in to get out. (*Pushes fingers toward center of trap and is then released.*) So sometimes surrender to control is a way to have more control.

ALYX: I don't see how that gives me *more* control!

THERAPIST: Fair enough. Let's make a hypothesis. Which do you suppose will be more freeing for you in this experiment, fighting against the trap or giving into it?

ALYX: I like to fight!

(*The therapist gives Alyx the trap and Alyx inserts her two index fingers into each end.*)

ALYX: This finger trap is scary, I don't like it.

THERAPIST: So Alyx, what happens when you pull against the trap?

ALYX: It gets tighter.

THERAPIST: Kinda like your parents' rules.

ALYX: Sort of.

THERAPIST: Sometimes the way out of a trap is to give in.

ALYX: I know what you are trying to get me to do.

THERAPIST: What's that?

ALYX: I should give in.

THERAPIST: Well, what was it like to fight against the trap?

ALYX: I didn't like it.

THERAPIST: And how about giving in?

ALYX: It was weird, kinda freaky.

THERAPIST: It was different for you.

ALYX: Giving in makes me feel bad about myself.

THERAPIST: You know a favorite song of mine by Cheap Trick has the lyric "surrender but don't give yourself away." How possible is it to keep your sense of who you are in place, yet still surrender?

ALYX: I never thought about it. Being a fighter is really how I see myself.

THERAPIST: You are a warrior. But is that what totally defines you?

ALYX: I don't know.

THERAPIST: Well, a fighter or a warrior tries to find ways to win. Maybe you can win the war by surrendering in some battles.

ALYX: (*Pause.*) How is surrendering good?

THERAPIST: OK, let's take a look at the advantages of giving in. What were the advantages of giving in to the finger trap?

ALYX: I got away.

THERAPIST: What else?

ALYX: Less stress.

THERAPIST: Anything else?

ALYX: Less wasted energy.

THERAPIST: So I guess there are some advantages to surrender. How do you put this new knowledge into action for you?

Alyx did not like being caught in the finger trap and surrender was an uncomfortable problem-solving strategy for her. Her therapist helped her reflect on her new experience (e.g., "Well, what was it like for you to fight against the trap?"; "And how about giving in?").

Empathy was used to amplify the experience (e.g., "It was different for you."). The therapist also explicitly tested Alyx's absolutistic view of herself ("You are a warrior. But is that what totally defines you?"). The therapist also worked with Alyx to see the advantages of surrender.

ONE-WORD STORY

Ages: 8–18 years.

Purpose: Teaching cooperation, reciprocity, and that no one is always in total control.

Materials Needed: None.

In One-Word Story (Bedore, 2004), an improvisational theater game, children stand or sit next to each other. They are instructed to take turns telling a story, but each storyteller only contributes one word during his or her turn. Bedore suggests that after the story you can ask each member if he or she guessed the story would end in the way it did. Thus, the experiment is followed by an evaluation of the results to assist with forming meaningful conclusions. Bedore cogently explained that this game teaches cooperation, reciprocity, and the reality that no one person is always in total control.

One-Word Story is good for children who have difficulty in reciprocal interaction and letting go of control. Like Counting on You, the game can readily be applied to family work. Power struggles will emerge in families battling with control issues. The game also preempts discounting any family members' contribution since everyone adds equally to the story.

Depression

Behavioral experiments are also applied to depressive spectrum disorders. Generally, these experiments test children's pessimistic beliefs about themselves, others, and the world. Behavioral experiments encourage patients to take action and carry the message that inertia contributes to greater depressed mood. Similarly to the other adventures in this chapter, these behavioral experiments provide children and adolescents with powerful disconfirming experiences. Below we describe two examples of working with depressed children.

Kareem was a 9-year-old boy who experienced ongoing depression and pessimism. He believed that he should never experience any sad moods and his happy moods should be "amazing." "Amazing" in Kareem's mind meant the happy feelings should be a 10 on a 1–10 scale and he should feel like characters in a Disney movie. Moreover, Kareem was certain that most if not all people shared this conviction. Kareem was trapped by a sort of emotional perfectionism and burdened by unrelenting absolutistic standards for his own happiness. Of course, the result of these rigid beliefs was persistent depression, sadness, anhedonia, and irritability.

We set up a survey experiment with Kareem. He selected a variety of people to survey and asked them how happy they believed they should feel each day and, on average, how happy they actually felt each day. Figure 7.1 shows the results of Kareem's survey and the following dialogue illustrates how the experiment was processed.

THERAPIST: Kareem, let's look at your data.

KAREEM: I asked a lot of other people.

THERAPIST: You did. What do you notice in the "How happy I should feel" column?

KAREEM: I don't know. They are all high?

THERAPIST: How many 10's are there?

KAREEM: One.

THERAPIST: While many of them are high, only one is "amazing." What do you make of that?

KAREEM: Maybe I am the only one who thinks life must be amazing.

FIGURE 7.1. Kareem's happiness survey.

Person	How happy I should feel	How happy I actually feel
Edgar (friend)	8	7
Maurice (friend)	9	7
Chelsea (friend)	8	7
Jacqui (friend)	10	8
Tomas (friend)	9	6
Al (friend)	8	8
Luke (friend)	8	8
Mother	8	8
Father	8	7
Brother	9	8
Uncle	8	8
Aunt	8	8
Cousin	8	8
Cousin	7	7

Conclusions:

It's not reasonable to always expect things to be "amazing."

People are about as happy as they expect.

It's not reasonable to expect everything to be amazing when you don't believe things have to be amazing. The numbers are really close and you feel satisfied.

THERAPIST: So?

KAREEM: Well, it's probably not always reasonable to expect things to be amazing.

THERAPIST: Let's write that down on paper. Now, what do you get from the second column?

KAREEM: Most people feel less happy than they guess they should.

THERAPIST: And what does that mean to you?

KAREEM: People's hopes for happiness don't come true.

THERAPIST: Do the numbers say that?

KAREEM: I guess not.

THERAPIST: How close are the two numbers in each column to each other?

KAREEM: Really close.

THERAPIST: What do you take from that?

KAREEM: People are not as happy as they expect.... Nobody's feeling amazing.

THERAPIST: How do you put this all together?

KAREEM: It's not reasonable to expect everything to be always amazing. The numbers are really close to each other.

THERAPIST: How much does that set you up to feel satisfied with feeling good most of the time?

KAREEM: Really satisfied.

The work with Kareem illustrates the systematic way you can process the survey experiment. The dialogue included both abstract and concrete Socratic questions ("What do you make of that?"; "Do the numbers say that?"; "How many 10's are there?"; "How close are the two numbers in each column to each other?"; "How much does that set you up to feel satisfied with feeling good most of the time?"). Finally, Kareem recorded his conclusions in writing.

Many adolescents are convinced that they must enjoy something in order to do the task or activity. Indeed, this rigid belief system reflects emotional reasoning (prisoner of feeling). Behavioral experiments are especially useful in disconnecting youth from this distortion. Claire was a depressed 14-year-old girl who stubbornly resisted doing anything she did not find entirely satisfying and enjoyable. The activities in the not enjoyable category included attending certain classes, talking about her thoughts and feelings in therapy, practicing soccer, doing household chores, and telling her parents her weekend plans. Not surprisingly, Claire skipped school, refused school homework, broke curfew, and preferred silence to communicating in therapy.

After identifying her beliefs in a self-monitoring task, we set up an experiment to test her beliefs. She agreed to test out the beliefs "I cannot do things I do not enjoy" and "Nothing comes out of doing things I should do." A key element in the process was facilitating Claire's curiosity ("Let's see if this hypothesis holds up. If you have to enjoy an activity to do it, what would the numbers show?"). Her assignment was at least to attempt and at best to complete heretofore avoided activities/tasks. Claire then rated her level of enjoyment. Figure 7.2 shows the results from Claire's therapeutic adventure. The following dialogue with Claire illustrates how the experiment was processed.

THERAPIST: Claire, what do you see in the numbers on your chart?

CLAIRE: Now you get to see how much my life sucks and is full of crap.

THERAPIST: What makes you say that?

CLAIRE: Look at the numbers, dumbass. They are 0–2.

THERAPIST: Thanks for directing my attention to that. Huh, it is curious.

CLAIRE: What is so curious?

THERAPIST: I see that there was not much enjoyment, but what was the belief we were testing?

CLAIRE: (*Quietly.*) I have to like something to do it.

THERAPIST: And your prediction?

CLAIRE: I couldn't do things I don't enjoy.

THERAPIST: Do the numbers bear that out?

CLAIRE: You are so smart. You figure it out.

THERAPIST: OK, I will. Let's see ... if the belief is true, there should be just a few things attempted and fewer things completed. How many were attempted?

FIGURE 7.2. Claire's behavioral experiment.

Activity	Attempted	Completed	Level of enjoyment
History class	X	X	2
Algebra homework	X		0
Spanish homework	X	X	2
Chemistry homework	X	X	0
Therapy assignment	X	X	1
Call re plans	X	X	0
Clean bathroom	X		0
Dishes	X	X	1

Conclusions:
I can do things I don't enjoy.
Something good comes out of doing things I don't enjoy but have to do.

CLAIRE: Everything.

THERAPIST: And completed?

CLAIRE: Six.

THERAPIST: And you filled this out honestly?

CLAIRE: Are you calling me a liar? Of course I did!

THERAPIST: So what do you make of that?

CLAIRE: I don't know.

THERAPIST: You attempted everything and completed most things. Would that happen if you had to enjoy things to complete them?

CLAIRE: Stop being a smartass. I hate being told I am wrong.

THERAPIST: Just one more thing. ... Did anything good happen that you enjoyed as a result of your doing the things on your paper?

CLAIRE: My parents let me go to the Maroon 5 concert and sleep over at Arielle's.

THERAPIST: Huh, so something good came out of doing things you have to do but don't enjoy?

CLAIRE: I guess.

THERAPIST: Let's write down what we found out.

Claire's irritability contributed to her prickly approach to processing the experiment. The therapist tolerated Claire's emotionally provocative statements ("Look at the numbers, dumbass."; "Stop being a smartass.") and kept the focus on the therapeutic target. The dialogue included concise questions ("And completed?"; "And your prediction?") in order to avoid long verbalizations and lecturing. This is particularly important with patients who are as emotionally reactive as Claire.

Eating Disorders

Waller et al. (2007) recommended a number of experiments for eating disorders. Planning and cooking a meal, trying on various clothes in changing rooms, looking at self in a mirror, and adding a small snack without exercising are excellent examples. Cooper, Whitehead, and Boughton (2004) designed many inventive exposures to test thoughts in patients with eating disorders. They developed an experiment for testing eating-disordered patients' overevaluation of eating and control. For example, they experimented with beliefs such as "Eating will help me feel better/make the pain go away" or "Not eating will stop me from feeling bad." Patients tested these beliefs by recording how the duration and intensity of negative feelings changed as a function of their overeating, healthy eating, and restriction. Further, Cooper et al. also used a survey experiment to test whether eating certain foods was unhealthy. For instance, a patient can survey peers and check to see if they think it is healthy to add a slice of cheese to her lunch.

Family meals are at the heart of several approaches to eating disorders (Lock et al., 2001; Minuchin & Fishman, 1974). These adventures fit very nicely into our cognitive-behavioral work with patients with eating disorders. Interaction patterns, interpersonal strategies, and belief systems reveal themselves in this context.

FAMILY MEALS

Ages: 5–18 years.

Purpose: Testing inaccurate beliefs, practicing new family interaction patterns.

Materials Needed:

- Table for eating meal, brought in by the family.
- Meals.
- Paper, pen, or pencil.

The Family Meals experiment begins with family members' predictions. For instance, Skylar, a 14-year-old girl with anorexia, hypothesized: "Mom will get frustrated and force food on me. Dad will withdraw and get depressed. They'll start fighting. Prentiss [Skylar's sister] will make jokes and be the center of attention. I'll get anxious and angry and lose my appetite." Skylar's mother guessed that, left on her own, Skylar would not eat enough, Dad will give up, Skylar will become "willful and stubborn," and Prentiss will feel left out. The mother believed she herself would feel depressed and be seen as incompetent. For his part, Skylar's father predicted he would be left out and his wife would criticize any type of involvement. He further hypothesized that Skylar and his wife would get into a conflict where they would "get into each other's faces and dig in their heels." Prentiss would get upset and try to cheer everyone up. Prentiss guessed that Dad would joke with her and talk about her softball. Skylar would get jealous because she has not played much recently because of her excessive food restriction. Mom and Skylar would fight over how much Skylar ate "because they are so much alike and me and my dad are the same."

Once the hypotheses are aired, the family meal is scheduled. The family brings in a meal and the session takes place. The therapist observes the interaction. When a clinically significant moment occurs, the therapist intervenes. The family then is invited to experiment with a different way of acting, interacting, or thinking.

Skylar's family brought in the meal and sat down for lunch. Skylar's mother initially unwrapped Skylar's BLT sandwich for her. The therapist seized the moment and asked Skylar and her mother what was running through their minds. Skylar said, "Here we go again. She's treating me like a baby. I hate this." Mom wrote, "I need to set up the food right so she will eat it. She will pull it into little pieces and it will look too gross to eat." The therapist then coached both Skylar and her mother through a new way of relating to each other around the food. Mom tried to let Skylar prepare her own plate and Skylar experimented with being assertive ("Mom, pass me the sandwich, please."). After the new behavior took place, the therapist asked Skylar and her mother for their thoughts. Her mother said, "I can't believe it! She's doing good!" Skylar wrote, "She's going to make me put more mayo on the sandwich. I'll never do anything good enough for her." The discrepancy between Skylar's prediction (criticism and control) and the actual occurrence (mother's surprise and acceptance) was subsequently processed through Socratic dialogue.

The meal continued for several minutes. As Skylar ate normally, Prentiss became very animated and attention seeking ("Hey, look outside. It's the new roller coaster at the amusement park! Remember when we went there last year, and you all got mad at Skylar? Remember when I got this big bruise at soccer?"). When her mother and father began responding to Prentiss, Skylar started to look rather grim and said, "Will you shut up? You are a drama queen." Their mother and father almost in unison replied, "Skylar, shut up and eat." The experiment thus yielded another potentially productive moment.

The therapist asked Prentiss what was going through her mind ("This is boring. Nothing's happening. I want time to talk."). On her thought record, Skylar wrote "Prentiss is a little bitch. She brings these things up to Mom and Dad to bring me down. They prefer that little princess to me. I'll never live up to their expectations. I'm left out of their world." This interaction provided an opportunity for additional experimentation. The therapist referred back to the family's hypotheses and brought the data together with the present interaction ("It seems like you all worry about being left out. Let's try experimenting with talking and focusing on a nonconflictual topic that everyone can make a contribution to.").

PICTURE PERFECT

Ages: 8–18 years.

Purpose: Decreasing all-or-none thinking about beauty, worth, and/or attractiveness.

Materials Needed:

- Cut-outs of models' faces from popular teen magazines.
- Paper or whiteboard.
- Marker.

Picture Perfect is an experiment developed for children and adolescents who believe weight absolutely determines their beauty, worth, and attractiveness. Picture Perfect takes advantage of youngsters' infatuation with teen magazines and their tendency to compare themselves to models in the magazines. Additionally, Picture Perfect works to disrupt and derail their excessive attention to body images and any physical flaw. While we do these adventures in groups, they can also be used with individuals.

The therapist prepares for the exercise by cutting out models' faces from popular teenage magazines. It is important to vary the type of faces and include different ethnicities. The patients are then given the task of sorting the models' pictures into three categories such as "pretty," "OK," and "unattractive." After sorting, the patients are asked to make explicit their decision rules for placing the pictures in each category. Each rule is written on a whiteboard or paper. After these "data" from the experiment are recorded, the children and the therapist process the information and form conclusions.

There are several key turning points in the exercise. First, placing any airbrushed model in the "unattractive" category for any reason is a curious result. Indeed, this reflects eating-disordered patients' excessive attention to any negative detail (e.g., "Her earrings were too large."). The Socratic question "How do you explain the fact that you found models in a teen magazine unattractive?" often leads to treatment-enhancing conclusions (e.g., "I blow small flaws out of proportion."). Further, comparing the frequency count in each category often yields productive results. For instance, in a recent group session seven pictures were put in the pretty category, nine were OK, and nine were in the unattractive category. The therapist then asked the group members to reflect on their experience (e.g., "What do you make of the fact that you placed 72% of models and celebrities in the average to below-average range?"). The group members concluded "I guess we are overly strict judges of appearance."

The third key point is found in the "attractive" column. The therapist refers the patients to their decision rules for inclusion in the pretty category. In a recent group, the eating-disordered patients listed makeup, hair, complexion, smile, eyes, and accessories as their criteria for beauty. Body and weight were nowhere on the list. The therapist then asked, "What do you make of the fact that weight is not on the list?" The girls were shocked and paused before remarking, "We're confused." The therapist then followed with, "If weight was such a determining factor, how can it be left out?" The girls countered with "We just forgot." If this occurs in your encounters with patients, it works just to add weight to the list and ask, "We have 10 items with 1 being weight. How can weight absolutely determine beauty if it is 1 out of 10?" Finally, in the last stage of unpacking the data, the question "If weight was an absolutely determining factor, how could any of these pictures be put in a beautiful category?" could be asked.

Obsessive–Compulsive Disorder

OCD is another disorder that traditionally responds well to behavioral experiments. Typically, these experiments take the form of exposure/response prevention procedures (ERP). Generally, the process is initiated with an *in vivo* or imaginal exposure to the obsessive fear while coaching the child to prevent or delay the compulsive/neutralizing behavior as long as possible (Piacentini et al., 2006). Like most other exposure-based procedures, ERP proceeds in a graduated, systematic manner. In this section, we present several therapeutic adventures with different children challenged by OCD.

Liam was a 9-year-old boy who saw his 4-year-old sister as a "disease carrier." Anything his sister came into contact with became immediately contaminated. Liam either carefully avoided these contaminants or cleansed himself by repeated washing. Liam had not hugged, kissed, or held his sister's hand in over 2 years. He predicted that if he did not cleanse himself immediately he would instantaneously become very ill, pass out, have a seizure, swallow his tongue, and die.

We challenged Liam with several adventures combining traditional ERP. Liam prepared for his series of experiments with coping thoughts developed through various cognitive restructuring (Chapter 5) and rational analysis techniques (Chapter 6). Liam's adventures with his "contaminated" sister included graduated steps. Early in the process, Liam touched surfaces following his sister's contact with them, while preventing the washing response. Then he gave his sister a high-five, which involved fleeting contact, and was coached to not wash his hands. A handshake and walking down the hall hand in hand followed the high-five. Finally, hugging his sister without his cleansing ritual was the final step.

We have encountered an interesting subset of patients with OCD where anger is the contaminant. Patients see anger as a source of danger and their own anger as potentially uncontrollable and infecting others in a viral way. Being angry is a "bad thought" and the product of a "diseased mind" are common assumptions for these patients. Frequently, these children and adolescents live in families where anger is prohibited and even forbidden. One mother remarked, "Anger is an emotion that I wish was purged from the range of human emotional experience." The FEAR effect (Barrett et al., 1996) helps explain the phenomenon.

The "FEAR effect" refers to Family Enhancement of Avoidant Responses. When it is in place, parents believe that negative affect damages or ruptures relationships. Family interaction patterns perpetuate the rules and implicit codes regarding cognitions, emotions, and behaviors (Waters & Barrett, 2000). From our standpoint, the sense that anger is contagious is a function of both the FEAR effect and its concomitant overprotectiveness and enmeshment in the family system. Enmeshment (Hansen & L'Abate, 1982; Minuchin & Fishman, 1974; Nichols, 1996) is characterized by excessive intrusiveness (talking for other members), shared identity (she's just like me), and a common survival mechanism to maintain the existing family system. There is a sense of reciprocal dependency in which there is a belief that each member feels what the other feels. One child clearly defined this pattern by saying, "I feel what Mommy feels. When Mommy feels sad, I feel sad too. It makes us be close to each other."

Ronnie was a high-functioning 16-year-old boy who was an excellent student and varsity athlete. He suffered from rather severe OCD, which was marked by several cleansing rituals (hand sanitizing, showering, daily laundering routines, and repeated cleansing of surfaces with Clorox) and avoidance of other people because he carried a contaminant within himself. After several self-monitoring procedures, Ronnie remained unable to clarify the contaminant other than to express his vague sense that "I have a virus or disease that will make my family very sick to their stomach."

Several traditional ERP procedures were modestly successful with Ronnie's symptoms, but most symptoms stubbornly persisted. Then, in a family session where there was open conflict between Ronnie and his parents, Ronnie demonstrated the forbidden anger. Both parents were aghast and stated that anger was a most unwelcome emotion in their family. They believed anger was "destructive," that it "soils" the family, and that it "contaminated" relationships. Ronnie's father also confessed that "anger makes me sick to my stomach." Indeed, the content of these beliefs were directly linked to Ronnie's contamination fears.

The ERP process began with Ronnie writing down his angry thoughts ("My dad is a control demon. My mother is a bitch. They treat me like a fucking baby."). After writing down the thoughts, Ronnie described his urge to wash as 70%. He read and reread the thoughts until his urge decreased to 30%, and at 30%, he was able to resist the urge to wash.

The next step was sharing his anger with his parents in session. His tasks included making predictions about what would happen, observing the true results, and resisting the urge to wash. Ronnie made predictions about his parents' reactions to his anger (e.g., "They'll think I'm bad"; "They'll see me as out of line"; "They'll think I am out of control"; "They'll think there's something wrong with me"; "They'll see me as ruining the family."). His parents were invited into the session, but Ronnie's specific predictions were not initially shared with them.

Ronnie then shared various things that made him angry about his parents with them in session. He began with things that made him moderately angry (5- on a 10-point scale). After Ronnie expressed his annoyance with his folks, the therapist elicited the parents' reactions ("What was it like for you to hear Ronnie's anger?"; "What ran through your mind?"). Ronnie then checked his predictions against his parents' actual reactions and noted whether they disconfirmed or confirmed his hypotheses.

It is important to note that some of Ronnie's predictions were accurate (e.g., both mother and father said they saw his anger as a sign of loss of emotional control and as a burden to the family). For this reason, therapists should take care to initially try this experiment in session so they can help the family process predictions that are confirmed. In this particular case, the therapist applied a test of evidence to the parents' belief that anger is a sign of loss of control. Further, the therapist also used reattribution to help Ronnie's parents craft a new explanation for his anger (e.g., "What's another explanation of anger other than ruining a family?"; "How is your family functioning preserved by extinguishing all anger?"; "What are the advantages of expressing anger in your family?"; "What make you guess that your family will be better off with Ronnie's OCD rather than his anger?").

Marvelle was a 16-year-old male who was an outstanding student, leader, and athlete in high school. However, he suffered from debilitating OCD with rather unusual symptoms. He was certain that unless he avoided casual contact with other people, he would lose his abilities and distinctive personality. He feared if he did not physically brush off after contact, he would transform into the other person and consequently lose himself. He avoided bumping into others in the hall and even dodged pats on the back and high-fives. After his predictions were clearly elicited, an experiment was conducted.

Marvelle was a genuine history buff and enjoyed history trivia tests. The therapist presented the idea of Marvelle taking a history trivia test, then having appropriate physical contact with others, not brushing them off, and then retaking the quiz. The therapist asked Marvelle to predict his performance on the second trivia test. He predicted that his performance after the contact would suffer.

Marvelle took a history trivia test found online in the therapist's office. He obtained a 30% correct score. Then two staff members sat on a couch in the therapist's office.

There was also an empty chair to make the situation more optional, so Marvell had to choose to sit in the middle of the couch between the two staff members. Marvelle chose to sit in the middle and subsequently brushed up against the others. His reported SUDS level was a 10 on a 1–10 scale. After the contact, Marvell took the history trivia test again and obtained a 76% score.

The therapist asked Marvelle to compare his predicted results to what really happened. Marvell said the experience was "weird and confusing," which indicated that doubt was creeping into his thoughts, feelings, and behavior system. He concluded that contact was not harmful and could be positive, but more likely it was neutral. The therapist and Marvelle designed additional experiments examining the effect of optional contact on his ability and personality.

GERM SCAVENGER HUNT

Ages: 6–15 years.

Purpose: OCD treatment.

Mateials Needed:

- Paper.
- Markers or crayons.
- Scissors.

Germ Scavenger Hunt is a therapeutic adventure for children that combines graduated exposure, rational analysis, contingent rewards, and play. It is well suited to children with contamination fears. The game is implemented in several phases. In the first phase, the scavenger hunt idea is introduced. Different types of germs or contaminants are written or drawn on small slips of paper. As in Who's Got the Germ? (Chapter 6), young children could write a plus sign (+) to represent good germs that boost immunity, a minus sign (–) to signal an illness-producing germ, and use a blank slip to illustrate neutral germs (see Figure 7.3). The words or drawings can be made more complex and specific for older or more sophisticated patients. Then you place the germs in various places in your office and clinic. Since children with OCD fear touching various surfaces, this practice works well. We typically place the germs on handrails, counters, door knobs, and the like. You, the child, and the parents search and collect as many germs as possible. In order for the children to collect a germ, they must touch the surface. After all the germs are collected, the scores are tallied much like in Who's Got the Germ? The one with the most germs wins a small prize. Finally, the scavenger hunt process is summarized. The following dialogue illustrates the summary process with 9-year-old Desmond.

DESMOND: That was fun!

THERAPIST: Wow, who knew that collecting germs could be fun?

DESMOND: Not me!

THERAPIST: So let's count up what you have.

FIGURE 7.3. Example of germs for Germ Scavenger Hunt.

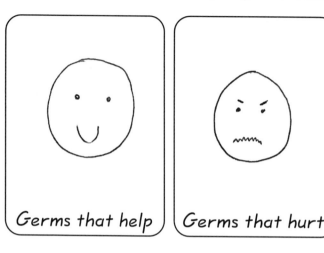

Germs that help | Germs that hurt | Germs that do not help or hurt

DESMOND: I have six pluses, four minuses, and four blanks.

THERAPIST: What does that mean about all germs being bad?

DESMOND: Not all germs are bad.

THERAPIST: That's sure the way your collection adds up. Where did you find all your germs?

DESMOND: All over the place: on the floor, the shelf, the stairs, and on stuff in the building.

THERAPIST: Kind of like where real germs live.

DESMOND: Yep.

THERAPIST: And you had to touch these things, right?

DESMOND: Right.

THERAPIST: How often did you wash your hands?

DESMOND: I didn't.

THERAPIST: So, what have you discovered about what OCD tells you?

DESMOND: He's full of crap, not all germs are bad, and I can touch things without washing.

THERAPIST: Let's write that down!

The summary process with Desmond illustrates several points. First, Desmond had fun! Second, the therapist walked through the summary with Desmond using specific and systematic questioning (e.g., "What does that mean about all germs being bad?"; "Where did you find all your germs?"). Finally, Desmond was able to respond to a concluding synthesizing question (e.g., "So, what have you discovered about what OCD tells you?").

MUSICAL CONTAMINANTS

Ages: 6–10 years.

Purpose: Multiple-player game for OCD treatment.

Materials Needed:

- "Contaminated" objects.
- Music.
- Chairs set in a circle.

Musical contaminants is a game-like exposure task for children with OCD and fears of contamination. It is based on the musical chairs game and is well suited to family and/or group work. Before the game begins, contaminated objects are scaled on a hierarchy. The lowest scoring object on the hierarchy is then passed around the room while the music is playing. The game's twist is that the person who has the object when the music is over is the winner. The winner of each round gets a small prize. The next higher object on the hierarchy is then passed around the room. The passing process is graduated exposure. It provides graded practice because the length of time the patient holds onto the object increases as the game continues. Additionally, most children will want to win, so they will hold onto the object longer as the game continues and the suspense builds toward when the music stops. After each round, the therapist should process the experience, help the child summarize findings, and punch the Ticket to Glide.

Lourdes, an 8-year-old girl suffering from OCD, was initially quite reluctant to engage in any exposure trials since she had had unfortunate experiences with exposure with two prior therapists. Musical contaminants provided a nonthreatening alternative to testing her contamination fears with stuffed animals and clothes. She believed her animals and clothes were "poisoned" with germs after they were touched by other children who were sick.

The family (mother, father, and brother) accompanied Lourdes to the session and brought the "diseased clothes and stuffed animals." The game was explained to the family. Fortunately, Lourdes and her brother, Miguel, enjoyed healthy sibling competition. In fact, at one point in the game, Miguel and Lourdes fought over the contaminated toy, with Lourdes eventually winning a tug of war. The following dialogue shows how to work through the summary process after the experiment ends.

THERAPIST: Lourdes, how many of the animals did you hold onto?

LOURDES: Pretty much all of them.

THERAPIST: How worried are you that you will get sick?

LOURDES: Not very much.

THERAPIST: How come?

LOURDES: It was fun. I didn't think about it.

THERAPIST: How much do you want to wash?

LOURDES: Not at all.

THERAPIST: Hmm ... How come?

LOURDES: No need to. I'm not feeling sick to my stomach and nobody looks like they are going to throw up. Miguel just has a stupid look on his face.

THERAPIST: So, if these things had bad sickness on them, is this what you would guess would happen?

LOURDES: No. They must be safe now.

The game added a reinforcing value to the therapeutic adventures ("It was fun."). Lourdes learned that after the contaminants were spread around, no disasters occurred. Finally, she was asked to derive a synthesizing conclusion ("So, if these things had bad sickness on them, is this what you would guess would happen?").

Perfectionism
SHARING THE PERSIAN FLAW

Ages: 5–18 years.

Purpose: Modifying beliefs that mistakes are terrible and completely visible to others.

Materials Needed:

- Paper with geometric shapes to color (see Figure 7.4).
- Crayons.

Sharing the Persian Flaw is a procedure designed to decrease perfectionism and fear of failure. It is based on the U.S. television series *Joan of Arcadia*, which aired from 2003 to 2005. During one episode, Joan is unnerved by her imperfection and her lack of control over others and events. Over the course of the show, Joan learns about Persian rug makers who purposefully make errors in their beautiful rugs. These errors are the artists' signatures and ways to express their humility. As defined in the program, the Persian flaw emphasizes the idea that life must be lived in its unpredictable and most imperfect reality. We adapted the Persian flaw for cognitive therapy with children in the following ways. The procedure begins with the therapist's explanation of the metaphor and then continues with the presentation of the task.

"Do you know what a Persian flaw is? Many people think Persian rugs are the most beautiful rugs in the world. But you know what? The rug makers make mistakes in the rug on purpose. They make mistakes as kind of a special signature. They think that mistakes are the things that make us especially human. Mistakes allow us to know ourselves and for others to know us as we truly are. They believe they should be shared rather than hidden. How does this sound?

"So we are going to do a craft. I want you to color in this design imperfectly. You make three mistakes but don't tell anyone what they are. Instead, write them on the back."

FIGURE 7.4. Example of Sharing the Persian Flaw shape.

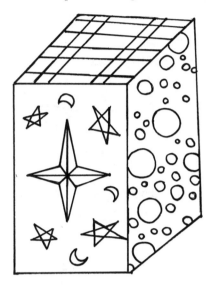

The task involves completing a geometric shape "imperfectly," recording the mistakes, rating the visibility and awfulness of the mistakes, and then sharing the artwork with others to survey whether their mistakes were noticeable and awful. Before the survey, patients record their predictions. After the survey, you and the child evaluate the results and derive a conclusion. The following dialogue illustrates Sharing the Persian Flaw with Avivah, a 10-year-old anxious girl. Figure 7.5 shows the results of Avivah's survey.

THERAPIST: Avivah, let's look at the results of your survey. How many people found all of your mistakes?

AVIVAH: None!

THERAPIST: That's curious. What do you make of that?

AVIVAH: It's weird.

THERAPIST: What did you guess would happen?

AVIVAH: Most people would see all my mistakes.

THERAPIST: So how does that make you feel?

AVIVAH: Weird. I didn't expect that.

THERAPIST: So you are confused. But what about?

AVIVAH: I thought my mistakes would be as clear to others as they are to me.

THERAPIST: Huh. But they weren't. Let's write that down. How about the ratings of the art? How many were less than 5?

AVIVAH: None.

THERAPIST: What did you predict?

FIGURE 7.5. Avivah's Sharing the Persian Flaw survey.

Predictions:

Most people will see all my mistakes.

They will see the drawing as just OK (5 or less).

Most people will see the mistakes as 7 or higher on the bad scale.

Person	Saw all mistakes (yes/no)	Rating of artwork	How bad were mistakes?
Mom	No	6	3
Dad	No	6	3
Brother	No	5	2
Carly	No	7	1
Rebekah	No	7	1
Zeke	No	8	2
Daisy	No	9	1
Sumi	No	8	2
Orin	No	7	2

Conclusions:

My mistakes aren't as clear to others as they are to me.

Even though I messed up, people still thought it was pretty good.

I think my mistakes are worse than they really are.

AVIVAH: Most people would see it as a 5 or less.

THERAPIST: What do you make of that?

AVIVAH: Weird again.

THERAPIST: How so?

AVIVAH: Even though I messed up, people thought it was pretty good.

THERAPIST: Seems like it. Let's write that down. Now let's look at how many people thought the mistakes were bad. How many 7's or higher were there?

AVIVAH: None!

THERAPIST: So what does that mean?

AVIVAH: I think my mistakes are worse than they really are. I'll write that one down!

Avivah's example makes several important points. First, specific and concrete questions yielded productive data ("How many people found all of your mistakes?"; "How many are greater than 5?"). Avivah's doubt crept in early and was repeated in the process ("It's weird."). The therapist modeled a scientific hypothesis-testing attitude throughout the task (e.g., "That's curious."; "What do you make of that?"; "So, what does that mean?").

PALM PRINT YOUR MISTAKES

Ages: 6–15 years.

Purpose: Decreasing conviction that mistakes are bad and must be avoided.

Materials Needed:

- Construction or butcher's paper.
- Finger paint.
- Paper towels.
- Pen, pencil, or marker.

Palm Print Your Mistakes is an exposure task for children who do not like to get messy and are afraid of making mistakes. The task involves the child dipping his or her palms into finger paint and placing the palm print on a sheet of construction or butcher paper. Then, in each palm print, patients will write down their mistakes. The palm print is a unique type of signature that represents the child's individuality, yet it will never be perfectly stamped on the paper. A palm print is rife with imperfections! Palm Print Your Mistakes brings together the experience that life is messy, errors are inevitable, and mistakes mark one's individuality.

Palm Print Your Mistakes occurs in several stages. An introduction to the metaphor is the first stage. For example, the therapist says:

Do you know what a fingerprint or handprint is? No two people have the same handprints or fingerprints. They mark you as a unique individual. What we are going to do is make your handprint with the finger paint. How does this sound?

In step two the children dip their hands in the finger paint. We recommend you use a nontoxic washable brand and, of course, keep several paper towels on hand or perhaps supply children with a smock or apron.

Once the handprint is made and dries, you move onto step three. In this phase, the child writes a flaw on each finger (e.g., "I disobey sometimes."). After all the flaws are recorded on the fingers, the child reads them aloud. In the concluding step, four, the therapist helps the child make sense of the experience. The following dialogue is with 12-year-old Odie.

THERAPIST: So, Odie, what do you make of this?

ODIE: It's a mess.

THERAPIST: I know, but what about all the mistakes written on your fingers?

ODIE: There are a lot of them.

THERAPIST: Well, can you have fingerprints without fingers?

ODIE: Of course not. That's stupid!

THERAPIST: And fingerprinting makes you uniquely human, right?

ODIE: Right.

THERAPIST: What's on the fingerprints?

ODIE: My mistakes.

THERAPIST: So how are your mistakes and fingerprints alike?

ODIE: You can't be human without them.

THERAPIST: Exactly. So what conclusion should we write here on the palm?

ODIE: I can't be human or me without mistakes.

In this dialogue, the therapist began and ended with abstract open-ended questions ("What did you make of this?"; "What conclusion should we write?"). The middle phase of the dialogue consisted of systematic concrete questions to guide Odie's discovery ("What about all the mistakes written on your fingers?"; "Can you have fingerprints without fingers?"; "What's on your fingerprints?"; "How are your mistakes and fingerprints alike?"). The process concluded with Odie recording his conclusion on the palm print.

Pervasive Developmental Disabilities/Sensory Sensitivities
COUNTING ON YOU

Ages: 6–18 years.

Purpose: Teaching listening, patience, and perspective taking, and noticing subtle cues associated with turn taking.

Materials Needed: None.

Counting on You (Bedore, 2004) is a good, simple game for children with PDD, social skills deficits, impulsivity, and excessive egocentrism. While the game was initially developed for groups of children, it can also be readily applied to family work.

In Counting on You, an improvisational theater game, children sit in a circle. The leader then explains that they must count together, one person at a time. The players are welcome to say the next number at any time, but if two members speak at once the counting returns to "1." The point of the game is to reach a high number. As Bedore (2004) notes, this game is ideal when players speak over each other and interrupt one another. The task requires listening, patience, perspective taking, and noticing subtle cues associated with turn taking. When family members intrude, interrupt, and have difficulty hearing each other, Counting on You is a fun experiment.

Children diagnosed with PDD often experience severe sensory sensitivities. Noises, tastes, textures, and sights may provoke anxiety, irritability, and even a heightened disgust response. With the next examples, we show how experiments helped four youngsters with PDD and a variety of sensory sensitivities.

Suri was an 8-year-old girl with high-functioning Asperger Syndrome who found denim, socks, and warm room temperatures highly aversive. She first constructed and practiced several coping thoughts via cognitive restructuring and rational analysis procedures (e.g., Master of Disaster). Then, in session, Suri's mom gradually raised the room temperature while Suri played. When Suri recognized the rising temperature, she was prompted to read her coping cards. Suri's mother's involvement in the session prepared her to conduct daily practice at "turning up the heat" at home between sessions. Suri learned to tolerate warm room temperatures without panicking or having tantrums.

Suri's aversion to tight socks was similarly treated with graduated experiments. Cognitive restructuring produced several coping cards. Then Suri and her mother enacted several experiments outside of the session. First, lightweight, loose-fitting socks were tried. Once Suri conquered this challenge, heavier, tighter socks were attempted.

Ari was a 10-year-old boy with PDD who detested unanticipated sounds and the smells of lemon and cinnamon. He demonstrated an exaggerated startle response to loud, unanticipated noises. This was particularly distressing for him because he lived in an urban environment where sirens and blaring car horns were everyday occurrences. Unannounced fire alarms in his elementary school were particularly traumatizing for him. If a fire drill occurred, he would scream wildly and run out of the room like a shot out of a cannon. Not surprisingly, this was quite disconcerting for school personnel.

Ari's treatment adventures were complex. His hierarchies combined type of noise, level of predictability, and degree of personal control, as seen in Figure 7.6. Like most experiments, cognitive restructuring and rational procedures prepared him for the adventures. The experiments started with balloon bursts varied by proximity and predictability. Then Ari habituated to the fire alarm sounds beginning with recordings at low volumes controlled by him and progressing to higher volumes controlled by others. We also used ear phones at medium volume to make the sound more "personal." Of course, we did not use high volumes with the ear phones to prevent harm to Ari's ears. Finally, the parents worked with the local fire station and school to "practice" using real alarms.

Josie was an 11-year-old with high-functioning autism who was "spooked" by mascots, clowns, and other characters in costumes whose faces were obscured. She experienced extreme anxiety whenever she anticipated seeing a mascot, costumed/masked character, or clown. Of course, this made family outings to amusement parks, circuses, ice shows, and sporting events very stressful. Josie's discomfort was especially problematic since her father was a high school football and basketball coach! Josie's belief about these characters included the perception that since the facial expressions were frozen and unchanging, the mascots were dangerous and unpredictable. Further, her magical thinking contributed to the sense that the human individual inside the costume was controlled by the character.

A series of therapeutic adventures were designed with Josie (Figure 7.7). First, Josie read the local entertainment and sports daily in search of stories about mascots, costumed characters, and clowns creating danger and harming others. Second, Josie watched TV shows with these characters in them (e.g., ice shows, clown cartoon shows, sporting events). Next, the parents taped the mascots performing at games. Viewing times were lengthened as Josie habituated to them. A fourth experiment involved her dad bringing the mascot costume home and Josie successfully approaching it. After successful experimentation with that adventure, Josie actually put the mascot head on her own head. The final experiments included graduated practices where Josie watched the mascot from far away in the gym doorway, then from sitting in the bleachers moderately close to the mascot, then from sitting in the bleachers behind the mascot, and ultimately, having her picture taken with the mascot.

FIGURE 7.6. Ari's graduated adventures.

Practice fire alarm at school

Practice alarm at firehouse

Practice alarm randomly controlled at medium volume with earphones

Practice alarm controlled by self at medium volume with earphones

Practice alarm at high volumes controlled by others

Practice alarm at high volumes controlled by self

Practice alarm at medium volumes controlled by others

Practice alarms at medium volumes controlled by self

Practice alarms at low volumes controlled by others

Practice alarms at low volumes controlled by self

Balloon burst behind a barrier without a warning

Balloon burst behind a barrier with a warning

Balloon burst close to him without a warning

Balloon burst close to him with warning

Balloon burst in office but in far corner without a warning

Balloon burst in office but in far corner with warning

Balloon burst outside of office door without a warning

Balloon burst outside of office door with a warning

Dayna was an 8-year-old child with PDD who was disgusted by the sensations of tags on clothes and by food textures such as pudding, milkshakes, cream-based soups, and Jell-o. She and her family experimented with wearing "tags" for increasingly longer periods of time until habituation occurred. Each step was explained to Dayna as setting a new "world record." Times began at 1 minute and were increased by 2 minutes when her SUDS rating (Chapter 2) decreased by 50% for two consecutive trials.

Dayna believed that thick liquids would cause her to choke or gag. She developed coping statements through cognitive restructuring (Chapters 5 and 6). Then she used the coping statements to navigate through increasingly challenging adventures. Experiments were graduated by the amount of liquid ingested (small sip, progressing to bigger swallows) and thickness of liquid (watered-down cream soup, thicker cream-based soup, watered down milkshake, thick shake). Like the other PDD cases described in this section, therapeutic adventures gave Dayna greater behavioral flexibility.

FIGURE 7.7. Josie's experiments.

Take a picture with the mascot

Increase proximity to mascot in live action

Increase proximity to costume; wearing mascot head

Watch videotapes of mascots at games

Watch mascots on TV

Search local newspapers for stories about dangerous mascots

Specific/Simple Phobias

Exposure treatments were initially used to treat a variety of simple phobias such as animal phobias, snake phobias, insect phobias, elevator phobias, and needle phobias. The focus is on the concrete object, stimulus, or situation children dread and avoid. Graded exposure hierarchies are established and patients work their way toward facing down increasingly strong fears. In this section, we describe work with several children who have various phobias: Jonas, an 11-year-old needle and physician phobic; Abraham, a 9-year-old elevator phobic; Cat, an 11-year-old girl who worried excessively about vomiting; and Molly, a 5-year-old girl who feared public toilets.

NEEDLE PHOBIA

Jonas was an 11-year-old boy who dreaded any type of injection. His fear of needles also generalized to physicians' offices and practitioners' white coats. This was particularly problematic because Jonas had a compromised immune system and needed a flu shot every fall, as well as regular follow-up visits to his pediatrician.

Jonas, his mother, and his therapist agreed to initially work on his fear of physicians and their offices and then progress toward injections. We developed the hierarchy shown in Figure 7.8. As the hierarchy indicates, we progressed slowly up from the bottom of the list. Initially, we borrowed a white coat from a child psychiatry resident in our clinic and simply draped it over a chair. Then we encouraged Jonas to try it on. Jonas clearly enjoyed this step and benefited from a sense of greater control.

The next two steps in the hierarchy (3 and 4) required the assistance of psychiatric residents in the clinic. We used them as "phobic stimuli" and varied their proximity to Jonas. Steps 5 and 6 in Jonas's adventures combined the white coat with noninvasive procedures performed by volunteer resident physicians. The final four steps prompted greater approach behavior toward the pediatric clinic. The step involving Jonas making his own appointment was added to further his sense of control.

We realize that not every clinician has access to resident physicians as helpers in their patients' adventures. However, a white lab coat could be purchased and worn by office staff. In fact, we encouraged Jonas and his mom to purchase a lab coat and practice at home. Since Jonas's fears complicated his medical treatment, his pediatrician

FIGURE 7.8. Jonas's physician hierarchy.

10. Well-child visit
9. Making an appointment for visit
8. Sitting in the waiting room without an appointment
7. Visiting the pediatrician's office and not having an appointment
6. Having blood pressure taken by physician in a white lab coat
5. Being weighed by a physician in a white lab coat
4. Being in the same room with the physician in a white lab coat
3. Seeing a physician in a white lab coat in the hall
2. Wearing a white lab coat
1. Seeing a white lab coat on the table

FIGURE 7.9. Jonas's flu shot hierarchy.

7. Get shot from pediatrician
6. Pediatrician holds syringe while close to Jonas
5. Sit in office with shot coming closer
4. Sit in pediatrician's office and talk about shot
3. Receive "fake" flu shot from staff
2. View video of flu shot/other injections
1. View and hold picture of needle

was extremely collegial and participated in his adventures. It is highly likely that most pediatricians in similar cases will be equally collaborative.

Jonas's fear of needles was treated in a similar fashion. A hierarchy was developed, as shown in Figure 7.9. The therapist and Jonas began with a picture of a needle and then moved up the ladder to videos of injections. Then a staff member dressed in a white coat administered a "flu shot" with a syringe from a toy doctor's kit. It is important to note that the staff member played the part of the pediatrician expertly. She swabbed the area with an alcohol patch and set up the injection with appropriate "doctor chat" (e.g., "The alcohol will feel cool, you might feel a little pinch").

Once these steps were accomplished, Jonas challenged himself with visits to the pediatrician's office. He sat in the office while they discussed flu shots, and the syringe was put gradually closer to him, until the pediatrician held it in her hand. The final step included the actual injection.

ELEVATOR PHOBIA

Abraham was the 9-year-old son of a very accomplished engineer. However, he was deathly afraid of elevators. He worried that the elevator car would become stuck, there would not be enough air in the car to support life, and he would suffocate. Not surprisingly, longer rides, smaller elevators, and crowded elevators were especially stressful for him.

Abraham's family was extremely supportive of him. They would take the stairs and escalators whenever he would become frightened. When they traveled to high-rise hotels, they took rooms on the lowest floors so Abraham could avoid the elevator as much as possible. However, as is the case with most anxious and phobic patients, Abraham came to therapy when avoidance was no longer possible. Abraham's father was offered a 2-year assignment that included living in the company's high-rise penthouse apartment on the 50th floor. Naturally, the stairs were no longer a compensatory option for Abraham!

A hierarchy for Abraham, shown in Figure 7.10, was collaboratively developed. The lower rungs of the hierarchy involved increasing proximity to the elevators. These experimental steps also involved observing the elevators to help Abraham habituate to them as well as evaluate the probability of elevators getting stuck. These steps were readily accomplished in a homework assignment between sessions.

The next several steps involved increasing Abraham's comfort entering the stationary elevator car with the door open. His attention was directed to the rescue factors within the elevator car. We then increased the number of people riding in the elevator. Interestingly, Abraham preferred to initially ride the elevator with the therapist rather than his family because he believed his parents would make him too nervous. Finally, in the last phase, Abraham rode elevators for increasingly longer times with more people onboard.

FEAR OF VOMITING

Graduated practice is well illustrated through the work with Cat, an 11-year-old girl with severe fears about vomiting. Cat became increasingly uncomfortable in school settings when there were unpleasant odors (other children with their shoes off, flatulence, food smells in the cafeteria) and if she experienced tightness in her throat, hiccups, burping, or a full mouth. She dreaded the possibility of vomiting and of seeing another child vomiting. She was disgusted by the sight, touch, smell, taste, and sound of vomiting. She feared the loss of control associated with the vomiting.

The therapist and Cat developed a hierarchy of graduated tasks for the vomiting phobia (see Figure 7.11). The first task included imaginal exposure. Cat and the therapist wrote a storybook about a child vomiting in school, which she titled "I hurl, you hurl." Special care was directed toward placing thoughts and feelings in thought bubbles over the characters' heads. Additionally, Cat and the therapist drew disgusting details in the vomit drawings using a variety of colors.

Then the therapist and Cat listened to sound effects of various people vomiting. The sounds were titrated from least to most disgusting using a SUDS (1–10) procedure. In this practice phase, Cat moved up the sound hierarchy when her SUDS decreased by 50% for five consecutive trials.

In her next adventures, Cat was systematically exposed to baby foods that looked like vomit and smelled bad (e.g., peas, squash). She began by habituating to the smell and progressed to tolerating small bits of the "vomit substance" on her fingers, smear-

FIGURE 7.10. Abraham's elevator hierarchy.

Ride 10+ floors at peak hours with parents

Ride 10+ floors at nonpeak hours with parents

Ride elevators 8–10 floors at peak hours with parents

Ride elevator 8–10 floors at nonpeak hours with parents

Ride 6 floors with family

Ride 6 floors with therapist

Ride 3 floors with mother, father, and two brothers

Ride 3 floors with therapist

Stay in elevator for 5 minutes with door open

Stay in car for 1 minute with the door open and eye alarm and phone

Step into the elevator car with the door open, count to 10, step out

Stand at edge of door while elevator door opens

Stand 5 yards from elevator

Sit in lobby with parent in local buildings near elevator banks

Stand approximately 10 yards from elevator

FIGURE 7.11. Cat's vomit hierarchy.

Practice "throwing up"
Drink carbonated beverage quickly
Hold water in mouth
Put baby food on cheeks
Smear baby food on hands
Touch small bits of baby food on finger tips
Smell baby food (green peas, ham)
Listen to vomit sound effects
Write the vomit book (I hurl, you hurl)

ing it all over her hands, and having the substance on her face. Therapy moved on when SUDs ratings decreased by 50% and length of time increased. Cat's goal was to keep her SUDS at 50% decline for 5 minutes for repeated trials.

In order to help her disconnect the sensation of tightness and fullness in her mouth from vomiting and catastrophe, additional practice tasks were developed. She held her breath for 30 seconds and held a small amount of water in her mouth for 10 seconds. Next, Cat needed to learn that burping did not catastrophically lead to vomiting. Therefore, she drank several sips of soda in rapid succession so that she could burp without disaster. Finally, Cat put it all together by pretending to vomit, while pouring the baby food or vomit substance in the toilet to simulate the sight and sound of vomiting.

FEAR OF PUBLIC TOILETS

Molly, age 5, feared public toilets. "They will swallow me up and I'll float away and be gone forever," she thought. While she had no problems using bathrooms in private residences and her preschool, public restrooms in restaurants, airports, department stores, and hospitals were assiduously avoided. Her fear was exacerbated by automatic flushing systems and particularly by loud flushing noises caused by strong water pressure. Behavioral experiments were constructed to address Molly's fears of the loud noises, unpredictability, and being swallowed up (see Figure 7.12).

The adventures began with listening to the noise. Flushing sounds were recorded off a sound-effects site on the Internet and played at various volumes controlled by Molly. Then the sounds were controlled and played unpredictably by the therapist in session and at home by the parents. Then Molly went into public bathrooms with her parents armed with a tape recorder and recorded the flushing sounds. She then listened to the sounds. The tape-recording process was also an experiment to help her gain greater proximity to the public restrooms.

After Molly inoculated herself to loud unanticipated flushing noises, we progressed to increasing her tolerance of public bathrooms. At the clinic, we designed a "Ride to Glory" that helped increase the reinforcement value of her bathroom trips and her exposure to institutional restrooms. In the Ride to Glory, Molly sat in the therapist's wheeled office chair, wore a crown, and was pushed around the clinic by her mother and/or the therapist. She waved regally to the office staff proclaiming, "I'm riding to the bathroom

FIGURE 7.12. Molly's graduated experiments with public toilets.

Sit and eliminate on automatic flush toilet

Sit and eliminate on manual flush toilet

Sit on toilet while flushing automatic toilet

Sit on toilet while flushing manual toilet

Flush water down toilet while standing

Ride to Glory

Listen to tape

Tape institutional toilets flushing

Listen to increasingly loud flushing sounds occurring unpredictably

Listen to increasingly loud flushing sounds controlled by self

on my adventure!" The praise and attention she received from the office staff was an excellent reward for her.

In the next set of adventures, Molly and her mother went into the bathroom with a cup of water, approached the commode, poured the water in the bowl, and flushed. She then sought out automatic flushing systems and did the same experiment for homework. Molly progressed to pouring the water in the bowl while sitting on the toilet seat. These experiments gave Molly the "evidence" that she would not be swallowed. Finally, Molly used the public restrooms during genuine "nature calls."

Selective Mutism

BATTLESHIP

Ages: 6–12 years.

Purpose: Experiential game for selective mutism.

Materials Needed:

- Grid-lined paper.
- Pencils or pens.

Or

- Commercial Battleship game.

The game Battleship is a creative choice for children with selective mutism (Bergman, 2006). Battleship is a fun game that is interactive but requires minimal verbal interaction. The players simply give a location ("B 6") and an outcome ("Hit," "Miss," "Sunk"). Thus, the game is fun and provides a pleasant context for initial verbal interaction. For the child struggling with more severe forms of selective mutism, the game might include whispering responses to a parent, increasing speaking volume to parent, whispering to the therapist, and speaking aloud to the therapist. Homework assignments might include playdates during which the patient plays Battleship with peers.

Separation Anxiety

Children troubled by separation also benefit from graduated adventures. They need to test mental equations such as "Without Mom, I'm weak" or "If I am apart from my parents, something bad will happen to them." Like most behavioral experiments for other disorders, adventures for youngsters with separation anxiety follow cognitive interventions (e.g., Handprint on Your Heart, Bad Math). *In vivo* experiments in the therapists' office are common next steps.

Judah was a 7-year-old who dreaded being apart from his mother. When separated, Judah's heart raced, his respiration rate increased, he "got sweaty," felt faint, and was dizzy. His extremities felt weak and he literally froze in place and cried. He believed that "without Mom, bad things are sure to happen. I can't cope on my own, no one will comfort me."

A traditional hierarchy for Judah was collaboratively developed for in-session exposures (see Figure 7.13). We called this "Judah's away from Mom" hierarchy. The adventures began with Mom sitting away from him and progressed to Judah staying in the session while his mother moved farther away from him until she waited for him in the waiting room.

HANSEL AND GRETEL TECHNIQUE

Ages: 5–10 years.

Purpose: Treatment of separation anxiety.

Materials Needed:

- Paper.
- Scissors.
- Markers.
- Photos.

The Hansel and Gretel Technique (Shapiro et al., 2005) is an innovative way to implement graduated practice with children with separation anxiety and may offer an alternative to a traditional hierarchy. We adapted this creative intervention so it becomes a behavioral experiment/exposure task. The adventure starts with an introduction reminding the children of the Hansel and Gretel story. The key point for children to get is that the way you can find your way back to caretaking figures is to follow the bread

FIGURE 7.13. Judah's away from Mom hierarchy.

Mom waiting in waiting room
Mom outside the office door, down the hall
Mom outside the office door with door closed
Mom outside the office door with door open
Mom at door
Mom on chair, Judah alone on couch

crumbs. Then the child and parent create self-instructional cues by cutting out paper bread crumbs. Photographs, drawings, and simple written messages representing comfort, confidence, and competence when separated from parents are placed on the crumbs. After the bread crumbs are made, the parent hides in the clinic but lays out a path of crumbs for the child to follow in order for the child to find him or her. The child then follows the bread crumbs, picking up each one while reading it aloud on route to discovering the parent. Generally, we repeat the procedure several times in a session. The family is encouraged to practice the exercise several times in their home between sessions.

Social Anxiety

Experiments and exposures are staples in treating social anxiety. They test children's predictions of negative evaluation, embarrassment, and humiliation. The types of experiments are almost endless and can be tailored to individuals' specific predictions and circumstances. Grover, Hughes, Bergman, and Kingery (2006) described a graduated experiment for a 12-year-old patient with social phobia who feared ordering meals at a restaurant. The clinician created a menu, set up a small table with chairs in the office, took down the order on a pad, and brought paper plates to the table when the order was completed.

Maya was a talented 17-year-old art student who attended a magnet school for fine arts. However, her social anxiety and accompanying fear of negative evaluation caused her to avoid sharing her work with the class. Since this was a course requirement, she was failing the class. After completing a variety of cognitive restructuring and rational analysis procedures, Maya was ready for her adventure. A classroom was set up in the clinic's group room. Maya was invited to bring a sample of her work to present to the "class." Various staff members were recruited to be "art critics." Several of the recruits were instructed to provide negative feedback to Maya. This provided Maya with a real-life circumstance to manage her emotional arousal and practice her coping thoughts in response to the negative evaluation. Returning a meal ordered at a restaurant because it is too cold or not prepared exactly right, asking for directions, calling someone by the wrong name, trying on many clothes in a dressing room and returning them to a clerk without purchasing any item are just a few examples of other experiments (Kendall et al., 2005). In this section, we describe a number of adventures completed by socially anxious children. Let's Go Shopping, Reading Allowed, and Museum Piece represent three examples.

LET'S GO SHOPPING

Ages: 5–10 years.

Purpose: Graded exposure for social anxiety.

Materials Needed:

- Paper.
- Markers.
- Scissors.
- Small prizes (erasers, stickers, candy, etc.).

Let's Go Shopping is a therapeutic adventure that is a fun way for socially anxious children to practice social skills, conversations, and encountering potentially embarrassing situations. The adventure has the added benefit of providing a naturally occurring reward (e.g., the thing the child purchases).

The adventure begins with the therapist and the patient making paper money. We then ask clinic staff to be storekeepers and stock them with small prizes (erasers, small arcade prizes, stickers, candy, etc.). Let's Go Shopping involves graded practice. Children are initially asked to perform a smaller skill (e.g., make eye contact, smile, ask the question "How much does this cost?", and say "Thank you."). As children gain practice, the task becomes more difficult and the child has to engage in more conversation with the store owner, return an item, make change, and so on.

READING ALLOWED

Ages: 7–18 years.

Purpose: Graded exposure for social anxiety.

Materials Needed:

- Reading materials.
- Audience members.

Reading Allowed is a therapeutic adventure for children with social anxiety, performance fears, and fears of negative evaluation. Reading Allowed offers opportunities for children to gain graded practice while making mistakes in front of others, problem solving, getting criticism and coping with it, having a successful experience, and managing their anxiety. Accordingly, there are several versions of Reading Allowed.

In one version, the child reads aloud relatively simple materials in front of varying numbers of different people. In each subsequent step, more people are added to the audience. This adventure is good for children who are bothered primarily by the amount and type (children, adults, etc.) of audience.

A second version involves the child reading gradually more challenging material in front of various people. This is apt for children who hold perfectionistic beliefs and fears of negative evaluation/humiliation. They dread revealing imperfections in front of others and worry they will be rejected, criticized, punished, and/or humiliated.

MUSEUM PIECE

Ages: 12–18 years.

Purpose: Decreasing performance and evaluation anxiety.

Materials Needed:

- Museum Piece Diary (Form 7.1).

Museum Piece is an experiential procedure for adolescents with performance and evaluation fears. Like many experiential techniques, Museum Piece combines elements from both ACT and CBT. It is similar to the chessboard metaphor espoused by Hayes and colleagues (1999). Unlike traditional ACT procedures, it also involves direct cognitive processing. Museum Piece involves imagery, rational analysis, and behavioral experimentation. Museum Piece begins with the explanation of the metaphor such as the following:

"A museum piece is something housed in a museum. Museums hold works of art. There are many works of art. There are many forms, shapes, and types of art in a museum. In fact, the degree of uniqueness often characterizes each museum piece. Just being in the museum is an achievement.

"Visitors come into the museum and view the pieces. They look at items and pass judgment on them. They like, dislike, or feel neutral toward the pieces. Some pieces they value, others they devalue and criticize, and still others they can take or leave. It is rare that every piece in a museum is valued by everyone always. However, once something is created and placed in the museum, it cannot be changed. It is judged as it is.

"It is kind of like that with people. People are who they are. People pass judgment on others and it is the rare person who is judged positively by everyone always. No one escapes negative judgments. Like museum pieces, people are worthy just by being who they are. However, being worthy does not prevent people from judging or criticizing.

"I would like you to try to experiment with taking a stance like a museum piece. Imagine you are like a work of art, which of course you are! Invite criticism and judgment, tolerate it, don't try to change yourself, and simply absorb it like a museum piece with full acceptance of the fact no one gets to hang out without judgment, disapproval, and criticism from others. How does this sound?"

Some teenagers may not respond to the museum metaphor. This is OK since you can readily change the metaphor to a movie, TV show, music, or athlete. After the metaphor is explained to the child, the experiment begins. This phase resembles traditional exposure-based approaches to social anxiety where the patient goes out and elicits criticism from other people. Simply, the adolescent keeps track of the criticism and may even ask for it, rates feelings, writes automatic thoughts, and then rationally talks back to the negative thoughts from the perspective of a museum piece. Form 7.1 is a Museum Piece Diary.

Pilar is a 17-year-old patient with an eating disorder who had severe performance and evaluation anxiety which accompanied her distorted body image. The following dialogue illustrates the Museum Piece procedure (see Figure 7.14 for her completed Museum Piece Diary).

THERAPIST: First, I have to congratulate you on getting this criticism.

PILAR: (*sarcastically*) Great! Now I know how little people think of me.

THERAPIST: What makes you say that?

PILAR: Look at all the criticisms! I got criticized every freaking day.

FIGURE 7.14. Pilar's Museum Piece Diary.

Date	Criticism	Feeling	Automatic thought	Response from the Museum Piece's perspective
Feb. 18	Mother criticized clothes.	Depressed (7) Anxious (7)	She thinks I have no taste. I must look ugly.	Everyone has his or her own opinion.
Feb. 19	Friend said "I looked pale and nervous."	Anxious (8)	She thinks I'm a freak. I'm ugly. Why can't I hide my feelings? She can see right through me.	Who is putting a negative label on looking pale and nervous? All it is is a description. If she can see through me, who says it is bad? She is just paying attention to me.
Feb. 20	Went on a date. Friend said I laughed quietly.	Anxious (9)	He doesn't think I am funny and have a good sense of humor.	Is there only one way to laugh? Who gets to set the rules on laughing?
Feb. 20	Had pizza on date. Date laughed during dinner. Said I was cute when I chewed.	Anxious (9)	He's watching me eat. He thinks I'm a fat pig who stuffs my face.	If this is true, who says his opinion is fact?
Feb. 20	Date didn't kiss me.	Depressed (8)	He's not into me.	Just because he didn't kiss me doesn't mean he's not into me. If he's not into me it's his loss.
Feb. 21	Mother said "I spew venom from my mouth" when I was sarcastic.	Anxious (8)	She thinks I'm rude and disrespectful.	She can have this feeling about me. It doesn't last long and she gets over it.
Feb. 21	Date called to hang out. Mother said I spent too much time on phone.	Anxious (8)	Mother thinks I spend too much time thinking about boys.	Everyone disapproves of someone sometimes. It is just life.
Feb. 22	Physics teacher gave me a 92 and said I was more careless than usual.	Anxious (9)	He thinks I'm slacking off.	Even if this is true, opinion isn't always fact.

THERAPIST: Yeah, wasn't that the point of the experiment? You faced criticism just like a museum piece.

PILAR: But it was so hard.

THERAPIST: I know it was. In fact, it is supposed to be hard. Handling real and/or perceived criticisms is a difficult thing. How many of the criticisms could you see from the museum piece's perspective?

PILAR: Three, the ones from my mother on the 18th and the 21st, and the one about Danny not kissing me. So I didn't do well with this.

THERAPIST: Well, let's talk about that some. You saw three from the museum's perspective, and how many of the other criticisms did you tolerate?

PILAR: All of them, I guess. But it was hard! I hated it!

THERAPIST: But you put yourself out there on display nonetheless! What do you think that means about you that although it was difficult and you hated it, you allowed yourself to be vulnerable to embarrassment and criticism?

PILAR: (*Pause.*) Maybe I am tougher than I think I am.

THERAPIST: Maybe ... we'll have to keep testing that. Do you think you'll be able to handle being on display better with greater practice with the Museum Piece?

PILAR: Maybe. I don't know.

THERAPIST: Are you willing to try?

PILAR: Willing but not wanting!

THERAPIST: Willing is good! Let's look at the other criticisms. Your friend said you looked pale and nervous and she could see right through you. Who's putting a negative spin on that?

PILAR: You know, that's a good question. I never thought about that.

THERAPIST: So write that down. How is it that Steph can see right through you?

PILAR: She's just really tuned into me. She pays so much attention to me. She's a good friend.

THERAPIST: And how is that bad?

PILAR: (*Laughs.*) OK, I get it!

THERAPIST: Let's move onto the date.

PILAR: Do we have to?

THERAPIST: Who makes the rules on laughing? Is there some code in your high school about laughing?

PILAR: OK. I know I'm stupid.

THERAPIST: It's not about being stupid or not. It's about trying to see it from the museum piece's perspective, which is different for you. Is different the same as stupid?

PILAR: Of course not!

THERAPIST: How can you apply this to the laughing?

PILAR: Just because I don't laugh like other people doesn't mean I'm a freak. There really are no rules. Everybody has different laughs.

THERAPIST: This next one is a tough one, I bet.

PILAR: The pizza situation was tough.

THERAPIST: It was. How is saying you are cute when you chew the same as saying you're a pig?

PILAR: It's like a cow chewing its cud. It's gross that he's looking at me that way.

THERAPIST: OK. I don't know if Danny is seeing you that way or not, but even if he does think your chewing is pig-like, how does his opinion equal absolute fact?

PILAR: It doesn't.

THERAPIST: We have three to go. How are you feeling now?

PILAR: Better. A bit more relieved from the criticisms. In fact, when I look over some of them, they don't seem like criticisms.

THERAPIST: Your mom said you spewed venom?

PILAR: Yeah, she doesn't like my sarcasm.

THERAPIST: And she disapproves.

PILAR: She does.

THERAPIST: So how do you tolerate her disapproval?

PILAR: I don't.

THERAPIST: How complete and long-lasting is it?

PILAR: It isn't. She gets over it. It's kind of the same with her disapproval about me being "boy-crazy." Everybody is disapproved of sometimes. It's just life. And you know what? I worked hard on that physics test. I can say him thinking I am a slacker is his opinion, not fact.

THERAPIST: So what does this mean?

PILAR: Maybe criticism isn't bad. It's just annoying and uncomfortable.

The dialogue with Pilar is marked by several important points. The therapist began with reinforcing Pilar for collecting and recording criticisms. Second, the therapist balanced validating Pilar's difficulties with criticism (e.g., "I know it was hard.") and challenging her tolerance for discomfort (e.g., "But you put yourself on display nonetheless!"). There was a mix of specific, concrete questions (e.g., "How many of the other criticisms did you tolerate?") and abstract synthesizing questions (e.g., "What do you think that means about you that although it was difficult and you hated it, you allowed yourself to be vulnerable to embarrassment and criticism?").

CONCLUSION

The techniques in this chapter illustrated the use of "doing" in a context of emotional arousal to provide a truly change-producing experience. To be most effective, exposures

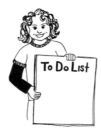

BOX 7.1 Summary Pad for Exposure and Experiments

- Be sure to educate and orient patients and families to exposure.
- Remember experiments and exposures are collaborative rather than prescriptive.
- Children, adolescents, and families lead the way in experiments and exposures.
- Tailor experiments to children, adolescents, and families.
- Align with children and adolescents against the distress.
- Graduated experiments and exposures are recommended.
- Exposure should be comprehensive and repeated, and make use of optimal emotional engagement.
- Experiments should not stop until arousal decreases.
- Add in cognitive processing of the exposure.
- Be sure to reward effort.
- Feel free to be creative and have fun with exposures.

and other behavioral experiments need to be individually designed, implemented in session, generalized to other settings, and followed up by evaluating the results with the patients. These behavioral experiments provide patients with opportunities to use the skills they have learned in therapy, including self-regulation and cognitive restructuring. The therapist needs to play an active role during these experiential interventions. Therapists and patients work collaboratively to design and complete the experiments, as well as to process the outcomes. Behavioral experiments are some of the most fun, engaging, and rewarding therapy interventions for many patients (and therapists!).

FORM 7.1

Museum Piece Diary

Date	Criticism	Feeling	Automatic thought	Response from the Museum Piece's perspective

CHAPTER 8

Final Points

This book reflects approximately 4 years of planning, clinical work, research, and writing. Deciding on our final words of advice was a difficult task because our work is ongoing. Nonetheless, in this epilogue, we chose to reinforce what we see as an important set of attitudes, try to encourage you to persist despite inevitable clinical challenges, and encourage you to return to the text like you would seek out a trusted colleague for support and guidance. Therefore, we offer seven attitudes to consider and remember.

INVOLVE AND ENGAGE THE CHILDREN AND THEIR FAMILIES IN THE PROCESS

Tell me and I'll forget. Show me and I may not
remember. Involve me and I'll understand.
—NATIVE AMERICAN PROVERB

Cognitive-behavioral psychotherapy is not a sterile intellectual exercise. It requires the patient's emotional involvement. Impersonal and abstract use of worksheets, forms, and other procedures rarely reaches children. Collaboration and partnering with children engages them in the process. When children are coarchitects of their interventions, the clinical work is more meaningful to them. Using this text is itself collaboration; we are partners in the treatment process. While we provide numerous techniques, you must involve and engage your patient in the process.

BE PATIENT WITH YOURSELF AND THE CHILDREN, ADOLESCENTS, AND FAMILIES YOU TREAT

Genius is eternal patience.
—MICHELANGELO

Clinical and supervisory experience tells us that psychotherapists recognize the awesome responsibility of taking care of child and adolescent patients. Psychotherapists place much internal pressure on themselves and their patients to get better. Often, there is a search for a "silver bullet method" that will alleviate distress in an almost immediate and complete way. In short, psychotherapists are often impatient beings.

Cognitive-behavioral psychotherapy is work, not magic. In our experience, change occurs due to the deliberate, systematic application of procedures within a context of a productive working alliance. In fact, rushing the patient has been shown to rupture treatment (Creed & Kendall, 2005). Accordingly, we encourage patience with those who you treat regarding the timeline for change. Therapeutic change frequently occurs in small, marginally noticeable degrees rather than in dramatic bursts of epiphany. Slow, small change reflects positive therapeutic momentum!

In conclusion, I (R. D. F.) fondly remember seminars at the Center for Cognitive Therapy—Newport Beach led by Dr. Christine A. Padesky and Dr. Aaron T. Beck. As postdocs, we would eagerly await Dr. Beck's visits from Philadelphia like teenagers standing in line for a rock concert. During one particularly meaningful session, Dr. Beck differentiated the notions of time-limited and time-efficient treatment. Time-limited treatment involves conducting psychotherapy within an arbitrary set of predetermined sessions regardless of acuity, severity, and/or contextual issues. Time-efficient treatment involves doing psychotherapy in the most effective way within the shortest time period for an individual given their circumstances. For some individuals, six sessions is time-efficient. For others, 40 sessions is time-efficient. This knowledge helped me become more patient in my work with children and adolescents.

REMAIN FLEXIBLE WITH TECHNIQUE AND PROCESS

Interrogate your hidden assumptions.
        —CORNEL WEST

Remaining flexible will help you responsibly address difficulties in a deliberate and calm manner. Rigid thinking and stereotyped practice close options and paint clinicians into tight corners. Looking at problems from multiple angles adds perspectives and fuels productive exploration.

Ethnocultural alertness also requires as well as enhances flexibility. While the literature is sound for CBT, the data is frequently plagued by a neglect of ethnocultural variables. Many studies do not report or include cultural issues (Weisz, Huey, & Weersing, 1998). However, recent research shows a welcome shift in attention (Cardemil & Battle, 2003; Cardemil, Reivich, Beevers, Seligman, & James, 2007; David-Ferdon & Kaslow, 2008; Eyberg, Nelson, & Boggs, 2008; Huey & Polo, 2008; Silverman, Pina, & Viswesvaran, 2008). Alertness to cultural vicissitudes broadens worldviews and conceptual paradigms, making cognitive therapy's tent a bigger place. Welcoming sometimes difficult dialogues about cultural issues in therapy makes all the procedures in the book more relevant. Cardemil and Battle (2003, p. 203) aptly noted, "In addition to actively learning about topics relevant to specific racial/ethnic minority status, one must make a shift in both attitude and behavior. This approach requires psychologists to acknowledge the limitations of their own worldview and to tolerate the anxiety that may accompany breaching these topics in psychotherapy."

CREATE AND INNOVATE

It may be hard for an egg to turn into a bird: It would be a jolly sight harder for it
to learn to fly while remaining an egg. We are like eggs at present. And you cannot
go on indefinitely being just an ordinary egg. We must be hatched or go bad.
                                                                    —C. S. LEWIS

While we hope this book gives you many treatment options for children and families, the text is a *starting* point rather than an end point. Feel free to adopt and modify
the procedures to suit your individual patients. Make the techniques your own through
active collaboration with children, a genuine understanding of the principles of CBT,
and creativity. There are limitless ways for you to innovate and place your own signature on the procedures.

USE THEORY AND RESEARCH TO GUIDE YOU

Look at every path closely and deliberately and then ask ourselves this crucial question:
does this path have heart? If it does, the path is good. If it doesn't, it is of no use.
                                                                    —CARLOS CASTENEDA

At the end of the day, psychotherapists may sometimes feel lost and alone after facing challenging clinical cases. Fortunately, CBT with children enjoys a rich empirical
tradition and the professional literature is filled with helpful information. In our experience, there is much comfort in a greater knowledge base. Rely on theoretical, clinical,
and empirical advances for direction. The state of professional knowledge provides a
map for you to use the procedures in the texts as well as a way of dealing with other
everyday dilemmas in clinical practice.

CONTINUE TO LEARN

Think left and think right and think low and think high.
Oh, the thinks you can think up if you try.
                                                                    —THEODOR GEISEL (DR. SEUSS)

Competency in CBT is a process rather than an ending point. Therefore, lifelong
learning is key in maintaining momentum. Fortunately, there are many opportunities
at professional conventions to attend clinical workshops and scientific sessions. The
annual meetings of the American Psychological Association, Association for Behavioral
and Cognitive Therapies, American Psychiatric Association, and American Academy of
Child and Adolescent Psychiatry are loaded with offerings. The World Congress of Cognitive and Behaviour Therapy and the European Association for Behavioural and Cognitive Therapies showcase recent advances around the world. Indeed, cognitive therapy
is growing worldwide! The United Kingdom is a hotbed for CBT (*www.babcp.com*).
Additionally, the Brazilian Society for Cognitive Therapy (SBTC) is one example of a
very active national organization (*www.sbtc.orgbr*). There are opportunities for intensive training and getting regular supervision via onsite and distance learning at flag-

ship cognitive therapy centers in Philadelphia (*www.beckinstitute.org*) and Huntington Beach (*www.padesky.com*). These centers also offer valuable training videotapes and other resources. Continued professional growth makes all the procedures in this book even more exciting.

EMBRACE DIFFICULT MOMENTS AND MISTAKES

Great moments are born from great opportunity.
—HERB BROOKS

I (R. D. F.) remember with fondness Dr. Christine A. Padesky's supervisory axiom when I was a postdoc in 1987 that a stuck point in therapy is just another opportunity to ask a better question. To this day, her admonition inspires me to persist during difficult moments and mistakes. As mentioned in previous chapters, responding to immediacy in sessions is a staple in CBT. Frequently, children's and families' strong negative emotions erupt in the urgent context of the present moment. These eruptions present wonderful opportunities for practicing techniques in this book and should be welcomed rather than avoided. Calhoun, Moras, Pilkonis, and Rehm (1998, p. 159) reminded us, "Even EST's that are based on highly specific intervention instructions must be adapted in unpredictable ways on a moment to moment basis."

Friedberg, Gorman, and Beidel (2009) noted that therapists often hold absolutistic perfectionistic beliefs about their work. However, Padesky (2007) urged real-world clinicians to develop a greater tolerance for ambiguity. Indeed, practice requires action (Hayes, 2007). Treatment often cannot wait until all data is collected and everything is known. Therefore, effective clinical action begins in an ambiguous context and is commonly imperfect. The task of the cognitive-behavioral psychotherapist somewhat parallels that of a Marine officer (Fick, 2005). You have to take a reasonable, deliberate approach and mindfully adapt to changing, perhaps unforeseen, realities.

PERSONAL NOTES

What we remember from childhood we remember forever.
—CYNTHIA OZICK

While trying to live by the seven attitudes outlined above, I (J. M. M.) am reminded of how these principles apply not just to my professional life, but also to my personal life. I strive to "involve and engage" and to model the "be patient" attitude for my two young daughters. I work to include them in discussions about what I am spending my time doing, and why I have chosen psychotherapy as my vocation. Thus, they are sometimes quite curious about what I do, and will offer their own suggestions! During one of the more time-consuming portions of the book-writing process, I was explaining to my then 5- and 3-year-olds (Lydia and Juliana) that I was working on a book to guide other "feeling doctors" in helping children with their feelings. As a budding reader, Lydia was quite intrigued by this process. After further discussion she realized this text was of no interest to her, thought for a moment, and responded, "For your next book, you should write a bible!" These lofty expectations my young daughter set for me made me chuckle, and provided a good laugh for our parish priest, but also reminded me how our own children and the children we work with look to us as "experts" who inspire and model creativity and change. This is an awesome responsibility, but an even more awesome opportunity!

Persistence and hard work never goes out of style!
—BARBARA A. FRIEDBERG, MBA

My personal style consultant, Barbara A. Friedberg, shapes both my outer and inner world. Writing a book like this one requires considerable patience, frustration tolerance, attention to detail, determination, and creativity. There were many weekends after an exhausting work week that I was tempted to watch movies, NFL football, and Major League Baseball. However, the dual ethos of persistence and discipline enabled me to efficiently crank out the text and even enjoy my share of New York Giants and Mets games. The point for you as consumers of this book is that diligently managing frustration and maintaining theoretical and clinical self-discipline more often than not yields desired results. As we noted earlier, this book represents about 4 years of work, so it ends not with a period but rather with three periods (...), signifying looking expectantly forward to our next challenges and the horizons of our personal and professional growth....

References

Abramson, L. Y., Seligman, M. E. P., & Teasdale, J. D. (1978). Learned helplessness in humans: Critique and reformulation. *Journal of Abnormal Psychology, 87,* 49–74.

Achenbach, T. M. (1991a). *Manual for Child Behavior Checklist/4–18 and 1991 profile.* Burlington: University of Vermont, Department of Psychiatry.

Achenbach, T. M. (1991b). *Manual for the Teacher's Report Form and 1991 profile.* Burlington: University of Vermont, Department of Psychiatry.

Achenbach, T. M. (1991c). *Manual for Youth Self-Report and 1991 profile.* Burlington: University of Vermont, Department of Psychiatry.

Achenbach, T. M. (2007). Applications of the Achenbach System of empirically based assessment to children, adolescents, and their parents. In S. R. Smith & L. Handler (Eds.), *The clinical assessment of children and adolescents: A practitioner's handbook* (pp. 327–344). Mahwah, NJ: Erlbaum.

Addis, M. E. (2002). Methods for disseminating research products and increasing evidence-based practice: Promises, obstacles, and future directions. *Clinical Psychology: Science and Practice, 9,* 381–392.

Albano, A. M. (1995). Treatment of social anxiety in adolescents. *Cognitive and Behavioral Practice, 2,* 271–298.

Albano, A. M. (2000). Treatment of social phobia in adolescents: Cognitive behavior programs focused on intervention and prevention. *Journal of Cognitive Psychotherapy, 14,* 67–76.

Albano, A. M., Chorpita, B. F., & Barlow, D. H. (2003). Childhood anxiety disorders. In E. J. Mash & R. A. Barkley (Eds.), *Childhood psychopathology* (pp. 279–330). New York: Guilford Press.

Allen, J. L., & Rapee, R. M. (2005). Anxiety disorders. In P. J. Graham (Ed.), *Cognitive behavior therapy for children and families* (2nd ed., pp. 300–319). New York: Cambridge University Press.

Allers, R., & Minkoff, B. (Directors). (1994). *The lion king* [motion picture]. United States: Walt Disney Feature Animation.

Anderson, D. A., Lundgren, J. D., Shapiro, J. R., & Paulosky, C. A. (2004). Assessment of eating disorders: Review and recommendations for clinical use. *Behavior Modification, 28,* 763–782.

Anderson, S., & Morris, J. (2006). Cognitive behaviour therapy for people with Asperger syndrome. *Behavioural and Cognitive Therapy, 34,* 293–303.

Arnold, C., & Walsh, B. T. (2007). *Next to nothing*. New York: Oxford University Press.

Atchison, D. (Director). (2006). *Akeelah and the bee* [motion picture]. United States: Spelling Bee Productions.

Attwood, T. (2003). Frameworks for behavioral interventions. *Child and Adolescent Psychiatric Clinics of North America, 12*, 65–86.

Attwood, T. (2004). Cognitive behavior therapy for children and adults with Asperger's syndrome. *Behaviour Change, 21*, 147–161.

Azrin, N. H., & Nunn, R. G. (1973). Habit reversal: A method of eliminating nervous habits and tics. *Behaviour Research and Therapy, 11*, 619–628.

Bailey, V. (2001). Cognitive-behavioral therapies for children and adolescents. *Advances in Psychiatric Treatment, 7*, 224–232.

Ballard, C. (Director). (1996). *Fly away home* [motion picture]. United States: Columbia Pictures and Sand Dollar Productions.

Bancroft, T., & Cook, B. (Directors) (1998). *Mulan* [motion picture]. United States: Walt Disney Feature Animation.

Bandura, A. (1977a). Self-efficacy: Toward a unifying theory of behavior change. *Psychological Review, 84*, 191–215.

Bandura, A. (1977b). *Social learning theory*. Englewood Cliffs, NJ: Prentice-Hall.

Bandura, A. (1986). *Social foundations of thought: A social cognitive theory*. Englewood Cliffs, NJ: Prentice-Hall.

Barkley, R. A. (1995). *Taking charge of ADHD*. New York: Guilford Press.

Barkley, R. A. (1997). *Defiant children: A clinician's manual for parent training*. New York: Guilford Press.

Barkley, R. A., & Benton, C. M. (1998). *Your defiant child: Eight steps to better behavior*. New York: Guilford Press.

Barkley, R. A., Edwards, G. H., & Robin, A. L. (1999). *Defiant teens: A clinician's manual for assessment and family intervention*. New York: Guilford Press.

Barkley, R. A., Robin, A. L., & Benton, C. M. (2008). *Your defiant teen: 10 steps to resolve conflict and rebuild your relationship*. New York: Guilford Press.

Barlow, D. H. (1988). *Anxiety and its disorders: The nature and treatment of anxiety and panic*. New York: Guilford Press.

Barlow, D. H., Allen, L. B., & Choate, M. L. (2004). Toward a unified treatment for emotional disorders. *Behavior Therapy, 35*, 205–230.

Barlow, D. H., & Cerny, J. A. (1998). *Psychological treatment of panic*. New York: Guilford Press.

Barrett, P. M., Dadds, M. R., & Rapee, R. M. (1996). Family treatment of childhood anxiety: A controlled trial. *Journal of Consulting and Clinical Psychology, 64*, 333–342.

Bateson, G. (1972). *Steps to an ecology of mind*. New York: Dutton.

Baum, L. F. (1900). *The wizard of Oz*. New York: Schocken.

Beal, D., Kopec, A. M., & DiGiuseppe, R. (1996). Disputing patients' irrational beliefs. *Journal of Rational-Emotive and Cognitive-Behavioral Therapy, 14*, 215–229.

Beck, A. T. (1976). *Cognitive therapy and the emotional disorders*. New York: International Universities Press.

Beck, A. T. (1985). Cognitive therapy, behavior therapy, psychoanalysis, and pharmacotherapy: A cognitive continuum. In M. J. Mahoney & A. Freeman (Eds.), *Cognition and psychotherapy* (pp. 325–347). New York: Plenum Press.

Beck, A. T. (1996). *Beck depression inventory–II*. San Antonio, TX: Psychological Corporation.

Beck, A. T., & Clark, D. A. (1988). Anxiety and depression: An information processing perspective. *Anxiety Research, 1*, 23–36.

Beck, A. T., Emery, G., & Greenberg, R. L. (1985). *Anxiety disorders and phobias: A cognitive perspective*. New York: Plenum Press.

Beck, A. T., Rush, A. J., Shaw, B. F., & Emery, G. (1979). *Cognitive therapy for depression*. New York: Guilford Press.

Beck, A. T., Steer, R. A., & Brown, G. K. (1996). *Beck depression inventory manual* (2nd ed.). San Antonio, TX: Psychological Corporation.

Beck, A. T., Weissman, A., Lester, D., & Trexler, L. (1974). The measurement of pessimism: The Hopelessness Scale. *Journal of Consulting and Clinical Psychology, 42,* 861–865.

Beck, J. S. (1995). *Cognitive therapy: Basics and beyond.* New York: Guilford Press.

Beck, J. S., Beck, A. T., Jolly, J. (2001). *Beck Youth Inventories.* San Antonio, TX: Psychological Corporation.

Beck, J. S., Beck, A. T., Jolly, J. B., & Steer, R. A. (2005). *Beck Youth Inventories for children and adolescents* (2nd ed.). San Antonio, TX: Psychological Corp.

Becker, W. C. (1971). *Parents are teachers.* Champaign, Ill: Research Press.

Bedore, B. (2004). *101 Improv games for children and adults.* Alameda, CA: Hunter House.

Beidel, D. C., & Turner, S. M. (2006). *Shy children, phobic adults* (2nd ed.). Washington, DC: American Psychological Association.

Beidel, D. C., Turner, S. M., & Morris, T. L. (1995). A new inventory to assess childhood social anxiety and phobia: The Social Phobia and Anxiety Inventory for Children. *Psychological Assessment, 7,* 73–79.

Bennett, H. J. (2007). *It hurts when I poop: A story for children who are scared to use the potty.* Washington, DC: Magination Press.

Bennett-Levy, J., Westbrook, D., Fennell, M., Cooper, M., Rouf, K., & Hackmann, A. (2004). Behavioural experiments: Historical and conceptual underpinnings. In J. Bennett-Levy, G. Butler, M. Fennell, A. Hackmann, M. Mueller, & D. Westbrook (Eds.), *Oxford guide to behavioral experiments in cognitive therapy* (pp. 1–20). Oxford, UK: Oxford University Press.

Berg, B. (1986). *The assertiveness game.* Dayton, OH: Cognitive Counseling Resources.

Berg, B. (1989). *The anger control game.* Dayton, OH: Cognitive Counseling Resources.

Berg, B. (1990a). *The anxiety management game.* Dayton, OH: Cognitive Counseling Resources.

Berg, B. (1990b). *The depression management game.* Dayton, OH: Cognitive Counseling Resources.

Berg, B. (1990c). *The self-control game.* Dayton, OH: Cognitive Counseling Resources.

Berg, B. (1992a). *The conduct management game.* Los Angeles: Western Psychological Services.

Berg, B. (1992b). *The feelings game.* Los Angeles: Western Psychological Services.

Berg, B. (1992c). *The self-concept game.* Los Angeles: Western Psychological Services.

Bergman, R. L. (2006, October). Cognitive-behavioral therapy for selective mutism. In R. D. Friedberg (Chair), *From protocols to practice: Translating CBT research to clinical care.* Symposium conducted at the annual meeting of the American Academy of Child and Adolescent Psychiatry, San Diego, CA.

Bernard, M. E., & Joyce, M. R. (1984). *Rational–emotive therapy with children and adolescents.* New York: Wiley.

Berry, J. (1995). *Feeling scared.* New York: Scholastic.

Berry, J. (1996). *Feeling sad.* New York: Scholastic.

Bird, B. (Director). (2004). *The incredibles* [motion picture]. United States: Walt Disney Pictures and Pixar Animation.

Bird, H. R., Gould, M. S., & Staghezza, B. (1992). Aggregating data from multiple informants in child psychiatry epidemiological research. *Journal of the American Academy of Child and Adolescent Psychiatry, 31,* 78–85.

Birmaher, B., Khetarpal, S., Brent, D. A., Cully, M., Balach, L., Kaufman, J., et al. (1997). The Screen for Child Anxiety Related Emotional Disorders (SCARED): Scale construction and psychometric characteristics. *Journal of the American Academy of Child and Adolescent Psychiatry, 36,* 545–553.

Blenkiron, P. (2005). Stories and analogies in cognitive behavioral therapy: A critical review. *Behavioural and Cognitive Therapy, 33,* 45–59.

Boal, A. (2002). *Games for actors and non-actors* (2nd ed.). New York: Routledge.

Bose-Deakins, J. E., & Floyd, R. G. (2004). A review of the Beck Youth Inventories of emotional and social impairment. *Journal of School Psychology, 42,* 333–340.

Bouchard, S., Côté, S., & Richard, D. C. S. (2007). Virtual reality applications for exposure. In D. C. S. Richard & D. L. Lauterbach (Eds.), *Handbook of exposure therapies* (pp. 347–388). San Diego: Academic Press.

Boxmeyer, C. L., Lochman, J. E., Powell, N., Yaros, A., & Wojnaroski, M. (2007). A case study of the Coping Power Program for angry and aggressive youth. *Journal of Contemporary Psychotherapy, 37,* 165–174.

Brewin, C. R. (1988). *Cognitive foundations of clinical psychology.* London, UK: Erlbaum.

Brooks, S. J., & Kutcher, S. (2001). Diagnosis and measurement of adolescent depression: A review of commonly utilized instruments. *Journal of Child and Adolescent Psychopharmacology, 11,* 341–376.

Bunting, E. (1994). *Smoky night.* San Diego: Harcourt Brace.

Burns, D. D. (1980). *Feeling good.* New York: Springer.

Burum, B. A., & Goldfried, M. R. (2007). The centrality of emotion to psychological change. *Clinical Psychology: Science and Practice, 14,* 407–413.

Calhoun, K. S., Moras, K., Pilkonis, P. A., & Rehm, L. P. (1998). Empirically supported treatments: Implications for training. *Journal of Consulting and Clinical Psychology, 66,* 151–162.

Candy, C. M., & Fee. V. E. (1998). Underlying dimensions and psychometric properties of the Eating Behaviors and Body Image Test for adolescent girls. *Journal of Clinical Child Psychology, 27,* 117–127.

Cardemil, E. V., & Battle, C. L. (2003). Guess who's coming to therapy?: Getting comfortable with conversations about race and ethnicity in psychotherapy. *Professional Psychology, 34,* 278–286.

Cardemil, E. V., Reivich, K. J., Beevers, C. G., Seligman, M. E. P., & James, J. (2007). The prevention of depressive symptoms in low income, minority children: Two-year follow-up. *Behavior Research and Therapy, 45,* 313–327.

Carroll, K. M., & Nuro, K. F. (2002). One size cannot fit all: A stage model for psychotherapy manual development. *Clinical Psychology: Science and Practice, 9,* 396–406.

Cartledge, G. C., & Milburn, J. F. (Eds.). (1996). *Cultural diversity and social skills instruction: Understanding ethnic and gender differences.* Champaign, IL: Research Press.

Castonguay, L. G., Pincus, A. L., Agras, W. S., & Hines, C. E. (1998). The role of emotion in group cognitive-behavioral therapy for binge eating disorder: When things have to feel worse before they get better. *Psychotherapy Research, 8,* 225–238.

Caton-Jones, M. (Director). (1993). *This boy's life* [motion picture]. United States: Knickerbocker Films and Warner Brothers Pictures.

Chambless, D. L., & Ollendick, T. H. (2001). Empirically supported psychological interventions: Controversies and evidence. *Annual Review of Psychology, 52,* 685–716.

Chansky, T. E. (2000). *Freeing your child from obsessive–compulsive disorder.* New York: Three Rivers Press.

Chi, T. C., & Hinshaw, S. P. (2002). Mother–child relationships of children with ADHD: The role of maternal depressive symptoms and depression-related distortions. *Journal of Abnormal Child Psychology, 30,* 387–400.

Chorpita, B. F., Daleiden, E. L., & Weisz, J. R. (2005a). Identifying and selecting the common elements of evidence-based interventions: A distillation and matching model. *Mental Health Services Research, 7,* 5–20.

Chorpita, B. F., Daleiden, E. L., & Weisz, J. R. (2005b). Modularity in the design and application of therapeutic interventions. *Applied and Preventive Psychology, 11,* 141–156.

Chorpita, B. F., Tracey, S. A., Brown, T. A., Collica, T. J., & Barlow, D. H. (1997). Assessment of worry in children and adolescents: An adaptation of the Penn State Worry Questionnaire. *Behaviour Research and Therapy, 35,* 569–581.

Ciminero, A. R., & Drabman, R. S. (1977). Current advances in behavioral assessment of children. In B. B. Lahey & A. E. Kazdin (Eds.), *Advances in child clinical psychology* (pp. 47–82). New York: Plenum Press.

Clark, D. A. (1999). Cognitive-behavioral treatment of obsessive–compulsive disorder: A commentary. *Cognitive and Behavioral Practice, 6,* 408–415.

Clark, D. (2004). *Cognitive-behavioral therapy for OCD.* New York: Guilford Press.

Clark, D. M., Beck, A. T., & Alford, B. A. (1999). *Scientific foundations of cognitive theory and therapy of depression.* New York: Wiley.

Clark, L. (2005). *SOS: Help for parents* (3rd ed.). Bowling Green, KY: Parents Press and SOS Programs.

Clarke, G. N., DeBar, L. L., & Lewinsohn, P. M. (2003). Cognitive-behavioral group treatment for adolescent depression. In A. E. Kazdin & J. R. Weisz (Eds.), *Evidence-based psychotherapies for children and adolescents* (pp. 120–134). New York: Guilford Press.

Clarke, G. N., Lewinsohn, P. M., & Hops, H. (1990a). *Adolescent coping with depression course.* Eugene, OR: Castalia.

Clarke, G. N., Lewinsohn, P. M., & Hops, H. (1990b). *Student workbook: Adolescent coping with depression course.* Eugene OR: Castalia.

Clarke, G. N., Rohde, P., Lewinsohn, P. M., Hops, H., & Seeley, J. R. (1999). Cognitive-behavioral treatment of adolescent depression: Efficacy of acute group treatment and booster sessions. *Journal of the American Academy of Child and Adolescent Psychiatry, 38,* 272–279.

Clements, R., & Musker, J. (Directors). (1989). *Little mermaid* [motion picture]. United States: Silver Screen Partners IV, Walt Disney Feature Animation, and Walt Disney Pictures.

Clements, R., & Musker, J. (Directors). (1992). *Aladdin* [motion picture]. United States: Walt Disney Feature Animation.

Cohen, J. A., Deblinger, E., Mannarino, A. P., & Steer, R. (2004). A multi-site, randomized controlled trial for children with sex abuse-related PTSD symptoms. *Journal of the American Academy of Child and Adolescent Psychiatry, 43,* 393–402.

Cohen-Sandler, R. (2005). *Stressed-out girls: Helping them thrive in the age of pressure.* New York: Penguin Books.

Coie, J. D., & Dodge, K. A. (1998). Aggression and antisocial behavior. In W. Damon (Series Ed.) & N. Eisenberg (Vol. Ed.), *Handbook of child psychology: Vol. 3: Social, emotional, and personality development* (5th ed., pp. 779–862). New York: Wiley.

Connors, C. K. (2000). *Connors' Rating Scales—Revised: Technical manual.* North Tonawanda, NY: Multi Health Systems.

Cook, J. W., Taylor, L. A., & Silverman, P. (2004). The application of therapeutic storytelling techniques with preadolescent children: A clinical description with illustrative case study. *Cognitive and Behavioral Practice, 11,* 243–248.

Cooper, M. J., Rose, K. S., & Turner, H. (2005). Core beliefs and the presence or absence of eating disorders symptoms and depressive symptoms in adolescent girls. *International Journal of Eating Disorders, 38,* 60–64.

Cooper, M. J., Whitehead, L., & Boughton, N. (2004). Eating disorders. In J. Bennett-Levy, G. Butler, M. Fennell, A. Hackman, M. Mueller, & D. Westbrook (Eds.), *Oxford guide to behavioral experiments in cognitive therapy* (pp. 267–284). New York: Oxford University Press.

Cooper, Z., & Fairburn, C. G. (1987). The Eating Disorder Examination: A semi-structured interview for the assessment of the specific psychopathology of eating disorders. *International Journal of Eating Disorders, 6,* 9–16.

Corstorphine, E., Mountford, V., Tomlinson, S., Waller, G., & Meyer, C. (2007). Distress tolerance in the eating disorders. *Eating Behaviors, 8,* 91–97.

Cosby, B. (1997). *The meanest thing to say.* New York: Scholastic.

Cotterell, N. B. (2005, May). *Extramural training seminar.* Paper presented at the Beck Institute for Cognitive Therapy and Research, Philadelphia.

Craske, M. G., & Barlow, D. H. (2001). Panic disorder and agoraphobia. In D. H. Barlow (Ed.), *Clinical handbook of psychological disorders: A step-by-step treatment manual* (3rd ed., pp. 1–59). New York: Guilford Press.

Creed, T. A., & Kendall, P. C. (2005). Therapist alliance building within a cognitive behavioral treatment for anxiety in youth. *Journal of Consulting and Clinical Psychology, 73,* 498–505.

Crick, N. R., & Dodge, K. A. (1996). Social information processing mechanisms in reactive and proactive aggression. *Child Development, 67,* 993–1002.

Curry, J. F., & Wells, K. C. (2005). Striving for effectiveness in the treatment of adolescent depression: Cognitive behavioral therapy for multisite community intervention. *Cognitive and Behavioral Practice, 12,* 177–185.

Dattilio, F. M. (1998). Cognitive behavioral family therapy. In F. M. Dattilio (Ed.), *Case studies in couples and family therapy* (pp. 62–84). New York: Guilford Press.

Dattilio, F. M. (1997). Family therapy. In R. L. Leahy (Ed.), *Practicing cognitive therapy: A guide to interventions* (pp. 409–450). New York: Aronson.

Dattilio, F. M. (2000). Families in crisis. In F. M. Dattilio & A. Freeman (Eds.), *Cognitive behavior strategies in crisis intervention* (2nd ed., pp. 316–338). New York: Guilford Press.

Dattilio, F. M. (2001). Cognitive behavior family therapy: Contemporary myths and misconceptions. *Contemporary Family Therapy, 23,* 3–18.

Dattilio, F. M. (2002). Homework assignments in couple and family therapy. *Journal of Clinical Psychology, 58,* 535–547.

David-Ferdon, C., & Kaslow, N. J. (2008). Evidence-based psychosocial treatments for child and adolescent depression. *Journal of Clinical Child and Adolescent Psychology, 37,* 62–104.

Davis, N., & Pickard, B. (2008). The healing power of music. In L. C. Rubin (Ed.), *Popular culture in counseling, psychotherapy, and play-based interventions* (pp. 63–80). New York: Springer.

Dayton, J., & Faris, V. (Directors). (2006). *Little Miss Sunshine* [motion picture]. United States: Big Beach Films.

Deblinger, E., Behl, L. E., & Glickman, A. R. (2006). Treating children who have experienced sexual abuse. In P. C. Kendall (Ed.), *Child and adolescent therapy: Cognitive-behavioral procedures* (3rd ed., pp. 383–416). New York: Guilford Press.

Deblinger, E., & Heflin, A. H. (1996). *Treating sexually abused children and their non-offending parents: A cognitive behavioral approach.* Thousand Oaks, CA: Sage Publications.

De Los Reyes, A., & Kazdin, A. E. (2005). Informant discrepancies in the assessment of childhood psychopathology: A critical review, theoretical framework, and recommendations for future study. *Psychological Bulletin, 131,* 483–509.

DePino, C. (2004). *Blue cheese breath and stinky feet.* Washington, DC: Magination Press.

D'Eramo, K. S., & Francis, G. (2004). Cognitive-behavioral psychotherapy. In T. L. Morris & J. S. March (Eds.), *Anxiety disorders in children and adolescents* (pp. 305–328). New York: Guilford Press.

DiClemente, C. C. (2003). *Addictions and change.* New York: Guilford Press.

Dodge, K. A. (1985). Attributional bias in aggressive children. In P. C. Kendall (Ed.), *Advances in cognitive-behavioral research and therapy* (Vol. 4, pp. 73–110). New York: Academic Press.

Dozois, D. J. A., & Covin, R. (2004). The Beck Depression Inventory-II, Beck Hopelessness Scale, and Beck Scale for Suicidal Ideation. In M. Hersen (Series Ed.), & D. L. Segal & M. Hilsenrotn (Vol. Eds.), *Comprehensive handbook of psychological assessment: Vol. 2. Personality assessment and psychopathology.* New York: Wiley.

Dozois, D. J. A., & Dobson, K. S. (2001). Depression. In M. M. Antony & D. H. Barlow (Eds.), *Handbook of assessment and treatment for psychological disorders* (pp. 259–299). New York: Guilford Press.

Dozois, D. J. A., Dobson, K. S., & Ahnberg, J. L. (1998). A psychometric evaluation of the Beck Depression Inventory–II. *Psychological Assessment, 10,* 83–89.

Eder, R. A. (1994). Comments on children's self-narratives. In U. Neisser & R. Fivush (Eds.), *The remembering self: Construction and accuracy in the self-narrative* (pp. 180–190). Melbourne, Australia: Cambridge University Press.

Edwards, D. J. A., Dattilio, F. M., & Bromley, D. B. (2004). Developing evidence-based practice: The role of case-based research. *Professional Psychology: Research and Practice, 6,* 589–597.

Einstein, D. A., & Menzies, R. G. (2006). Magical thinking in obsessive–compulsive disorder, panic disorder, and the general community. *Behavioural and Cognitive Psychotherapy, 34,* 351–357.

Eisen, A. R., & Engler, L. B. (2006). *Helping your child overcome separation anxiety or school refusal.* Oakland, CA: New Harbinger.

Elkind, D. (1981). *The hurried child: Growing up too fast too soon.* Boston: Addison Wesley.

Elkind, D. (1984). *All grown up and no place to go: Teenagers in crisis.* Boston: Addison Wesley.

Elliott, J. (1991). Defusing conceptual fusions: The just because technique. *Journal of Cognitive Psychotherapy, 5,* 227–229.

Erdlen, R. J., & Rickrode, M. R. (2007). Social skills groups with youth: A cognitive-behavioral perspective. In R. W. Christner, J. L. Stewart, & A. Freeman (Eds.), *Handbook of cognitive-behavior group therapy with children and adolescents* (pp. 485–506). New York: Routledge.

Evans, D. L., & Andrews, L. W. (2005). *If your adolescent has depression or bipolar disorder.* New York: Guilford Press.

Eyberg, S. M. (1974). *Eyberg Child Behavior Inventory.* Odessa, FL: Psychological Assessment Resources.

Eyberg, S. M. (1992). Parent and teacher behavior inventories for the assessment of conduct behavior problems in children. In L. Vandecreek, S. Knapp, & T. L. Jackson (Eds.), *Innovations in clinical practice: A Sourcebook* (Vol. 11, pp. 261–270). Sarasota, FL: Professional Resource Press.

Eyberg, S. M., Nelson, M. N., & Boggs, S. R. (2008). Evidence-based psychosocial treatments for children and adolescents with disruptive behavior. *Journal of Clinical Child and Adolescent Psychology, 37,* 215–237.

Fairburn, C. G., & Cooper, Z. (1996). The eating disorder examination (12th ed.). In C. G. Fairburn & G. T. Wilson (Eds.), *Binge eating: Nature, assessment, and treatment* (pp. 361–404). New York: Guilford Press.

Faust, J. (2000). Integration of family and cognitive behavioral therapy for treating sexually abused children. *Cognitive and Behavioral Practice, 7,* 361–368.

Feindler, E. L., & Ecton, R. B. (1986). *Adolescent anger control: Cognitive behavioral techniques.* New York: Pergamon Press.

Feindler, E. L., Ecton, R. B., Kingsley, D., & Dubey, D. R. (1986). Group anger control training for institutionalized psychiatric male adolescents. *Behavior Therapy, 17,* 109–123.

Feindler, E. L., & Guttman, J. (1994). Cognitive behavioral anger control training. In C. W. LeCroy (Ed.), *Handbook of child and adolescent treatment manuals* (pp. 170–199). New York: Lexington Books.

Feindler, E. L., Marriott, S. A., & Iwata, M. (1984). Group anger control training for junior high delinquents. *Cognitive Therapy and Research, 8,* 299–311.

Fennell, M. J. V. (1989). Depression. In K. Hawton, P. M. Salkvoskis, J. Kirk, & D. M. Clark (Eds.), *Cognitive-behaviour therapy for psychiatric problems: A practical guide* (pp. 169–234). Oxford, UK: Oxford Medical.

Fick, N. (2005). *One bullet away: The making of a Marine officer.* Boston: Houghton Mifflin.

Fidaleo, R. A., Friedberg, R. D., Dennis, G., & Southworth, S. (1996). Imagery, internal dialogue, and action: An alternative treatment for PTSD. *Crisis Intervention, 3,* 143–155.

Finamore, D. (2008). *Little Miss Sunshine* and positive psychology as a vehicle for change in adolescent depression. In L. C. Rubin (Ed.), *Popular culture in counseling, psychotherapy, and play-based interventions* (pp. 123–140). New York: Springer.

Flannery-Schroeder, E. (2004). Generalized anxiety disorder. In T. L. Morris & J. S. March (Eds.), *Anxiety disorders in children and adolescents* (pp. 125–140). New York: Guilford Press.

Flannery-Schroeder, E., & Kendall, P. C. (2000). Group and individual cognitive behavioral treatments for youth with anxiety disorders: A randomized clinical trial. *Cognitive Therapy and Research, 24,* 251–278.

Fleck, R. (Director). (2006). *Half nelson* [motion picture]. United States: Hunting Lane Films, Journeyman Pictures, Silverwood Films, Original Media, Traction Media.

Fleming, V. (Director). (1939). *The wizard of Oz* [motion picture]. United States: Metro Goldwyn-Mayer Loew's.

Foa, E. B., & Andrews, L. W. (2006). *If your adolescent has an anxiety disorder.* New York: Oxford University Press.

Ford, E., Liebowitz, M., & Andrews, L. W. (2007). *What you must think of me.* Oxford, UK: Oxford University Press.

Forehand, R. L., & McMahon, R. J. (1981). *Helping the noncompliant child: A clinician's guide to parent training.* New York: Guilford Press.

Forsyth, J. P., Barrios, V., & Acheson, D. T. (2007). Exposure therapy and cognitive interventions:

Overview and newer third-generation perspectives. In D. C. S. Richard & D. L. Lauterbach (Eds.), *Handbook of exposure therapies* (pp. 61–108). San Diego: Academic Press.

Foster, J. (Director). (1991). *Little man Tate* [motion picture]. United States: Orion Pictures.

Frank, J. D. (1961). *Persuasion and healing: A comparative study of psychotherapy.* New York: Schocken Books.

Freeman, A., Pretzer, J., Fleming, B., & Simon, K. M. (1990). *Clinical applications of cognitive therapy.* New York: Plenum Press.

Friedberg, R. D. (1996). Cognitive behavioral games and workbooks: Tips for school counselors. *Elementary School Guidance and Counseling, 31,* 11–20.

Friedberg, R. D. (2006). A cognitive behavioral approach to family therapy. *Journal of Contemporary Psychotherapy, 36,* 159–165.

Friedberg, R. D., Friedberg, B. A., & Friedberg, R. J. (2001). *Therapeutic exercises with children: Guided self-discovery through cognitive behavior techniques.* Sarasota, FL: Professional Resource Press.

Friedberg, R. D., & Gorman, A. A. (2007). Integrating psychotherapeutic processes with cognitive behavioral procedures. *Journal of Contemporary Psychotherapy, 37,* 185–193.

Friedberg, R. D., Gorman, A. A., & Beidel, D. C. (2009). Training psychologists for cognitive-behavioral therapy in the raw world: A rubric for supervisors. *Behavior Modification, 33,* 104–123.

Friedberg, R. D., Mason, C., & Fidaleo, R. A. (1992). *Switching channels: A cognitive behavioral work journal for adolescents.* Sarasota, FL: Psychological Assessment Resources.

Friedberg, R. D., & McClure, J. M. (2002). *Clinical practice of cognitive therapy with children and adolescents: The nuts and bolts.* New York: Guilford Press.

Friedberg, R. D., & Wilt, L. H. (in press). Metaphors and stories in cognitive behavior therapy with children. *Journal of Rational Emotive and Cognitive Behavioral Therapy.*

Fristad, M. A., Emery, B. L., & Beck, S. J. (1997). Use and abuse of the Children's Depression Inventory. *Journal of Consulting and Clinical Psychology, 65,* 699–702.

Fristad, M. A., & Goldberg-Arnold, J. S. (2003). Family interventions for early-onset bipolar disorder. In B. Geller & M. P. DelBello (Eds.), *Bipolar disorder in childhood and adolescence* (pp. 295–313). New York: Guilford Press.

Fristad, M. A., & Goldberg-Arnold, J. S. (2004). *Raising a moody child.* New York: Guilford Press.

Gallo-Lopez, L. (2008). Marcia, Marcia, Marcia: The use and impact of television themes, characters, and images in psychotherapy. In L. C. Rubin (Ed.), *Popular culture in counseling, psychotherapy, and play-based interventions* (pp. 243–256). New York: Springer.

Galvin, M. (1989). *Clouds and clocks: A story for children who soil.* Washington, DC: Magination Press.

Garner, D. M. (1991). *Eating Disorder Inventory–2 manual.* Odessa, FL: Psychological Assessment Resources.

Garner, D. M., & Garfinkel, P. E. (1979). The Eating Attitudes Test: An index of the symptoms of anorexia nervosa. *Psychological Medicine, 12,* 871–878.

Garner, D. M., & Parker, P. P. (1993). Eating disorders. In T. H. Ollendick & M. Hersen (Eds.), *Handbook of Child and Adolescent Assessment* (pp. 384–399). Boston, MA: Allyn & Bacon.

Geddie, L. (1992). *Dinosaur relaxation script.* Unpublished manuscript, University of Oklahoma Health Sciences Center, Oklahoma City, OK.

Geller, J., & Drab, D. L. (1999). The Readiness and Motivation Interview: A symptom-specific measure of readiness for change in the eating disorders. *European Eating Disorders Review, 7,* 259–278.

Ginsburg, G. S., Grover, R. L., Cord, J. J., & Ialongo, N. (2006). Observational measures of parenting in anxious and nonanxious mothers: Does type of task matter? *Journal of Clinical Child and Adolescent Psychology, 35,* 323–328.

Ginsburg, G. S., & Kingery, J. N. (2007). Evidence-based practice for childhood anxiety disorders. *Journal of Contemporary Psychotherapy, 37,* 123–132.

Ginsburg, G. S., Siqueland, L., Masia-Warner, C., & Hedtke, K. A. (2004). Anxiety disorders in children: Family matters. *Cognitive and Behavioral Practice, 11,* 28–43.

Glatzer, R., & Westmoreland, W. (Directors). (2006). *Quinceanera* [motion picture]. United States: Cinetic Media and Kitchen Sink Entertainment.

Goldberg-Arnold, J. A., & Fristad, M. A. (2003). Psychotherapy for children with bipolar disorder. In B. Geller & M. P. DelBello (Eds.), *Bipolar disorder in childhood and early adolescence* (pp. 272–294). New York: Guilford Press.

Goldfried, M. R. (2003). Cognitive-behavior therapy: Reflections on the evolution of a therapeutic orientation. *Cognitive Therapy and Research, 27, 53–69.*

Goldfried, M. R., & Davila, J. (2005). The role of relationship and technique in therapeutic change. *Psychotherapy: Theory, Research and Practice, 42, 421–430.*

Goldfried, M. R., & Davison, G. C. (1976). *Clinical behavior therapy.* New York: Holt, Rinehart, & Winston.

Goodman, W. K., Price, L. H., Rasmussen, S. A., Mazure, C., Fleischmann, R. L., Hill, C. L., et al. (1989). The Yale–Brown Obsessive–Compulsive Scale. *Archives of General Psychiatry, 46, 1006–1016.*

Gosch, E. A., Flannery-Schroeder, E., Mauro, C. F., & Compton, C. N. (2006). Principles of cognitive-behavioral therapy for anxiety disorders in children. *Journal of Cognitive Psychotherapy, 20, 247–262.*

Gotham, H. J. (2006). Advancing implementation of evidence-based practices into clinical practices: How do we get there from here. *Professional Psychology: Research and Practice, 6, 606–613.*

Grave, J., & Blissett, J. (2004). Is cognitive behavior therapy developmentally appropriate for young children?: A critical review of the evidence. *Clinical Psychology Review, 24, 399–420.*

Greenberg, L. (2006). Emotion-focused therapy: A synopsis. *Journal of Contemporary Psychotherapy, 36, 87–93.*

Greenberg, L. S., & Paivio, S. C. (1997). *Working with emotions: Changing core schemes.* New York: Guilford Press.

Greenberg, L. S., & Paivio, S. C. (2002). *Working with the emotions in psychotherapy.* New York: Guilford Press.

Greenberger, D., & Padesky, C. A. (1995). *Mind over mood: Changing how you feel by changing the way you think.* New York: Guilford Press.

Greene, R. W. (2001). *The explosive child: A new approach for understanding and parenting easily frustrated, chronically inflexible children* (2nd ed.). New York: HarperCollins.

Greenspan, S. (1993). *Playground politics.* Reading, MA: Addison Wesley.

Greenspan, S., & Greenspan, N. T. (1985). *First feelings.* New York: Penguin Books.

Greenspan, S., & Greenspan, N. T. (1989). *The essential partnership.* New York: Penguin Books.

Gross. J. J. (2002).Emotion regulation: Affective, cognitive, and social consequences. *Psychophysiology, 39, 281–291.*

Gross, J. J., & John, O. P. (2003). Individual differences in two emotion processes: Implications for affect, relationships, and well-being. *Journal of Personality and Social Psychology, 64, 970–986.*

Grover, R. L., Hughes, A. A., Bergman, R. L., & Kingery, J. N. (2006). Treatment modification based on childhood anxiety diagnosis: Demonstrating the flexibility in manualized treatment. *Journal of Cognitive Psychotherapy, 20, 275–286.*

Guidano, V. F., & Liotti, G. (1983). *Cognitive processes and emotional disorders: A structural approach to psychotherapy.* New York: Guilford Press.

Guidano, V. F., & Liotti, G. (1985). A constructionalist foundation for cognitive therapy. In M. J. Mahoney & A. Freeman (Eds.), *Cognition and psychotherapy* (pp. 101–142). New York: Plenum Press.

Hall, B. (Creator). (2003). *Joan of Arcadia* [television series]. United States: Sony Pictures Television, CBS Productions, and Barbara Hall Productions.

Hammen, C., & Zupan, B. A. (1984). Self-schemas, depression, and the processing of personal information in children. *Journal of Experimental Child Psychology, 37, 598–608.*

Hansen, J. C., & L'Abate, L. (1982). *Approaches to family therapy.* New York: Macmillan.

Hardwicke, C. (Director). (2003). *Thirteen* [motion picture]. United States: Michael London Pictures, Working Title Films, Antidote Films, and Sound for Film.

Hayes, A. M., & Strauss, J. L. (1998). Dynamic systems theory as a paradigm for the study of change in psychotherapy: An application of cognitive therapy for depression. *Journal of Consulting and Clinical Psychology, 66,* 939–947.

Hayes, S. C. (1994). Content, context, and types of psychological acceptance. In S. C. Hayes, N. S. Jacobson, V. M. Follette, & M. J. Dougher (Eds.), *Acceptance and change: Context and content in psychotherapy* (pp. 13–32). Reno, NV: Context Press.

Hayes, S. C. (2007, July). ACT case conceptualization: Using RFT to correct flaws of traditional functional analysis. In M. Fennell (Chair), *Cognitive behavioral case formulation: Is the emperor clothed?* Panel presentation presented at the 5th World Congress of Behavioural and Cognitive Therapies, Barcelona, Spain.

Hayes, S. C., Strosdahl, K. D., & Wilson, K. G. (1999). *Acceptance and commitment therapy.* New York: Guilford Press.

Heffner, M., Sperry, J., Eifert, G. H., & Detweiler, M. (2002). Acceptance and commitment therapy in the treatment of an adolescent female with anorexia nervosa: A case example. *Cognitive and Behavioral Practice, 9,* 232–236.

Hembree, E. A., & Cahill, S. P. (2007). Obstacles to successful implementation of exposure therapy. In D. C. S. Richard & D. L. Lauterbach (Eds.), *Handbook of exposure therapies* (pp. 389–408). San Diego: Academic Press.

Hembree, E. A., Rauch, S. A. M., & Foa, E. B. (2003). Beyond the manual: The insider's guide to prolonged exposure to PTSD. *Cognitive and Behavioral Practice, 10,* 22–30.

Hesley, J. W., & Hesley, J. G. (2001). *Rent two films and let's talk in the morning.* New York: Wiley.

Hirai, M., Vernon, L. L., & Cochran, H. (2007). Exposure for phobias. In D. C. S. Richard & D. L. Lauterbach (Eds.), *Handbook of exposure therapies* (pp. 247–270). San Diego: Academic Press.

Hoffman, M. (1991). *Amazing grace.* New York: Dial.

Huebner, D. (2006). *What to do when you worry too much: A kid's guide to overcoming anxiety.* Washington, DC: Magination Press.

Huebner, D. (2007a). *What to do when you grumble too much: A kid's guide to overcoming negativity.* Washington, DC: Magination Press.

Huebner, D. (2007b). *What to do when your brain gets stuck: A kid's guide to overcoming OCD.* Washington, DC: Magination Press.

Huebner, D. (2008). *What to do when your temper flares.* Washington, DC: Magination Press.

Huey, S. J., & Polo, A. J. (2008). Evidence-based psychosocial treatments for ethnic minority youth. *Journal of Clinical Child and Adolescent Psychology, 37,* 262–301.

Hughes, J. (Director). (1985). *The breakfast club* [motion picture]. United States: A & M Films and Universal Pictures.

Huppert, J. D., & Baker-Morissette, S. L. (2003). Beyond the manual: The insider's guide to panic control treatment. *Cognitive and Behavioral Practice, 10,* 2–13.

Ilardi, S. S., & Feldman, D. (2001). The cognitive neuroscience paradigm: A unifying metatheoretical framework for the science and practice of clinical psychology. *Journal of Clinical Psychology, 57,* 1067–1088.

Ingram, R. E., & Kendall, P. C. (1986). Cognitive clinical psychology: Implications of an information processing perspective. In R. E. Ingram (Ed.), *Information-processing approaches to clinical psychology* (pp. 3–21). Orlando, FL: Academic Press.

Irwin, C., Evans, D. L., & Andrews, L. W. (2007). *Monochrome days.* Oxford, UK: Oxford University Press.

Jacobson, E. (1938). *Progressive relaxation.* Chicago, IL: University of Chicago Press.

Jamieson, P. E., with Rynn, M. A. (2006). *Mind race.* New York: Oxford University Press.

Jolly, J. B. (1993). A multi-method test of the cognitive content-specificity hypotheses in young adolescents. *Journal of Anxiety Disorders, 7,* 223–233.

Jolly, J. B., & Dykman, R. A. (1994). Using self-report data to differentiate anxious and depressive symptoms in adolescents: Cognitive content specificity and global distress. *Cognitive Therapy and Research, 18,* 25–37.

Jolly, J. B., & Kramer, T. A. (1994). The hierarchical arrangement of internalizing cognitions. *Cognitive Therapy and Research, 8,* 1–14.

Jones, J. V. & Lyddon, W. J. (2000). Cognitive therapy and empirically validated treatments. *Journal of Cognitive Psychotherapy, 14,* 337–345.

Kamphaus, R. W., VanDeventer, M. C., Brueggemann, A., & Barry, M. (2006). Behavior Assessment System for Children—2nd Edition. In S. R. Smith & L. Handler (Eds.), *The clinical assessment of children and adolescents* (pp. 311–326). New York: Routledge.

Kanfer, F. H., Karoly, P., & Newman, A. (1975). Reduction of children's fear of the dark by competence-related and situation threat-related verbal cues. *Journal of Consulting and Clinical Psychology, 27,* 146–155.

Kant, J., Franklin, M., & Andrews, L. W. (2008). *The thought that counts.* New York: Oxford University Press.

Kapalka, G. M. (2007). *Parenting your out of control child.* Oakland, CA: New Harbinger.

Kashdan, T. B., Barrios, V., Forsyth, J. P., & Steger, M. F. (2006). Experiential avoidance as a generalized psychological vulnerability comparison with coping and regulation strategies. *Behaviour Research and Therapy, 54,* 1301–1320.

Kaslow, N. J., Stark, K. D., Printz, B., Livingston, R., & Tsai, S. L. (1992). Cognitive Triad Inventory for Children: Development and relation to depression and anxiety. *Journal of Clinical Child Psychology, 4,* 339–347.

Kaslow, N. J., Tanenbaum, R. L., & Seligman, M. E. P. (1978). *The KASTAN: A children's attributional style questionnaire.* Unpublished manuscript, University of Pennsylvania.

Kazdin, A. E. (2001). *Behavior modification in applied settings.* Belmont, CA: Wadsworth.

Kazdin, A. E., Colbus, D., & Rodgers, A. (1986a). Assessment of depression and diagnosis of depressive disorder among psychiatrically disturbed inpatient children. *Journal of Abnormal Child Psychology, 14,* 499–515.

Kazdin, A. E., Rodgers, A., & Colbus, D. (1986b). The Hopelessness Scale for Children: Psychometric characteristics and concurrent validity. *Journal of Consulting and Clinical Psychology, 54,* 241–245.

Kearney, C. A. (2007). *Getting your child to say "yes" to school.* New York: Guilford Press.

Kearney, C. A., & Albano, A. M. (2000). *Therapist's guide for school refusal behavior.* San Antonio, TX: Psychological Corporation.

Kearney, C. A., & Silverman, W. K. (1993). Measuring the function of school refusal behavior: The School Refusal Assessment Scale. *Journal of Clinical Child Psychology, 22,* 85–96.

Keegan, K., with Moss, H. B. (2008). *Chasing the high.* New York: Oxford University Press.

Kelley, M. L. (1990). *School–home notes: Promoting children's classroom success.* New York: Guilford Press.

Kendall, P. C. (2006). Guiding theory for therapy with children and adolescents. In P. C. Kendall (Ed.), *Child and adolescent therapy: Cognitive-behavioral procedures* (3rd ed., pp. 3–30). New York: Guilford Press.

Kendall, P. C., Aschenbrand, S. G., & Hudson, J. L. (2003). Child-focused treatment of anxiety. In A. E. Kazdin & J. R. Weisz (Eds.), *Evidence-based psychotherapies for children and adolescents* (pp. 81–100). New York: Guilford Press.

Kendall, P. C., Chansky, T. E., Kane, M. T., Kim, R. S., Kortlander, E., Ronan, K., et al. (1992). *Anxiety disorders in youth: Cognitive-behavioral interventions.* Boston, MA: Allyn & Bacon.

Kendall, P. C., Chu, B., Gifford, A., Hayes, C., & Nauta, M. (1998). Breathing life into a manual. *Cognitive-Behavioral Practice, 5,* 89–104.

Kendall, P. C., Flannery-Schroeder, E., Panichelli-Mindel, S. M., Southam-Gerow, M., Henin, A., & Warman, M. (1997). Therapy for youths with anxiety disorders: A second randomized trial. *Journal of Consulting and Clinical Psychology, 65,* 366–380.

Kendall, P. C., & MacDonald, J. P. (1993). Cognition in the psychopathology of youth and implications for treatment. In K. S. Dobson & P. C. Kendall (Eds.), *Psychopathology and cognition* (pp. 387–430). San Diego, CA: Academic Press.

Kendall, P. C., Robin, J. A., Hedtke, K. A., Suveg, C., Flannery-Schroeder, E., & Gosch, E. (2005).

Considering CBT with anxious youth?: Think exposures. *Cognitive and Behavioral Practice, 12*, 136–148.

Kendall, P. C., & Suveg, C. (2006). Treating anxiety disorders in youth. In P. C. Kendall (Ed.), *Child and adolescent therapy: Cognitive behavioral procedures* (3rd ed., pp. 243–294). New York: Guilford Press.

Kennedy-Moore, E., & Watson, J. C. (1999). *The expression and nonexpression of emotion.* New York: Guilford Press.

Kingery, J. N., Roblek, T. L., Suveg, C., Grover, R. L., Sherrill, J. T., & Bergman, R. L. (2006). They're not just "little adults": Developmental considerations for implementing cognitive behavioral therapy with anxious youth. *Journal of Cognitive Psychotherapy, 20*, 263–273.

Klein, D. N., Dougherty, L. R., & Olino, T. M. (2005). Toward guidelines for evidence-based assessment of depression in children and adolescents. *Journal of Clinical Child and Adolescent Psychology, 34*, 412–432.

Koch, E. I., Gloster, A. T., & Waller, S. A. (2007). Exposure treatments for panic disorder with and without agoraphobia. In D. C. S. Richard & D. L. Lauterbach (Eds.), *Handbook of exposure therapies* (pp. 221–247). San Diego: Academic Press.

Koeppen, A. S. (1974). Relaxation training for children. *Journal of Elementary School Guidance and Counseling, 9*, 14–21.

Kovacs, M. (1985). The Children's Depression Inventory. *Psychopharmacology Bulletin, 21*, 995–998.

Kovacs, M. (1992). *Children's Depression Inventory.* New York: Multi-Health Systems.

Kraemer, S. (2006). Something happens: Elements of therapeutic change. *Clinical Child Psychiatry and Psychology, 11*, 239–248.

Krain, A. L., & Kendall, P. C. (2000). The role of parental emotional distress in parent report of child anxiety. *Journal of Clinical Child Psychology, 29*, 328–335.

Kraus, J. R. (2006). *Annie's plan.* Washington, DC: Magination Press.

Kronenberger, W. G., & Meyer, R. G. (2001). *The child clinician's handbook* (2nd ed.). Norton, MA: Allyn & Bacon.

Kuehlwein, K. (2000). Enhancing creativity in cognitive therapy. *Journal of Cognitive Psychotherapy, 14*, 175–187.

Kuiper, N. A., Olinger, L. J., & MacDonald, M. R. (1988). Vulnerability and episodic cognitions in a self-worth contingency model of depression. In L. B. Alloy (Ed.), *Cognitive processes in depression* (pp. 289–309). New York: Guilford Press.

Kumar, G., & Steer, R. A. (1995). Psychosocial correlates of suicidal ideation in adolescent psychiatric inpatients. *Suicide and Life Threatening Behavior, 25*, 339–346.

Kumar, G., Steer, R. A., Teitelman, K. B., & Villacis, L. (2002). Effectiveness of Beck Depression Inventory-II subscales in screening for major depressive disorders in adolescent psychiatric inpatients. *Assessment, 9*, 164–170.

Kuyken, W., Padesky, C. A., & Dudley, R. A. (2009). *Collaborative case conceptualization.* New York: Guilford Press.

LaGreca, A. M., & Lopez, N. (1998). Social anxiety among adolescents: Linkages with peer relations and friendships. *Journal of Abnormal Child Psychology, 26*, 83–94.

LaGreca, A. M., & Stone, W. L. (1993). Social Anxiety Scale for Children—Revised: Factor structure and concurrent validity. *Journal of Clinical and Child Psychology, 22*, 7–27.

Lam, K. S. L., & Aman, M. G. (2007). The Repetitive Behavior Scale—Revised: Independent validation in individuals with autism spectrum disorders. *Journal of Autism and Developmental Disorders, 37*, 855–866.

Lamb-Shapiro, J. (2000). *The bear who lost his sleep.* Plainview, NY: Childswork/Childsplay.

Lamb-Shapiro, J. (2001). *The hyena who lost her laugh: A story about changing your negative thinking.* Plainview, NY: Childswork/Childsplay.

Landy, R. J. (2008). *The couch and the stage.* New York: Aronson.

Larson, J., & Lochman, J. E. (2002). *Helping school children cope with anger: A cognitive behavioral intervention.* New York: Guilford Press.

Last, C. G. (2006). *Help for worried kids*. New York: Guilford Press.

Laurent, J., & Stark, K. D. (1993). Testing the cognitive content specificity hypothesis with anxious and depressed youngsters. *Journal of Abnormal Psychology, 102*, 226–237.

Lauterbach, D., & Reiland, S. (2007). Exposure therapy and post-traumatic stress disorder. In D. C. S. Richard & D. L. Lauterbach (Eds.), *Handbook of exposure therapies* (pp. 127–152). San Diego: Academic Press.

Leahy, R. L. (2007). Emotion and psychotherapy. *Clinical Psychology: Science and Practice, 14,* 353–357.

LeCouteur, A., Rutter, M., Lord, C., Rios, P., Robertson, S., Holdgrafer, M., et al. (1989). Autism Diagnostic Interview: A standardized investigator-based instrument. *Journal of Autism and Developmental Disorders, 19*, 363–387.

Lee, S. (Director). (1994). *Crooklyn* [motion picture]. United States: 40 Acres and a Mule Filmworks.

Leitenberg, H., Yost, L. W., & Carroll-Wilson, M. (1986). Negative cognitive errors in children: Questionnaire development, normative data, comparisons between children with and without self-reported symptoms of depression, low self-esteem, and evaluation of anxiety. *Journal of Consulting and Clinical Psychology, 54*, 528–536.

Lerner, J., Safren, S. A., Henin, A., Warman, M., Heimberg, R. G., & Kendall, P. C. (1999). Differentiating anxious and depressive self-statements in youth: Factor structure of the Negative Affect Self-Statement Questionnaire among youth referred to an anxiety disorder clinic. *Journal of Clinical Child Psychology, 28*, 82–93.

LeRoi, A., & Rock, C. (Creators). (2005). *Everybody hates Chris* [television series]. United States: Chris Rock Entertainment, 3 Art Entertainment, CBS Paramount Network Television, and Paramount Network Television.

Lezine, D. A., & Brent, D. (2008). *Eight stories up*. New York: Oxford University Press.

Linehan, M. M. (1993a). *Cognitive behavioral treatment for borderline personality disorder*. New York: Guilford Press.

Linehan, M. M. (1993b). *Skills training manual for healing BPD*. New York: Guilford Press.

Linehan, M. M., Cochran, B. N., & Kehrer, C. A. (2001). Dialectical behavioral therapy for BPD. In D. H. Barlow (Ed.), *Clinical handbook of psychological disorders* (3rd ed., pp. 470–522). New York: Guilford Press.

Lochman, J. E., Barry, T. D., & Pardini, D. A. (2003). Anger control training for aggressive youth. In A. E. Kazdin, & J. E. Weisz (Eds.), *Evidence-based psychotherapies for children and adolescents* (pp. 263–281). New York: Guilford Press.

Lochman, J. E., Fitzgerald, D. P., & Whidby, J. M. (1999). Anger management with aggressive children. In C. Schaefer (Ed.), *Short-term psychotherapy groups for children* (pp. 301–349) Northvale, NJ: Aronson.

Lochman, J. E., & Wells, K. C. (2002a). Contextual social cognitive mediators and child outcome: A test of the theoretical model in the Coping Power Program. *Development and Psychopathology, 14*, 945–967.

Lochman, J. E., & Wells, K. C. (2002b). The Coping Power program at middle school transition: Universal and indicated prevention effects. *Psychology of Addictive Behaviors, 16*, 540–554.

Lock, J. (2002). Treating adolescents with eating disorders in the family context: Empirical and theoretical considerations. *Child and Adolescent Psychiatry Clinics of North America, 11*, 331–342.

Lock, J., & Fitzpatrick, K. K. (2007). Evidence-based treatments for children and adolescents with eating disorders: Family therapy and family-facilitated cognitive-behavioral therapy. *Journal of Contemporary Psychotherapy, 37*, 145–156.

Lock, J., & le Grange, K. (2005). *Help your teenager beat an eating disorder*. New York: Guilford Press.

Lock, J., le Grange, D., Agras, W. S., & Dare, C. (2001). *Treatment manual for anorexia nervosa: A family-based approach*. New York: Guilford Press.

Lockshin, S. B., Gillis, J. M., & Romanczyk, R. G. (2005). *Helping your child with autism spectrum disorder: A step by step workbook for families.* Oakland, CA: New Harbinger.

Loeber, R., Green, S. M., Lahey, B. B., & Stouthamer-Loeber, M. (1991). Differences and similarities between children, mothers, and teachers as informants on disruptive child behavior. *Journal of Abnormal Child Psychology, 19,* 75–95.

Lonczak, H. (2007). *Mookey the monkey gets over being teased.* Washington, DC: Magination Press.

Lopez, R., & Marx, J. (Music and Lyrics). (2003). *Avenue Q.* United States: Kevin McCollum, Robyn Goodman, Jeffrey Seller, Vineyard Theatre, and New Group (producers).

Lord, C., Rutter, M., Goode, S., Heemsbergen, J., Jordan, H., Mawhood, L., et al. (1989). Autism Diagnostic Observation Schedule: A standardized observation of communicative and social behavior. *Journal of Autism and Developmental Disorders, 19,* 185–212.

Madison, L. (2002). *The feelings book: The care and keeping of your emotions.* Middleton, WI: American Girl Books.

Maier, I. M. (2005a). *When Fuzzy was afraid of big and loud things.* Washington, DC: Magination Press.

Maier, I. M. (2005b). *When Fuzzy was afraid of losing his mother.* Washington, DC: Magination Press.

Maier, I. M. (2005c). *When Lizzy was afraid of trying new things.* Washington, DC: Magination Press.

Maloney, M. J., McGuire, J. B., & Daniels, S. R. (1988). Reliability testing of a children's version of the eating disorder test. *Journal of the American Academy of Child and Adolescent Psychiatry, 27,* 541–543.

Mansueto, C. S., Golomb, R. G., Thomas, A. M., & Stemberger, R. M. T. (1999). A comprehensive model for behavioral treatment of trichotillomania. *Cognitive and Behavioral Practice, 6,* 23–43.

March, J. S. (1997). *Multidimensional Anxiety Scale for Children.* New York: Multi-Health Systems.

March, J. S., with Benton, C. M. (2007). *Talking back to OCD.* New York: Guilford Press.

March, J. S., & Franklin, M. E. (2006). Cognitive-behavioral therapy for pediatric OCD. In B. O. Rothbaum (Ed.), *Pathological anxiety: Emotional processing in etiology and treatment* (pp. 147–165). New York: Guilford Press.

March, J. S., & Mulle, K. (1998). *OCD in children and adolescents.* New York: Guilford Press.

March, J. S., Parker, J. D. A., Sullivan, K., Stallings, P., & Conners, K. (1997). The Multidimensional Anxiety Scale for Children (MASC): Factor structure, reliability, and validity. *Journal of the American Academy of Child and Adolescent Psychiatry, 40,* 780–786.

March, J. S., Sullivan, K., & James, P. (1999). Test–retest reliability of the Multidimensional Anxiety Scale for Children. *Journal of Anxiety Disorders, 13,* 349–358.

Marcus, L. M., & Schopler, E. (1993). Pervasive developmental disorder. In T. H. Ollendick & M. Hersen (Eds.), *Handbook of child and adolescent assessment* (pp. 346–353). Boston: Allyn & Bacon.

Markus, H. (1990). Unresolved issues of self-representation. *Cognitive Therapy and Research, 14,* 241–253.

Mash, E. J., & Dozois, D. J. A. (2003). Child psychopathology: A developmental-systems perspective. In E. J. Mash, & R. A. Barkley (Eds.), *Child psychopathology* (2nd ed., pp. 3–71). New York: Guilford Press.

Mattis, S. G., & Ollendick, T. H. (1997). Children's cognitive responses to the somatic symptoms of panic. *Journal of Abnormal Child Psychology, 25,* 47–57.

McCurry, S., & Hayes, S. C. (1992). Clinical and experimental perspectives on metaphorical talk. *Clinical Psychology Review, 12,* 763–785.

McHolm, A. E., Cunningham, C. E., & Vanier, M. K. (2005). *Helping your child with selective mutism: Practical steps to overcome a fear of speaking.* Oakland, CA: New Harbinger.

McMahon, R. J., & Kotler, J. S. (2006). Conduct problems. In D. A. Wolfe & E. J. Mash (Eds.), *Behavioral and emotional disorders in adolescents* (pp. 153–225). New York: Guilford Press.

Mendlowitz, S. L., Manassis, K., Bradley, S., Scapillato, D., Miezitis, S., & Shaw, B. F. (1999). Cognitive-behavioral group treatment in childhood anxiety disorders: The role of parental involvement. *Journal of the American Academy of Child and Adolescent Psychiatry, 38,* 1223–1229.

Menendez, R. (Director). (1988). *Stand and deliver* [motion picture]. United States: American Playhouse.

Merlo, L., Storch, E. A., & Geffken, G. R. (2007). Assessment of pediatric obsessive–compulsive disorder. In E. A. Storch, T. K. Murphy, & G. R. Geffken (Eds.), *Handbook of child and adolescent obsessive–compulsive disorder* (pp. 67–108). Mahwah, NJ: Erlbaum.

Merlo, L. J., Storch, E. A., Murphy, T. K., Goodman, W. K., & Geffken, G. R. (2005). Assessment of pediatric obsessive–compulsive disorder: A critical review of current methodology. *Child Psychiatry and Human Development, 36,* 195–214.

Miller, W. R., & Rollnick, S. (1991). *Motivational interviewing: Preparing people for change.* New York: Guilford Press.

Miltenberger, R. G., Fuqua, R. W., & Woods, D. W. (1998). Applying behavior analysis to clinical problems: Review and analysis of habit reversal. *Journal of Applied Behavioral Analysis, 3,* 447–469.

Mineka, S., & Thomas, C. (1999). Mechanisms of change in exposure therapy for anxiety disorders. In T. Dagleish & M. Power (Eds.), *Handbook of cognition and emotion* (pp. 747–764). New York: Wiley.

Minuchin, S., & Fishman, H. C. (1974). *Family therapy techniques.* Cambridge, MA: Harvard University Press.

Morris, R. J., & Kratochwill, T. R. (1998). Childhood fears and phobias. In R. J. Morris & T. R. Kratochwill (Eds.), *The practice of child therapy* (3rd ed., pp. 91–131). Boston: Allyn & Bacon.

Moses, E. B., & Barlow, D. H. (2006). A new unified treatment approach for emotional disorders based on emotion science. *Current Directions in Psychological Science, 15,* 146–150.

Muris, P., Merckelbach, H., Van Brakel, A., & Mayer, B. (1999). The revised version of the Screen for Child Anxiety Related Emotional Disorders (SCARED-R): Further evidence for its reliability and validity. *Anxiety, Stress, and Coping, 12,* 411–425.

Murrell, A. R., Coyne, L. W., & Wilson, K. G. (2005). ACT with children, adolescents, and their parents. In S. C. Hayes & K. Strosdahl (Eds.), *Acceptance and commitment therapy: A clinician's guide* (pp. 249–271). New York: Springer.

Myers, K., & Winters, N. C. (2002). Ten-year review of rating scales: II. Scales for internalizing disorders. *Journal of the American Academy of Child and Adolescent Psychiatry, 41,* 634–659.

Myles, B. S. (2003). Behavioral forms of stress management for individuals with Asperger syndrome. *Child and Adolescent Psychiatric Clinics of North America, 12,* 123–141.

Najman, J. M., Williams, G. M., Nikles, J., Spence, S., Bor, W., & O'Callaghan, M. (2000). Mothers' mental illness and child behavior problems: Cause–effect association or observation bias? *Journal of the American Academy of Child and Adolescent Psychiatry, 39,* 592–602.

Nass, M. (2000). *The lion who lost his roar.* Plainview, NY: Childswork/Childsplay.

Nass, M. (2004). *The rabbit who lost his hop.* Plainview, NY: Childswork/Childsplay.

Nava, G. (Director). (1995). *Mi familia, my family* [motion picture]. United States: American Playhouse.

Nava, G. (Creator). (2002). *American family* [television series]. United States: 20th Century Fox Television, El Norte Productions, KCET, and the Greenblatt Janollan Studio.

Nelson, W. M., & Finch, A. J. (2000). *Children's Inventory of Anger (CHIA): Manual.* Los Angeles, CA: Western Psychological Services.

Nelson-Gray, R. O. (2003). Treatment utility of psychological assessment. *Psychological Assessment, 15,* 521–531.

Nichols. W. C. (1996). *Treating people in families.* New York: Guilford Press.

Novaco, R. W. (2003). *The Novaco Anger Scale and Provocation Inventory (NAS-PI).* Los Angeles, CA: Western Psychological Services.

Ollendick, T. H. (1983). Reliability and validity of the Revised Fear Survey Schedule for Children—R. *Behaviour Research and Therapy, 21,* 395–399.

Ollendick, T. H. (1998). Panic disorder in children and adolescents: New developments, new directions. *Journal of Clinical Child Psychology, 27,* 234–245.

Ollendick, T. H., & Cerny, J. A. (1981). *Clinical behavior therapy with children.* New York: Plenum Press.

Ollendick, T. H., King, N. J., & Frary, R. B. (1989). Fears in children and adolescents: Reliability and generalizability across gender, age, and nationality. *Behaviour Research and Therapy, 27,* 19–26.

Otto, M. (2000). Stories and metaphors in cognitive behavior therapy. *Cognitive and Behavioral Therapy, 7,* 166–172.

Overholser, J. C. (1993). Elements of the Socratic method, Part 2: Inductive reasoning. *Psychotherapy, 30,* 75–85.

Overholser, J. C. (1994). Elements of the Socratic method, Part 3: Universal definitions. *Psychotherapy, 31,* 286–293.

Padesky, C. A. (1988). *Intensive training series in cognitive therapy.* Workshop series presented at Newport Beach, CA.

Padesky, C. A. (1994). Schema change processes in cognitive therapy. *Clinical Psychology and Psychotherapy, 1,* 267–278.

Padesky, C. A. (2004). Behavioral experiments: At the crossroads. In J. Bennett-Levy, G. Butler, M. Fennell, A. Hackmann, M. Mueller, & D. Westbrook (Eds.,). *Oxford guide to behavioral experiments in cognitive therapy* (pp. 433–438). Oxford, UK: Oxford University Press.

Padesky, C. A. (2007, July). *The next frontier: Building positive qualities with cognitive behaviour therapy.* Invited address presented at the 5th World Congress of Behavioural and Cognitive Therapies, Barcelona, Spain.

Palansky, M. (Director). (2008). *Penelope* [motion picture]. United States: Stone Village Picutres, Type A Films, Grosvenor Park Productions, Tatira, and Zephyr Films.

Palmer, R., Christie, M., Condle, C., Davies, D., & Kenwick, J. (1987). The Clinical Eating Disorders Rating Instrument (CEDRI): A preliminary description. *International Journal of Eating Disorders, 6,* 9–16.

Patterson, G. R. (1976). *Living with children.* Champaign, IL: Research Press.

Patterson, G. R., & Forgatch, M. (1987). *Parents and adolescents living together.* Champaign, IL: Research Press.

Pelham, W. E., Fabiano, G. A., & Massetti, G. M. (2005). Evidence-based assessment of attention deficit hyperactivity disorder in children and adolescents. *Journal of Clinical Child and Adolescent Psychology, 34,* 449–476.

Pellegrino, M. W. (2002). *Too nice.* Washington, DC: Magination Press.

Perrin, S., Smith, P., & Yule, W. (2000). Practitioner review: The assessment and treatment of posttraumatic stress disorder in children and adolescents. *Journal of Child Psychology and Psychiatry, 41,* 277–289.

Persons, J. B. (1989). *Cognitive therapy in practice.* New York: Norton.

Persons, J. B. (1995, November). *Cognitive-behavioral case formulation.* Workshop presented at the annual meeting of the Association for the Advancement of Behavior Therapy, Washington, DC.

Persons, J. B. (2008). *The case formulation approach to cognitive-behavioral therapy.* New York: Guilford Press.

Peterson, L., & Sobell, L. C. (1994). Research contributions to clinical assessment. *Behavior Therapy, 25,* 523–531.

Piacentini, J., & Bergman, R. L. (2001). Developmental issues in cognitive therapy for childhood anxiety disorders. *Journal of Cognitive Psychotherapy, 15,* 165–182.

Piacentini, J. C., & Langley, A. K. (2004). Cognitive-behavior therapy for children who have obsessive–compulsive disorder. *Journal of Clinical Psychology, 60,* 1181–1194.

Piacentini, J. C., Cohen, P., & Cohen, J. (1992). Combining discrepant information from multiple sources: Are complex algorithms better than simple ones? *Journal of Abnormal Child Psychology, 20,* 51–63.

Piacentini, J. C., Langley, A. K., & Roblek, T. (2007a). *Cognitive-behavioral treatment of childhood OCD: It's only a false alarm (Therapist guide).* New York: Oxford University Press.

Piacentini, J. C., Langley, A. K., & Roblek, T. (2007b). *Cognitive-behavioral treatment of childhood OCD: It's only a false alarm (Workbook).* New York: Oxford University Press.

Piacentini, J. C., March, J. S., & Franklin, M. E. (2006). Cognitive-behavioral therapy for youth with obsessive–compulsive disorder. In P. C. Kendall (Ed.), *Child and adolescent therapy: Cognitive-behavioral procedures* (3rd ed., pp. 297–321). New York: Guilford Press.

Pliszka, S. R., Carlson, C. L., & Swanson, J. M. (1999). *ADHD with comorbid disorders: Clinical assessment and management.* New York: Guilford Press.

Pos, A., & Greenberg, L. S. (2007). Emotion-focused therapy: The transforming power of affect. *Journal of Contemporary Psychotherapy, 37,* 25–31.

Probst, M., Vandereycken, W., Van Coppenolle, H., & Vanderlinden, J. (1995). The Body Attitude Test for patients with an eating disorder: Psychometric characteristics of a new questionnaire. *Eating Disorders, 3,* 133–144.

Prochaska, J. O. (1979). *Systems of psychotherapy: A transtheoretical analysis.* Homewood, IL: Dorsey Press.

Prochaska, J. O., & DiClemente, C. C. (1992). Stages of change in the modification of problem behaviors. In M. Hersen, R. M. Eisler, & P. M. Miller (Eds.), *Progress in behavior modification* (pp. 184–214). Sycamore, IL: Sycamore Press.

Prochaska, J. O., DiClemente, C. C., & Norcross, J. C. (1992). In search of how people change. *American Psychologist, 47,* 1102–1114.

Quinn, P. O., & Stern, J. M. (1993). *The putting on the brakes activity book for young people with ADHD.* Washington, DC: Magination Press.

Rapee, R. M., Wignall, A. M., Hudson, J. L., & Schniering, C. A. (2000). *Treating anxious children and adolescents: An evidence-based approach.* Oakland, CA: New Harbinger.

Raskin, R. (2005). *Feeling better: A kid's book about therapy.* Washington, DC: Magination Press.

Reiner, R. (Director). (1986). *Stand by me* [motion picture]. United States: Act III, Act III Communications, Columbia Pictures Corporation, and The Body.

Reitman, J. (Director). (2007). *Juno* [motion picture]. United States: Fox Searchlight, Mandate Pictures, and Mr. Mudd.

Resick, P. A., & Calhoun, K. S. (2001). Posttraumatic stress disorder. In D. H. Barlow (Ed.), *Clinical handbook of psychological disorders* (3rd ed., pp. 60–113). New York: Guilford Press.

Reynolds, C. R., & Kamphaus, R. W. (2004). *Behavior Assessment System for Children–2 (BASC-2).* Circle Pines, MN: American Guidance Service.

Reynolds, C. R., & Richmond, B. O. (1985). *Revised Children's Manifest Anxiety Scale: Manual.* Los Angeles: Western Psychological Services.

Reynolds, W. M. (1987). *Suicidal Ideation Questionnaire.* Odessa, FL: Psychological Assessment Resources.

Reynolds, W. M. (1988). *Suicidal Ideation Questionnaire: A professional manual.* Odessa, FL: Psychological Assessment Resources.

Reynolds, W. M. (1993). Self-report methodology. In T. H. Ollendick & M. Hersen (Eds.), *Handbook of child and adolescent assessment* (pp. 98–123). Boston: Allyn & Bacon.

Richard, D. C. S., Lauterbach, D., & Gloster, A. T. (2007). Description, mechanisms of action, and assessment. In D. C. S. Richard & D. Lauterbach (Eds.), *Handbook of exposure therapies* (pp. 1–28). New York: Academic Press.

Robertie, K., Weidenbenner, R., Barrett, L., & Poole, R. (2008). Milieu multiplex: Using movies in the treatment of adolescents with sexual behavior problems. In L. C. Rubin (Ed.), *Popular culture in counseling, psychotherapy, and play-based interventions* (pp. 99–122). New York: Springer.

Robins, C. J., & Hayes, A. M. (1993). An appraisal of cognitive therapy. *Journal of Consulting and Clinical Psychology, 61,* 205–214.

Rogers, G. M., Reinecke, M. A., & Curry, J. F. (2005). Case formulation in TADS CBT. *Cognitive and Behavioral Practice, 12,* 198–208.

Ronan, K. R., Kendall, P. C., & Rowe, M. (1994). Negative affectivity in children: Development and validation of a self-statement questionnaire. *Cognitive Therapy and Research, 18,* 509–528.

Rooyackers, P. (1998). *101 Drama games for children.* Alameda, CA: Hunter House.

Rouf, K., Fennell, M., Westbrook, D., Cooper, M., & Bennett-Levy, D. (2004). Devising effective behavioral experiments. In J. Bennett-Levy, G. Butler, M. Fennell, A. Hackmann, M. Mueller, & D. Westbrook (Eds.), *Oxford guide to behavioral experiments in cognitive therapy* (pp. 1–20). Oxford, UK: Oxford University Press.

Rubin, L. C. (Ed.). (2007). *Using superheroes in counseling and play therapy.* New York: Springer.

Safran, J. D., & Muran, J. C. (2001). A relational approach to training and supervision in cognitive psychotherapy. *Journal of Cognitive Psychotherapy, 15,* 3–16.

Saigh, P. A. (1987). The use of an in vitro flooding package in the treatment of traumatized adolescents. *Journal of Developmental and Behavioral Pediatrics, 10,* 17–21.

Saigh, P. A., Yule, W., & Inamdar, S. C. (1996). Imaginal flooding of traumatized children and adolescents. *Journal of School Psychology, 34,* 163–183.

Samoilov, A., & Goldfried, M. R. (2000). Role of emotion in cognitive-behavior therapy. *Clinical Psychology: Science and Practice, 7,* 373–385.

Schniering, C. A., & Rapee, R. M. (2002). Development and validation of a measure of children's automatic thoughts: The Children's Automatic Thoughts Scale. *Behaviour Research and Therapy, 40,* 1091–1109.

Schopler, E., Reichler, R. J., & Renner, B. R. (1986). *The Childhood Autism Rating Scale.* Los Angeles: Western Psychological Services.

Schroeder, C. S., & Gordon, C. S. (2002). *Assessment and treatment of childhood problems: A clinician's guide* (2nd ed.). New York: Guilford Press.

Schulte, D., Bochum, R. U., & Eifert, G. H. (2002). What to do when manuals fail?: The dual model of psychotherapy. *Clinical Psychology: Science and Practice, 9,* 312–328.

Schwartz, S. (2003). *Wicked.* Araca Group, Jon Platt, & David Stone (Producers). New York: Marc Platt, Universal Pictures.

Seligman, M. E. P. (1995). The effectiveness of psychotherapy: The *Consumer Reports* study. *American Psychologist, 50,* 965–974.

Seligman, M. E. P., Peterson, C., Kaslow, N. J., Tanenbaum, R., Alloy, L., & Abramson, L. Y. (1984). Attributional style and depressive symptoms among children. *Journal of Abnormal Psychology, 93,* 235–238.

Seligman, M. E. P., Reivich, K., Jaycox, L., & Gillham, J. (1995). *The optimistic child.* Boston: Houghton Mifflin.

Shafran, R., Frampton, I., Heyman, I., Reynolds, M., Teachman, B., & Rachman, S. (2003). The preliminary development of a new self-report measure for OCD in young people. *Journal of Adolescence, 26,* 137–142.

Shapiro, J. E., Friedberg, R. D., & Bardenstein, K. K. (2005). *Child and adolescent therapy.* New York: Wiley.

Shapiro, L. (2004). *The chimp who lost her chatter.* Plainview, NY: Childswork/Childsplay.

Shapiro, L. (2006a). *The horse who lost her herd.* Plainview, NY: Childswork/Childsplay.

Shapiro, L. (2006b). *The koala who wouldn't cooperate.* Plainview, NY: Childswork/Childsplay.

Shaw, J., & Barzvi, A. (2005). *Who invented lemonade?: The power of positive perspective.* New York: Universe Inc.

Shenk, J. (1993, January). *Cognitive-behavioral therapy of obsessive–compulsive disorder.* Grand Rounds presentation at Mesa Vista Hospital, San Diego, CA.

Shirk, S. R. (2001). Development and cognitive therapy. *Journal of Cognitive Psychotherapy, 15,* 155–164.

Shirk, S. R., & Karver, M. (2003). Prediction of treatment outcome from relationship variables in child and adolescent therapy: A meta-analysis review. *Journal of Consulting and Clinical Psychology, 71,* 452–464.

Shirk, S. R., & Karver, M. (2006). Process issues in cognitive behavioral therapy for youth. In P. C. Kendall (Ed.), *Child and adolescent therapy: Cognitive behavioral procedures* (3rd ed., pp. 465–491). New York: Guilford Press.

Shyer, C. (Director). (1991). *Father of the bride* [motion picture] United States: Sandollar Productions, Touchstone Pictures, and Touchwood Pacific Partners I.

Silverman, W. K., & Ollendick, T. H. (2005). Evidence-based assessment of anxiety and its disorders in children and adolescents. *Journal of Clinical Child and Adolescent Psychology, 34,* 380–411.

Silverman, W. K., Pina, A. A., & Viswesvaran, C. (2008). Evidence-based psychosocial treatments for phobic and anxiety disorders in children and adolescents. *Journal of Clinical Child and Adolescent Psychology, 37,* 105–130.

Silverman, W. K., & Rabian, B. (1999). Rating scales for anxiety and mood disorders. In D. Shaffer, C. P. Lucas, & J. E. Richters (Eds.), *Diagnostic assessment in child and adolescent psychopathology* (pp. 127–166). New York: Guilford Press.

Slater, S., & Sheik, D. (2006). *Spring awakening.* New York: Atlantic Theatre.

Smith, P. A., Perrin, S., & Yule, W. (1999). Cognitive behavior for posttraumatic stress disorder. *Child Psychology and Psychiatry Review, 4*(4), 177–182.

Snood, E. D., & Kendall, P. C. (2007). Assessing anxious self-talk in youth: The Negative Affectivity Self-Statement Questionnaire Anxiety Scale. *Cognitive Therapy and Research, 31,* 603–619.

Snyder, K., Gur, R., & Andrews, L. (2007). *Me, myself, and them.* Oxford, UK: Oxford University Press.

Sobel, M. (2000). *The penguin who lost her cool.* Plainview, NY: Childswork/Childsplay.

Sofronoff, K., Attwood, T., & Hinton, S. (2005). A randomized controlled trial of CBT intervention for anxiety in children with Asperger syndrome. *Journal of Child Psychology and Psychiatry, 46,* 1152–1160.

Sokol, L. (2005, May). *Extramural training seminar.* Presented at the Beck Institute for Cognitive Therapy and Research, Philadelphia.

Southam-Gerow, M. (2004). Some reasons that mental health treatments are not technologies: Toward treatment development and adaptation outside labs. *Clinical Psychology: Science and Practice, 11,* 186–189.

Spence, S. H. (1998). A measure of anxiety symptoms among children. *Behaviour Research and Therapy, 36,* 545–566.

Spiegler, M. D., & Guevremont, D. C. (1998). *Contemporary behavior therapy* (3rd ed.). Pacific Grove, CA: Brooks/Cole.

Spielberger, C. D. (1988). *Manual for the State–Trait Anger Expression Inventory (STAXI).* Odessa, FL: Psychological Assessment Resources.

Stallard, P. (2002). *Think good, feel good: A cognitive behaviour workbook for children and young people.* Chichester, UK: Wiley.

Stallard, P. (2005). Cognitive behaviour therapy with prepubertal children. In P. Graham (Ed.), *Cognitive behaviour therapy for children and families* (2nd ed., pp. 121–135). Cambridge, UK: Cambridge University Press.

Stallard, P. (2007). Early maladaptive schemas in children: Stability and differences between a community and a clinic refused sample. *Clinical Psychology and Psychotherapy, 14,* 10–18.

Stallard, P., & Rayner, R. (2005). The development and preliminary evaluation of a Schema Questionnaire for Children (SQC). *Behavioural and Cognitive Psychotherapy, 33,* 217–224.

Stark, K. D. (1990). *Childhood depression: School-based depression.* New York: Guilford Press.

Stark, K. D., Swearer, S., Kurowski, C., Sommer, D., & Bowen, B. (1996). Targeting the child and family: A holistic approach to treating child and adolescent depressive disorders. In E. D. Hibbs & P. S. Jensen (Eds.), *Psychosocial treatment for child and adolescent disorders: Empirically-based strategies for clinical practice* (pp. 207–238). Washington, DC: American Psychological Association.

Steer, R. A., Kumar, G. T., & Beck, A. T. (1993a). Hopelessness in adolescent psychiatric inpatients. *Psychology Reports, 72,* 559–564.

Steer, R. A., Kumar, G. T., & Beck, A. T. (1993b). Self-reported suicidal ideation in adolescent psychiatric inpatients. *Journal of Consulting and Clinical Psychology, 61,* 1096–1099.

Steer, R. A., Kumar, G. T., Beck, A. T., & Beck, J. S. (2005). Dimensionality of the Beck Youth Inventories with child psychiatric outpatients. *Journal of Psychopathology and Behavioral Assessment, 27,* 123–131.

Steer, R. A., Kumar, G. T., Ranieri, W. F., & Beck, A. T. (1998). Use of the Beck Depression Inventory-II with adolescent psychiatric outpatients. *Journal of Psychopathology and Behavioral Assessment, 20,* 127–137.

Stemberger, R. M. T., McCombs-Thomas, A., MacGlashan, S. G., & Mansueto, C. S. (2000). Cognitive behavioral treatment of trichotillomania. In M. Hersen & M. Biaggio (Eds.), *Effective brief therapies* (pp. 319–334). San Diego: Academic Press.

Stewart, A. (2005). Disorders of eating control. In P. Graham (Ed.), *Cognitive-behavioral therapy for children and families* (2nd ed., pp. 359–384). New York: Cambridge University Press.

Storch, E. A., Geffken, G., & Murphy, T. (2007). *Handbook of child and adolescent obsessive-compulsive disorder.* New York: Routledge.

Storch, E. A., Murphy, T. K., Adkins, J. W., Lewin, A. B., Geffken, G. R., Johns, N. B., et al. (2006). The Children's Yale–Brown Obsessive–Compulsive Scale: Psychometric properties of child and parent-report formats. *Journal of Anxiety Disorders, 20,* 1055–1070.

Storch, E. A., Murphy, T. K., Geffken, G. R., Soto, O., Sajid, M., Allen, P., et al. (2004). Psychometric evaluation of the Children's Yale–Brown Obsessive–Compulsive Scale. *Psychiatry Research, 129,* 91–98.

Sutter, J., & Eyberg, S. M. (1984). *Sutter–Eyberg Student Behavior Inventory.* Odessa, FL: Psychological Assessment Resources.

Suveg, C., Kendall, P. C., Comer, J. S., & Robin, J. (2006). Emotion-focused cognitive-behavioral therapy for anxious youth: A multiple-baseline evaluation. *Journal of Contemporary Psychotherapy, 36,* 77–86.

Suveg, C., Southam-Gerow, M. A., Goodman, K. L., & Kendall, P. C. (2007). The role of emotion theory and research in child therapy development. *Clinical Psychology: Science and Practice, 14,* 358–371.

Suveg, C., & Zeman, J. (2004). Emotion regulation in children with anxiety. *Journal of Clinical Child and Adolescent Psychology, 33,* 750–759.

Swanson, J. M. (1992). *School based assessment and intervention for ADD students.* Irvine, CA: K. C. Publishing.

Swanson, J. M., Sandman, C. A., Deutsch, C. K., & Baren, M. (1983). Methylphenidate hydrochloride given with or before breakfast: I. Behavioral, cognitive, and electrophysiologic effects. *Pediatrics, 72,* 49–55.

Sze, K. M., & Wood, J. J. (2007). Cognitive behavioral treatment of co-morbid anxiety disorders and social difficulties in children with high functioning autism: A case report. *Journal of Contemporary Psychotherapy, 37,* 133–144.

Taylor, L., & Ingram, R. E. (1999). Cognitive reactivity and depressotypic processing in children of depressed mothers. *Journal of Abnormal Psychology, 108,* 202–210.

Thompson, T. L. (2002). *Loud lips Lucy.* Citrus Heights, CA: Savor Publishing House.

Thompson, T. L. (2003). *Worry wart Wes.* Citrus Heights, CA: Savor Publishing House.

Thompson, T. L. (2004a). *Catchin cooties Consuelo.* Citrus Heights, CA: Savor Publishing House.

Thompson, T. L. (2004b). *In grown Tyrone.* Citrus Heights, CA: Savor Publishing House.

Thompson, T. L. (2007). *Busy body Bonita.* Citrus Heights, CA: Savor Publishing House.

Thorpe, G. L., & Olson, S. C. (1997). *Behavior therapy* (2nd ed.). Needham Heights, MA: Allyn & Bacon.

Trousdale, G., & Wise, K. (Directors). (1991). *Beauty and the beast* [motion picture]. United States: Silver Screen Partners IV, Walt Disney Animation, and Walt Disney Pictures.

Turk, J. (2005). Children with developmental disabilities and their parents. In P. Graham (Ed.). *Cognitive behavior therapy for children and their families* (pp. 244–262). New York: Guilford Press.

Vacc, N. A., & Rhyne, M. (1987). The Eating Attitudes Test: Development of an adapted language form for children. *Perceptual and Motor Skills, 65,* 335–336.

Van Brunt, D. L. (2000). Modular cognitive-behavioral therapy: Dismantling validated treatment programs into self-standing treatment plan objectives. *Cognitive and Behavioral Practice, 7,* 156–165.

Van Sant, G. (Director). (1997). *Good Will Hunting* [motion picture]. United States: Be Gentlemen Limited Partnership, Lawrence Bender Productions, and Miramax.

Van Sant, G. (Director). (2000). *Finding Forrester* [motion picture]. United States: Columbia Pictures Corporation, Fountainbridge Films, and Laurence Mark Productions.

Vernon, A., & Al-Mabuk, R. (1995). *What growing up is all about.* Champaign, IL: Research Press.

Viorst, J. (1972). *Alexander and the terrible, horrible, no good, very bad day.* New York: Atheneum.

Wachtel, J. R., & Strauss, C. C. (1995). Separation anxiety disorder. In A. R. Eisen, C. A. Kearney, & C. E. Schaefer (Eds.), *Clinical handbook of anxiety disorders in children and adolescents* (pp. 53–81). Northvale, NJ: Aronson.

Wagner, A. P. (2000). *Up and down the worry hill.* Rochester, NY: Lighthouse Press.

Waller, G., Cordery, H., Corstorphine, E., Hinrichsen, H., Lawson, R., Mountford, V., et al. (2007). *Cognitive behavioral therapy for eating disorders: A comprehensive guide.* Cambridge, UK: Cambridge Press.

Walsh, B. T., & Cameron, V. L. (2005). *If your adolescent has an eating disorder.* New York: Oxford University Press.

Warfield, J. R. (1999). Behavioral strategies for hospitalized children. In L. Vandecreek, S. Knapp, & T. L. Jackson (Eds.), *Innovations in clinical practice: A sourcebook* (Vol. 17, pp. 169–182). Sarasota, FL: Professional Resource Press.

Washington, D. (Director). (2002). *Antwone Fisher* [motion picture]. United States: Fox Searchlight Pictures and Mondy Lane Entertainment.

Waters, T. L., & Barrett, P. M. (2000). The role of the family in childhood obsessive–compulsive disorder. *Clinical Child and Family Psychology Review, 3,* 173–184.

Waters, V. (1979). *Color us rational.* New York: Institute for Rational Living.

Waters, V. (1980). *Rational stories for children.* New York: Institute for Rational-Emotive Therapy.

Wedding, D., & Niemiec, R. M. (2003). The clinical use of films in psychotherapy. *Journal of Clinical Psychology, 59,* 207–213.

Weierbach, J., & Phillips-Hershey, E. (2008). *Mind over basketball.* Washington, DC: Magination Press.

Weisz, J. R. (2004). *Psychotherapy for children and adolescents: Evidence-based treatments and case examples.* New York: Cambridge University Press.

Weisz, J. R., Huey, S. J., & Weersing, V. R. (1998). Psychotherapy with children and adolescents: The state of the art. In T. H. Ollendick & R. J. Prinz (Eds.), *Advances in clinical child psychology* (Vol 20, pp. 49–91). New York: Plenum Press.

Weisz, J. R., Southam-Gerow, M. A., Gordis, E. B., & Connor-Smith, J. (2003). Primary and secondary control training for youth depression: Applying the deployment-focused model of treatment development and testing. In A. E. Kazdin & J. R. Weisz (Eds.), *Evidence-based psychotherapies for children and adolescents* (pp. 165–186). New York: Guilford Press.

Weisz, J. R., Thurber, C., Sweeney, L., Proffitt, V. D., & LeGagnoux, G. L. (1997). Brief treatment of mild to moderate child depression using primary and secondary control enhancement training. *Journal of Consulting and Clinical Psychology, 65,* 703–707.

Wellburn, K., Coristine, M., Dagg, P., Pontefract, A., & Jordan, S. (2002). The Schema Questionnaire—Short Form: Factor analysis and relationship between schemas and symptoms. *Cognitive Therapy and Research, 26,* 519–530.

Wells, A. (1997). *Cognitive therapy of anxiety disorders: A practice manual and conceptual guide.* New York: Wiley.

Wexler, D. B. (1991). *The PRISM workbook: A program for innovative self-management.* New York: Norton.

Wilfrey, D. E., Passi, V. A., Cooperberg, J., & Stein, R. I. (2006). Cognitive-behavioral therapy for youth with eating disorders and obesity. In P. C. Kendall (Ed.), *Child and adolescent therapy: Cognitive-behavioral procedures* (3rd ed., pp. 322–365). New York: Guilford Press.

Wilson, G. T., & Smith, D. (1989). Assessment of bulimia nervosa: An evaluation of the Eating Disorder Examination. *International Journal of Eating Disorders, 8,* 173–179.

Wolpe, J. (1958). *Psychotherapy by reciprocal inhibition.* Stanford, CA: Stanford University Press.

Wood, J. J., & McCleod, B. M. (2007). *Child anxiety disorders: A family-based treatment manual for practitioners.* New York: Norton.

Woods, D. W., & Miltenberger, R. G. (1995). Habit reversal: A review of applications and variations. *Journal of Behavioral Therapy and Experimental Psychiatry, 26,* 123–131.

Woods, J. E., & Luiselli, J. K. (2007). Habit reversal of vocal motor tics in child with Tourette's syndrome. *Clinical Case Studies, 6,* 181–189.

Yontef, G. (2007). The power of the immediate moment in gestalt therapy. *Journal of Contemporary Psychotherapy, 37,* 17–23.

Young, J. E. (1994). *Cognitive therapy for personality disorders: A schema-focused approach.* Sarasota, FL: Professional Resource Exchange.

Young, J. E. (1998). *Young Schema Questionnnaire—Short Form.* New York: Cognitive Therapy Center.

Youngstrom, E., Loeber, R., & Stouthamer-Loeber, M. (2000). Patterns and correlates of agreement between parent, teacher, and male adolescent ratings of internalizing and externalizing problems. *Journal of Consulting and Clinical Psychology, 68,* 1038–1050.

Zaillian, S. (Director). (1993). *Searching for Bobby Fischer* [motion picture]. United States: Mirage Entertainment.

Zeckhausen, D. (2008). *Full mouse, empty mouse: A tale of food and feelings.* Washington, DC: Magination Press.

Zinbarg, R. E. (2000). Comment on "Role of emotion in cognitive behavior therapy": Some quibbles, a call for greater attention to motivation for change, and implications of adopting a hierarchical model of emotion. *Clinical Psychology: Science and Practice, 7,* 394–399.

Index

f following a page number indicates a figure; *t* following a page number indicates a table

Achenbach Scales (ASCBA), 23*t*, 24
Activity Scheduling Grab-Bag technique, 98, 99*f*, 114*t*
Affective education, 65–70, 67*t*. *see also* Psychoeducation
  techniques for
    Naming the Enemy technique, 69–70
    Volcano technique, 68–69
Agenda setting, 7*t*
Aggression, 28–29, 251, 253–254
All-or-none thinking, 223–228, 224*f*, 263–264
Analogy, exposure and, 243–244
Anger
  assessment and, 22–23, 22*t*
  automatic thoughts and, 28–29
  behavioral experiments and, 241
  cognitive restructuring techniques and, 136–138, 138*f*, 152–161, 153*f*, 155*f*, 159*f*
  exposure and experiential learning techniques for, 251, 253–254
Anger Control Training program, 122–123
Anger Coping Program, 123
Anxiety
  assessment and, 19–22, 20*t*
  cognitive restructuring techniques and, 162–164, 164*f*
  pleasant activity scheduling and, 99–100
  social skills training and, 91
Anxiety hierarchy
  exposure and experiential learning techniques and, 277–281, 277*f*, 278*f*, 279*f*, 280*f*, 281*f*, 282–283, 282*f*
  systematic desensitization and, 87–89
Anxiety symptoms, 13, 15*f*
Are You Ready for Some Changes? technique, 139–142, 141*f*, 177*f*

Asperger syndrome, 123, 274–276, 276*f*
Assessment
  in the initial session, 13–16, 15*f*
  modular approach to intervention and, 2–3, 3*f*
  ongoing monitoring, 16, 17*f*
  overview, 12
  self-report and other-report measures, 17–31, 18*t*, 20*t*, 22*t*, 23*t*, 26*t*, 27*t*, 29*t*
  session structure and, 7*t*
  structure and, 6
Attainment, 240–242
Attentional refocusing, 123–124
Attention-deficit/hyperactivity disorder (ADHD), 13, 13–14, 15*f*, 25
Autistic Diagnostic Interview (ADI), 26, 26*t*
Autistic Diagnostic Observation Schedule (ADOS), 25, 26*t*
Automatic thoughts, 28–30, 29*t*. *see also* Cognitive restructuring
Avoidance, 91–92, 172–174, 173*f*

B

Back Up! technique, 102–104, 103*f*, 114*t*
Background information, 13
Barb Technique, 252*t*, 253–254
Battleship technique, 252*t*, 281
Beck Anger Inventory for Youth (BANI-Y), 22*t*, 23
Beck Depression Inventory–II (BDI-II), 13, 17–19, 18*t*
Beck Disruptive Behavior Inventory (BDBI), 23*t*, 24–25
Beck Disruptive Behavior Inventory for Youth (BDBI-Y), 25
Beck Hopelessness Scale (BHS), 13, 18*t*, 19

Beck Self-Concept Inventory, 29t, 31
Beck Youth Anxiety Scale (BYAS), 19–20, 20t
Beck Youth Depression Scale (BYDS), 17–19, 18t
Behavior Assessment Scale for Children–2 (BASC-2), 23t, 24
Behavioral charts, 36–38, 39f, 51f
Behavioral distress tolerance skills, 104, 104t
Behavioral experiments. *see also* Behavioral interventions
  cognitive restructuring techniques and, 172–174, 173f
  forms for, 290f
  metaphors and, 191
  overview, 240–242, 288–289, 289f
  session structure and, 7t
  techniques for, 251–288, 252t, 259f, 261f, 268f, 271f, 272f, 276f, 277f, 278f, 279f, 280f, 281f, 282f, 286f
  types of, 247–251
Behavioral hierarchies, 39, 40–45, 41f, 43f, 44f
Behavioral interventions. *see also* Behavioral experiments
  contingency contracting, 104–111, 106f
  distress tolerance skills, 104, 104t
  forms for, 115f–120f
  habit reversal, 101–104, 103f
  modeling, 86–87
  overview, 3f, 4, 79, 111–112, 112f, 113t–114t
  pleasant activity scheduling, 96–101, 97f, 99f, 100f
  relaxation techniques, 80–86, 81t, 83t, 85f
  social skills training, 89–96
  systematic desensitization, 87–89
Behavioral problems, 13–14
Behavioral rehearsal, 249–250
Behavioral self-monitoring techniques, 36–45, 39f, 40f, 41f, 43f–44f, 52f
  File My Fears Away technique, 40–42, 41f, 43f, 52f
  Keeping' My Stats technique, 38–39, 40f
  Up, Up, and Away technique, 42, 44f, 45, 113t
Behavioral tasks, structure and, 6
"Best-friend role play", 122
Body Attitude Test (BAT), 27t, 28
Books, affective education and, 66–68, 67t
Brain functioning, hot cognitions and, 9
Bull's-Eye Ball game, 249, 252t, 254
Bus Driver metaphor, 192t, 195–198, 196f, 197f, 230f

C

Calming Cue Cards technique, 81t, 84–86, 113t
Calming-Down Kits technique, 81t, 82–83, 83t, 85f

Caring or Control technique, 124t, 134–136, 135f
Case conceptualization, 2, 4–5, 5–6, 9, 10f, 13
Catastrophizing
  cognitive restructuring techniques and, 162–164, 164f
  rational analysis techniques and, 202–205, 204f, 218–221, 220f
Cat's Meow metaphor, 192t
Cave metaphor, exposure and, 244
Child Autism Rating Scale (CARS), 25, 26t
Child Behavior Checklist (CBCL), 24
Child Depression Inventory (CDI), 13
Child report of problems, 13–14
Children's Attributional Style Questionnaire (CASQ), 29t, 30
Children's Automatic Thoughts (CATS), 29t, 30
Children's Depression Inventory (CDI), 17–19, 18t
Children's Florida Obsessive–Compulsive Inventory (C-FOCI), 20t
Children's Inventory of Anger (ChIA), 22, 22t
Children's Negative Cognitive Error Questionnaire (CNCEQ), 29–30, 29t
Children's Obsessive–Compulsive Inventory (ChOCI), 20t, 21–22
Children's Yale–Brown Obsessive–Compulsive Scale (CY-BOCS), 21
Chinese Finger Trap technique, 252t, 256–257
Circle of Criticism technique, 252t, 253
Clean Up Your Thinking technique, 146–149, 148f, 179f
Clinical Eating Disorder Rating Instrument (CEDRI), 27, 27t
Clinical interviews, 13–14
Cognitive distortions, 70–74, 74f. *see also* Cognitive restructuring
Cognitive model, 70–74, 74f, 75f
Cognitive products, assessment and, 28–31, 29t
Cognitive restructuring
  exposure and, 245
  forms for, 176f–188f
  interventions, 123–174, 124t, 127f, 133f, 135f, 138f, 141f, 144f, 148f, 151f, 153f, 155f, 159f, 162f, 164f, 166f, 168f, 170f, 173f, 174f
  overview, 3f, 4, 121–123, 175
  rational analysis techniques and, 202–205, 204f
  session structure and, 7t
  social skills training and, 91
  structure and, 6
  techniques for
    Are You Ready for Some Changes? technique, 139–142, 141f, 177f
    Caring or Control technique, 124t, 134–136, 135f
    Clean Up Your Thinking technique, 146–149, 148f, 179f
    Coping Necklace technique, 124t, 129–130

Cut the Knot technique, 165–169, 166*f*, 168*f*
DARE (Don't Avoid, Rather Engage)
    technique, 172–174, 173*f*
En Fuego technique, 154–157, 155*f*, 183*f*
Fair or What I Want? technique, 136–138,
    138*f*
Handprint on Your Heart technique, 124*t*,
    130–131, 176*f*
Hot Shots, Cool Thoughts technique,
    152–154, 153*f*, 182*f*
It's Me, Not OCD technique, 145–146
Mad at 'Em Balm technique, 157–161, 159*f*,
    184*f*, 185*f*, 186*f*
For Now or Forever? technique, 124*t*,
    131–134, 133*f*
Rank Your Worries technique, 162–164, 164*f*,
    187*f*
Superhero Cape technique, 124–126, 124*t*
Swat the Bug technique, 149–150, 180*f*
Taming the Impulse Monster technique,
    161–162, 162*f*
Thought Crown technique, 124*t*, 126–128,
    127*f*
Toss Across technique, 124*t*, 128–129
Trash Talking technique, 150–152, 151*f*, 181*f*
Trick or Truth technique, 142–143, 144*f*, 178*f*
Wanting Versus Willing technique, 169–172,
    170*f*, 188*f*
Cognitive self-monitoring techniques, 45–49, 47*f*,
    48*f*, 53*f*, 54*f*
    My World technique, 49
    What's Bugging' You technique, 46–47, 47*f*, 53*f*
    Your Brainstorm technique, 47–48, 48*f*, 54*f*
Cognitive Triad Inventory for Children (CTIC),
    29*t*, 30
Collaboration
    exposure and, 242–243
    metaphors and, 191
    ongoing monitoring and, 16, 17*f*
    overview, 6, 244–245, 291
    psychoeducation and, 55–56
    sharing assessment results and, 15–16
Conduct disorder, 24–25
Connors' Parent and Teacher Rating Scales—
    Revised (CRS-R), 23–24, 23*t*
Connors' Parent Rating Scales (CPRS), 13
Connors' Teaching Ratings Scales (CTRS), 13
Consequences, 105. *see also* Reinforcement
Content in psychotherapy, 6, 7*t*
Contingency management
    cognitive restructuring techniques and, 165–169,
        166*f*, 168*f*
    contracting, 104–111, 106*f*
        Puzzle Pieces technique, 105–107, 106*f*, 114*t*
    habit reversal and, 101
    overview, 104–105, 114*t*

psychoeducation regarding, 120*f*
rational analysis techniques and, 221–223, 222*f*
Continuing education, 293–294
Control, 254–258. *see also* Rational analysis
Control Dice game, 200–202, 229*t*
Cool Kids Program, self-talk and, 121
Cooperation, 257–258
Coping Cats, 32, 45, 121, 122
Coping Koalas, 32, 45, 121, 122
Coping Necklace technique, 124*t*, 129–130
Coping skills, 128–130
Coping with Depression for Adolescents (CWD-A)
    program, 122
Count Dreadula Says technique, 208–210, 209*f*,
    229*t*, 234*f*, 235*f*
Counting on You technique, 252*t*, 274–276, 276*f*
Critical self-definition, 205–207, 207*f*
Cultural context, 4, 292
Cut the Knot technique, 165–169, 166*f*, 168*f*

D

DARE (Don't Avoid, Rather Engage) technique,
    172–174, 173*f*
Decatastrophizing, 190, 202–205, 204*f*
Depression
    assessment and, 17–19, 18*t*
    automatic thoughts and, 28
    exposure and experiential learning techniques
        for, 258–261, 259*f*, 261*f*
    self-talk and, 122
Developmental factors, 4–5, 191
Disabilities, 123, 274–276, 276*f*
Disorders, psychoeducation regarding, 56–57, 57*t*
Disruptive behavior disorders, 23–25, 23*t*
Disruptive Behavior Disorders Rating Scales
    (DBDRS), 23*t*, 25
Distress tolerance skills
    cognitive restructuring and, 123–124
    cognitive restructuring techniques and, 169–
        172, 170*f*, 172–174, 173*f*
    overview, 104, 104*t*
Don't Avoid, Rather Engage (DARE) technique,
    172–174, 173*f*
A Dozen Dirty Tricks Your Mind Plays on You
    technique, 72–73, 76*f*–77*f*
DSM-IV, SNAP-IV and, 25

E

Eating Attitudes Test (EAT), 27, 27*t*
Eating Behaviors and Body Image Test (EBBIT),
    27, 27*t*
Eating Disorder Examination (EDE), 26, 27*t*

Eating Disorder Inventory–2 (EDI-2), 27, 27*t*
Eating disorders, 26–28, 27*t*, 123, 262–264
Egocentrism, 274–276, 276*f*
Emotional reasoning
  cognitive restructuring techniques and, 161–162,
    162*f*
  exposure and experiential learning techniques
    for, 260–261, 261*f*
  rational analysis techniques and, 218–221, 220*f*
Emotional self-monitoring techniques, 31–36, 35*f*,
    37*f*, 50*f*
  Feeling Compass technique, 35–36, 37*f*
  Watch, Warning, Storm! technique, 33–35,
    35*f*, 50*f*
En Fuego technique, 154–157, 155*f*, 183*f*
Encouragement, 123–124
Etch A Sketch technique, 94–95, 114*t*
Ethnocultural data, 5, 292
Evaluation, 12. *see also* Assessment
  overview, 3, 3*f*
Evaluation anxiety, 284–288, 286*f*
Examining the advantages and disadvantages, 190
Experiential learning. *see also* Exposure
  forms for, 290*f*
  overview, 288–289, 289*f*
  techniques for, 251–288, 252*t*, 259*f*, 261*f*, 268*f*,
    271*f*, 272*f*, 276*f*, 277*f*, 278*f*, 279*f*, 280*f*,
    281*f*, 282*f*, 286*f*
  types of, 247–251
Experiments, behavioral. *see* Behavioral
    experiments
Exposure
  cognitive restructuring techniques and, 172–
    174, 173*f*
  forms for, 290*f*
  overview, 3*f*, 4, 240–242, 242–247, 243*t*,
    288–289, 289*f*
  procedure of, 245–246
  structure and, 6, 7*t*
  techniques for, 251–288, 252*t*, 259*f*, 261*f*, 268*f*,
    271*f*, 272*f*, 276*f*, 277*f*, 278*f*, 279*f*, 280*f*,
    281*f*, 282*f*, 286*f*
    Barb Technique, 252*t*, 253–254
    Battleship technique, 252*t*, 281
    Bull's-Eye Ball game, 252*t*, 254
    Chinese Finger Trap technique, 252*t*,
      256–257
    Circle of Criticism technique, 252*t*, 253
    Counting on You technique, 252*t*, 274–276,
      276*f*
    Family Meals technique, 252*t*, 262–263
    Germ Scavenger Hunt technique, 252*t*,
      267–268, 268*f*
    Hansel and Gretel Technique, 252*t*, 282–283,
      282*f*

    Let's Go Shopping technique, 252*t*, 283–284
    Museum Piece technique, 252*t*, 284–288,
      286*f*, 290*f*
    Musical Contaminants technique, 252*t*,
      269–270
    One-Word Story technique, 252*t*, 257–258
    Palm Print Your Mistakes technique, 252*t*,
      273–274
    Picture Perfect technique, 252*t*, 263–264
    Pop-Up Monkeys technique, 252*t*, 254–255
    Reading Allowed technique, 252*t*, 284
    Sharing the Persian Flaw technique, 252*t*,
      270–272, 271*f*, 272*f*
  types of, 247–251
Exposure/response prevention procedures (ERP),
    264–267. *see also* Exposure
Externalizing behavior, 13–14, 91
Eyberg Child Behavior Inventory (ECBI), 23*t*, 24

F

Fair or What I Want? technique, 136–138, 138*f*
Fake Math technique, 221–223, 222*f*, 229*t*
Family crafts, 250–251
Family formats, 9–10, 11*f*
Family Meals technique, 252*t*, 262–263
FEAR acronym (Feeling Frightened, Expecting Bad
    Things to Happen, Attitudes and Actions
    That Help, and Results and Rewards), 121
FEAR effect (Family Enhancement of Avoidant
    Responses), 265
Fear Survey Schedule for Children—Revised
    (FSSC-R), 20*t*, 21
Feedback, 6, 7*t*
Feeling Compass technique, 35–36, 37*f*, 113*t*
Feeling Faces charts, 32
File My Fears Away technique, 40–42, 41*f*, 43*f*,
    52*f*
For Now or Forever? technique, 124*t*, 131–134,
    133*f*

G

Games
  exposure and, 243*t*, 249
  as psychoeducation, 63, 65, 65*t*
  rational analysis and, 198–202
Generalized anxiety disorder, 122
Germ Scavenger Hunt technique, 252*t*, 267–268,
    268*f*
Group formats, 9–10, 11*f*
Guessing Game technique, 98–101, 100*f*, 114*t*,
    117*f*

H

Habit reversal, 101–104, 103*f*, 114*t*
  technique for
    Back Up! technique, 102–104, 103*f*, 114*t*
Habituation, exposure and, 245
Half-Nelson metaphor, 192*t*, 193–195
Handprint on Your Heart technique, 124*t*,
    130–131, 176*f*
Hansel and Gretel Technique, 252*t*, 282–283,
    282*f*
Hierarchy construction
  exposure and experiential learning techniques
    and, 277–281, 277*f*, 278*f*, 279*f*, 280*f*, 281*f*,
    282–283, 282*f*
  systematic desensitization and, 87–89
Hopelessness Scale for Children (HSC), 13, 18*t*,
    19
Hot Shots, Cool Thoughts technique, 152–154,
    153*f*, 182*f*

I

Improvisational theater games, 249–250
Impulse control, 161–162, 162*f*, 274–276, 276*f*
Instant Message Role Plays technique, 92–94,
    114*t*, 115*f*
It's in the Bag technique, 71–72
It's Me, Not OCD technique, 145–146, 244

J

Journaling, as exposure, 251

K

Keeping' My Stats technique, 38–39, 40*f*

L

Learned helplessness, 131–134, 133*f*
Let's Go Shopping technique, 252*t*, 283–284

M

Mad at 'Em Balm technique, 157–161, 159*f*, 184*f*,
    185*f*
Magnificent Seven Guidelines for metaphor use,
    191
Making a Book technique, 90–92, 114*t*

Master of Disaster technique, 202–205, 204*f*,
    229*t*, 231*f*–232*f*
Maze metaphor, 192*t*
Media, affective education and, 66–68, 67*t*
Medication referrals, ongoing monitoring and,
    16
Metaphors in treatment, 190–198, 192*t*, 196*f*,
    197*f*, 243–244
Mirror, Mirror technique, 214–218, 215*f*, 229*t*,
    237*f*
Modeling, 86–87, 118*f*–120*f*, 245
Modular approach to intervention, 2–4, 3*f*, 10–11,
    10*f*
Mood check-in, session structure and, 6
Mood symptoms, 13, 15*f*
Motivation, 139–142, 141*f*
Motivational interviewing, 139–142, 141*f*
Multidimensional Anxiety Scale for Children
    (MASC), 13, 19, 20*t*
Museum Piece technique, 252*t*, 284–288, 286*f*,
    290*f*
Music, affective education and, 66–68, 67*t*
Musical Contaminants technique, 252*t*, 269–
    270
My Playlist of Pleasant Events technique, 96–98,
    97*f*, 114*t*, 116*f*
My World technique, 49

N

Naming the Enemy technique, 69–70, 244
Negative Affect Self-Statement Questionnaire
    (NASSQ), 29*t*, 30
Negative reinforcement, 107–108. *see also*
    Consequences; Reinforcement
Neuroscience, 9
Newton's Cradle technique, 226–228, 229*t*
Novaco Anger Scale and Provocation Inventory
    (NAS-PI), 22, 22*t*

O

Obesity, cognitive restructuring and, 123
Obsessive–compulsive disorder (OCD)
  assessment and, 21–22
  cognitive restructuring and, 122, 145–146
  exposure and experiential learning techniques
    for, 264–274, 268*f*, 271*f*, 272*f*
  rational analysis games and, 198–200
One-Word Story technique, 252*t*, 257–258
Oppositional defiant disorder, 24–25
Other-report measures, 17–31, 18*t*, 20*t*, 22*t*, 23*t*,
    26*t*, 27*t*, 29*t*

P

Palm Print Your Mistakes technique, 252*t*, 273–274
PANDY, 32, 45
Parenting
  cognitive restructuring techniques and, 134–138, 135*f*, 138*f*, 165–169, 166*f*, 168*f*
  contingency management and, 104–111, 106*f*
  time-outs, 109–110
Parents
  behavioral interventions and, 111
  exposure and, 242–245
  forms for, 118*f*–120*f*
  psychoeducation for, 55–62, 57–62, 57*t*, 61*t*–62*t*
  report of problems by, 13–14
Password technique, 95–96, 114*t*
Patience, 291–292
Peer relationships, social skills training and, 91
Penn State Worry Questionnaire for Children (PSWQC), 20*t*, 21
Performance, 240–242
Performance anxiety, 284–288, 286*f*
Performance attainment, 3*f*, 4
Performance evaluation, 123–124
Pervasive developmental disorders
  assessment and, 25–26, 26*t*
  distress tolerance skills, 104
  exposure and experiential learning techniques and, 274–276, 276*f*
  self-talk techniques and, 123
  social skills training, 89
Pessimism, 131–134, 133*f*, 208–210, 209*f*
Phobias, 277–281, 277*f*, 278*f*, 279*f*, 280*f*, 281*f*
Picture Perfect technique, 252*t*, 263–264
Playing Centerfield technique, 223–226, 224*f*, 229*t*, 239*f*
Pleasant activity scheduling, 96–101, 97*f*, 99*f*, 100*f*, 114*t*, 120*f*
  techniques for
    Activity Scheduling Grab-Bag technique, 98, 99*f*, 114*t*
    Guessing Game technique, 98–101, 100*f*, 114*t*, 117*f*
    My Playlist of Pleasant Events technique, 96–98, 97*f*, 114*t*, 116*f*
Pop-Up Monkeys technique, 252*t*, 254–255
Positive reinforcement, 107–108. *see also* Reinforcement; Reward systems
Posttraumatic stress disorder (PTSD), 122
Presenting problems, 4
Preventing stimulus satiation, 108–109
Primary and Secondary Control Enhancement Training (PASCET) program, 122
Problem solving, 118*f*, 190

Professional development, 293–294
Progressive muscle relaxation, 80–81, 81*t*, 113*t*. *see also* Relaxation techniques
Prompting, 118*f*–120*f*
Psychoeducation
  affective education, 65–70, 67*t*
  for children and adolescents, 63–65, 64*t*, 65*t*
  cognitive model and, 70–74, 74*f*, 75*f*
  exposure and, 242–245
  forms for, 118*f*–120*f*
  information for parents, 55–62, 57*t*, 61*t*–62*t*
  modular approach to intervention and, 2–3, 3*f*
  overview, 3–4, 55, 56*f*, 74–75, 75*t*
  structure and, 6
Psychotherapeutic processes, 6–8, 7*t*
Puzzle Pieces technique, 105–107, 106*f*, 110, 114*t*

R

Rank Your Worries technique, 162–164, 164*f*, 187*f*
Rational analysis
  games in, 198–202
  game techniques
    Control Dice game, 200–202, 229*t*
    Who's Got the Germ? game, 198–200, 229*t*
  metaphors in, 190–198, 192*t*, 196*f*, 197*f*
  metaphor techniques
    Bus Driver metaphor, 192*t*, 195–198, 196*f*, 197*f*, 230*f*
    Cat's Meow metaphor, 192*t*
    Half-Nelson metaphor, 192*t*, 193–195
    Maze metaphor, 192*t*
    Spidey Sense metaphor, 192*t*
  overview, 3*f*, 4, 189–190, 228, 228*f*, 229*t*
  structure and, 6
  techniques for, 202–228, 204*f*, 207*f*, 209*f*, 212*f*, 215*f*, 220*f*, 224*f*
    Count Dreadula Says technique, 208–210, 209*f*, 229*t*, 234*f*, 235*f*
    Fake Math technique, 221–223, 222*f*, 229*t*
    Master of Disaster technique, 202–205, 204*f*, 229*t*, 231*f*–232*f*
    Mirror, Mirror technique, 214–218, 215*f*, 229*t*, 237*f*
    Newton's Cradle technique, 226–228, 229*t*
    Playing Centerfield technique, 223–226, 224*f*, 229*t*, 239*f*
    Thought Prospector technique, 205–207, 207*f*, 229*t*, 233*f*
    3-D thinking technique, 218–221, 220*f*, 229*t*, 238*f*
    Whether Report technique, 210–214, 212*f*, 229*t*, 236*f*
Reading Allowed technique, 252*t*, 284

Reattribution, 189–190, 202–205, 204*f*, 221–223, 222*f*

Regarding the cognitive model techniques
A Dozen Dirty Tricks Your Mind Plays on You technique, 72–73, 76*f*–77*f*
It's in the Bag technique, 71–72
Spot the Dirty Trick Diary technique, 73–74, 74*f*, 78*f*

Reinforcement, 101, 107–108, 118*f*–120*f*. *see also* Reward systems

Relaxation Scripts technique, 81*t*, 82, 113*t*

Relaxation techniques
Calming Cue Cards technique, 81*t*, 84–86, 113*t*
Calming-Down Kits technique, 81*t*, 82–83, 83*t*, 85*f*
overview, 80–86, 81*t*, 83*t*, 85*f*, 113*t*
psychoeducation regarding, 118*f*–119*f*
Relaxation Scripts technique, 81*t*, 82, 113*t*
Survival Kits technique, 81*t*

Repetitive Behavior Scale—Revised, 26, 26*t*

Response cost, 110–111

Revised Children's Manifest Anxiety Scale (RCMAS), 20, 20*t*

Reward systems, 105–107, 106*f*, 110–111, 246–247. *see also* Reinforcement

Role playing, 249–250

S

Scaling the feeling techniques, 32–33

Schema Questionnaire for Children (SQC), 29*t*, 31

Schema Questionnaire—Short Form (SQ-SF), 29*t*, 31

Schemas, assessment and, 29*t*, 30–31

School Refusal Assessment Scale (SRAS), 20*t*, 21

Screen for Child Anxiety Related Emotional Disorders (SCARED), 13, 19, 20*t*

Selective mutism, 281

Self-definition, 205–207, 207*f*, 214–218, 215*f*

Self-disclosure of the therapist, 6, 244–245

Self-instructional methods
forms for, 176*f*–188*f*
interventions, 123–174, 124*t*, 127*f*, 133*f*, 135*f*, 138*f*, 141*f*, 144*f*, 148*f*, 151*f*, 153*f*, 155*f*, 159*f*, 162*f*, 164*f*, 166*f*, 168*f*, 170*f*, 173*f*, 174*f*
overview, 121–123, 175

Self-monitoring
behavioral self-monitoring techniques, 39*f*, 40*f*, 41*f*, 43*f*–44*f*
cognitive self-monitoring techniques, 45–49, 47*f*, 48*f*
emotional self-monitoring techniques, 31–36, 35*f*, 37*f*
forms for, 50*f*–54*f*
overview, 3, 3*f*

session structure and, 7*t*
structure and, 6
techniques for, 31–54, 32*t*, 35*f*, 37*f*, 39*f*, 40*f*, 41*f*, 43*f*–44*f*, 47*f*, 48*f*

Self-report measures
initial assessment and, 13–14
overview, 12, 17–31, 18*t*, 20*t*, 22*t*, 23*t*, 26*t*, 27*t*, 29*t*

Self-talk techniques
forms for, 176*f*–188*f*
interventions, 123–174, 124*t*, 127*f*, 133*f*, 135*f*, 138*f*, 141*f*, 144*f*, 148*f*, 151*f*, 153*f*, 155*f*, 159*f*, 162*f*, 164*f*, 166*f*, 168*f*, 170*f*, 173*f*, 174*f*
overview, 121–123, 175

Sensory sensitivities, 274–276, 276*f*

Separation anxiety disorder, 122, 130–131, 282–283

Sharing the Persian Flaw technique, 252*t*, 270–272, 271*f*, 272*f*

SKAMP, 23*t*, 25

SNAP-IV, 13, 23*t*, 25

Social anxiety, 122, 283–288, 286*f*

Social Anxiety Scale for Children—Revised (SASC-R), 20*t*, 21

Social Phobia and Anxiety Inventory for Children (SPAI-C), 20*t*, 21

Social skills training
exposure and experiential learning techniques and, 274–276, 276*f*
overview, 89–96, 114*t*
psychoeducation regarding, 119*f*–120*f*
structure and, 6
techniques for
Etch A Sketch technique, 94–95, 114*t*
Instant Message Role Plays technique, 92–94, 114*t*, 115*f*
Making a Book technique, 90–92, 114*t*
Password technique, 95–96, 114*t*

Spence Children's Anxiety Scale (SCAS), 20–21, 20*t*

Spidey Sense metaphor, 192*t*

Spot the Dirty Trick Diary technique, 73–74, 74*f*, 78*f*, 146

State–Trait Anger Expression Inventory (STAXI), 22*t*, 23

Stimulus satiation, preventing, 108–109

Stories in rational analysis, 190–198, 192*t*, 196*f*, 197*f*

Storybooks, as psychoeducation, 63, 64*t*

Subjective units of distress (SUDS), 39

Suicidal Ideation Questionnaire (SIQ), 18*t*, 19

Suicidal Ideation Questionnaire—Jr. (SIQ-Jr), 18*t*, 19

Suicide ideation, initial assessment and, 15*f*

Superhero Cape technique, 124–126, 124*t*

Supervision, 293–294

Survey experiments, 249, 258–261, 259f, 261f
Survival Kits technique, 81t, 82–83, 83t
Swat the Bug technique, 149–150, 180f
Systematic desensitization, 87–89, 99–100, 113t, 119f

T

Taming the Impulse Monster technique, 161–162, 162f, 186f
Teacher Report Form (TRF), 24
Teachers, 111, 118f–120f
Testing the evidence, 122, 189, 210–214, 212f, 249
Therapeutic alliance/relationship, 6, 244–245
Therapists, advice for, 291–295
Think Good, Feel Good (Stallard, 2002), 32
Thought Crown technique, 124t, 126–128, 127f
Thought diaries
    anger and, 154–157, 155f
    cognitive restructuring techniques and, 131–136, 133f, 135f, 142–143, 144f, 154–157, 155f
    overview, 45–49, 47f, 48f
Thought Prospector technique, 205–207, 207f, 229t, 233f
3-D thinking technique, 218–221, 220f, 229t, 238f
Ticket to Glide exercise, 246–247
Tics, habit reversal and, 102–104, 103f
Time-out, 109–110
Toss Across technique, 124t, 128–129
Training, 293–294
Trash Talking technique, 150–152, 151f, 181f
Trick or Truth technique, 142–143, 144f, 178f

U

Universal definitions process, 190
Up, Up, and Away technique, 42, 44f, 45, 113t

V

Volcano technique, 68–69

W

Wanting Versus Willing technique, 169–172, 170f, 188f, 243
Watch, Warning, Storm! technique, 33–35, 35f, 50f
Weight problems, cognitive restructuring and, 123
What's Bugging' You technique, 46–47, 47f, 53f
Whether Report technique, 210–214, 212f, 229t, 236f
Who's Got the Germ? game, 198–200, 229t
Worry, cognitive restructuring techniques and, 162–164, 164f
Wound metaphor, exposure and, 243–244
Writing, as exposure, 251

Y

Yale–Brown Obsessive–Compulsive Scale (YBOCS), 21
Your Brainstorm technique, 47–48, 48f, 54f
Youth Self-Report (YSR), 24